AF872302

The Yellow Emperor's Inner Classic

A Thematic Edition, with Translation and Commentary

黃帝內經

Zachery Chionch

Designed by Destiny and Alchemy (元遇五行館)

Tradition and modern understanding, woven into one thread:
the Way of Heaven, Earth, and the human being.

The Yellow Emperor's Inner Classic: A Thematic Edition, with Translation and Commentary

First edition, 2026. Published in Singapore by Zachery Chionch. Designed by Destiny and Alchemy (元遇五行館).

ISBN 978-981-94-7172-0 (paperback)

For enquiries, write to DestinyAndAlchemy@gmail.com.

Copyright © 2026 Zachery Chionch. All rights reserved. No part of this book may be reproduced, stored in a retrieval system, or transmitted in any form or by any means, electronic, mechanical, photocopying, recording, or otherwise, without the prior written permission of the publisher, except for brief quotations embodied in reviews and scholarly work.

The classical passages have been translated afresh from the original Chinese of public-domain sources for this volume, and checked against standard editions and the classical commentaries. The established scholarly translations are listed in the Sources and are warmly recommended to readers who wish to study the text in greater philological depth. What is original to this book, and what the author offers as its contribution, is the thematic arrangement, the commentary, and the reading of the classic from the standpoint of a practitioner of the Chinese metaphysical and healing tradition. This is a thematic edition, not a complete translation: it presents the essential passages of the *Inner Classic*, drawn from all one hundred and sixty-two treatises and arranged by theme with commentary, rather than a word-for-word rendering of the entire text.

This book presents a philosophical and cultural tradition. It is offered for study, reflection, and self-cultivation. It is not medical advice and is not a substitute for diagnosis or treatment by a qualified physician. Readers with health concerns should consult a licensed practitioner. The dietary, sexual, and self-cultivation practices described in the classical sources are recorded here for understanding of the tradition, not as prescriptions.

陰陽者，天地之道也，
萬物之綱紀，變化之父母。

Yin and yang are the Way of Heaven and Earth, the cord and net of the ten thousand things, the father and mother of all change.

SU WEN · THE GREAT TREATISE ON YIN, YANG, AND THE CORRESPONDENCE OF IMAGES

Contents

黃帝內經 · *the inner classic, a thematic edition*

The Eleven Gates 十一門

A Practical Close

Reference

PROLOGUE

The Lineage of the Way

盤古 · 伏羲 · 神農 · 黃帝

Before Heaven and Earth were divided, the old accounts tell, there was only a vast and formless dark, a single breath turning upon itself without shape or bound. Within that primordial chaos Pangu (盤古) took form, and as he grew he raised the clear and the light to become Heaven and pressed the heavy and the turbid down to become Earth, and so split the one into two (開天闢地).

Into the world between them came the sages who taught humankind to live in step with Heaven and Earth. Fuxi (伏羲) looked up to the heavens and down to the earth, and drew the eight trigrams, giving the people the Book of Change and the reading of the patterns of things. Shennong (神農), the Divine Farmer, tasted the hundred herbs, and from him came the knowledge of plants and the first medicine.

After them came Huangdi (黃帝), the Yellow Emperor, under whose name this classic stands, remembered as the one who gathered the learning of his teachers into a single teaching on the body, the Way, and the nurturing of life.

This book begins where that lineage points: not at medicine alone, nor at destiny or cultivation alone, but at the one Way from which Heaven, Earth, and the human being all descend.

PREFACE

The One Thread

There is an old habit, in our time, of cutting the world into separate rooms. Medicine sits in one room, and a person walks in only when something has already broken. Destiny sits in another, visited out of curiosity or fear. The shape of a home belongs to a third room, the calendar to a fourth, and the quiet inner work of meditation to a fifth that many never enter at all. Each room has its own door, its own expert, its own vocabulary, and the rooms rarely speak to one another.

The tradition this book draws from did not build those walls. To the physicians, Daoists, and scholars of early China, a human life was a single field of relationships. The food on the table, the season turning outside the window, the slope of the land behind the house, the feelings moving through the chest at night, the year of one's birth, and the breath rising and falling in stillness were not five subjects. They were five views of one thing: the movement of *qi* (氣), the living breath that flows through Heaven, Earth, and the human being and binds them into one body.

At the centre of that field of thought stands one book. The *Huangdi Neijing* (黃帝內經), the *Inner Classic of the Yellow Emperor*, is the oldest and most influential text of Chinese medicine, and it is at the same time one of the great books of Daoist thought. It does not read like a manual. It reads like a long conversation between a ruler and his teachers about how to live in keeping with the way things are. The aim is simple: that the body stays whole, the spirit stays clear, and a person reaches the full span of years Heaven allotted. Health, in this book, is never separate from time, weather, emotion, conduct, and the cultivation of the inner life. It is the visible sign that a person is in tune with a much larger order.

This volume takes the *Inner Classic* as its spine. Around that spine it gathers the traditions that grew from the same root and never truly parted from it: the cosmology of the *Daodejing* and the *Zhuangzi*; the art of reading time and fate that became the Eight Characters and the Purple Star; the reading of land and dwelling that became Feng Shui; the divinatory mathematics of the *Yijing*, the *Book of Change*; and the inner alchemy of the Daoist adepts, who turned the physician's language of essence, breath, and spirit into a path of transformation. These are usually taught as separate disciplines. Here they are treated as what an older eye saw them to be: dialects of one language.

The claim is not a modern invention laid over the past. The sources say it plainly. The Tang physician Sun Simiao held that no one could be called a great doctor who had not also read widely. The true healer, he said, must know the classics, the histories, and the works of Laozi and Zhuangzi, and must have learned the waxing and waning of the five phases and the motions of the heavens. The Ming master Zhang Jingyue wrote that medicine and the *Yi* share one source, because Heaven and the human being share one principle, and that principle is yin and yang. When the great geomancer's manual defines its art, it describes the same single *qi* that the physician feels at the wrist, dividing into yin and yang and branching into the five phases. The unity was assumed. What was rare, and prized, was the person who could hold the whole of it in one mind.

That is the reader this book hopes to serve, and the reader it hopes to help form. Its purpose is not only to explain techniques, though it explains a good many. It is to cultivate a way of seeing in which destiny, health, environment, spirit, virtue, timing, method, energy, and the inner work of cultivation are recognised as facets of one process of alignment. A person who sees this way reads a pulse and a year and a landscape with the same underlying grammar. They treat the cause rather than chase the symptom. They understand that to change a life is often to change a habit of breath, a relationship to a season, or a stance of the heart.

For each major idea, the chapters move through the same arc. They begin with the classical understanding, drawn as far as possible from the texts themselves rather than from later summaries. They set out the philosophical ground beneath the idea. They show how it joins Heaven, Earth, and the human being, and how it touches health, destiny, energy, place, and cultivation. They bring the idea into the conditions of modern life, where most readers actually live. And where it helps, they include the voice of practice: the small, hard-won observations that physicians and adepts have passed down, which no theory quite replaces.

A reader may come to this book as a student of medicine, a diviner, a person drawn to cultivation, or simply someone who senses that these were never really separate pursuits. To each, the invitation is the same. Follow the one thread. It runs through everything.

THE WIDER TRADITION

The Five Arts

There is an old way of dividing the Chinese arts of life into five, the *wu shu* (五 術), the Five Arts. They are usually given as Mountain, Medicine, Destiny, Divination, and Physiognomy, and though they are studied today as if they were five trades, the tradition regarded them as five applications of one knowledge. This book is, in the end, a book of the Five Arts, gathered around the classic that lies nearest their common root. It is worth naming them at the outset, so that the reader can see the whole field of which the *Inner Classic* is the centre.

Mountain (山 , *shan*) is the art of self-cultivation, named for the mountain hermits who pursued it. It covers the disciplines of breath, stillness, posture, and diet; the guarding and refining of essence, breath, and spirit; and the inner alchemy that returns them toward their source. It is taken up in the gate on cultivation and in the closing chapters on the inner elixir and on stillness and return, and is the quiet ground of all the rest.

Medicine (醫 , *yi*) is the art of healing the body: the reading of pulse and colour, the channels and the needle, the herbs and the regimens of nourishing life. The *Inner Classic* is its foundation, and so it is the largest presence in these pages, running through both the Basic Questions and the Spiritual Pivot and the interpretive essays woven among them.

Destiny (命 , *ming*) is the art of reading the pattern a life is born with. The Eight Characters of the Four Pillars and the chart of the Purple Star set out the moment of a birth as a map of the five phases and the stars, one to be understood and worked with rather than simply endured. It is the subject of the chapter on reading a life.

Divination (卜 , *bu*) is the art of reading the pattern of a present moment, so as to act with the way it is already tending rather than against it. It casts and reads the hexagrams of the *Book of Change* , and the finer methods built on the same view of the cosmos: the plum-blossom numerology, and the art of the hidden formations, Qi Men Dun Jia, which sets a question against the pattern of time and direction. It shares its whole grammar with the medicine, as the chapter on the *Yi* and medicine shows.

Physiognomy (相 , *xiang*), the art of reading forms, is wider than its English name suggests. It is the reading of the face and the hand, in which character and fortune are read from the body's outward signs. This is the same reading of the surface for the inner state that the physician makes when he reads the five organs in the five features of the face. And it is the reading of the form of land and dwelling, which is Feng Shui, taken up among the wider arts in the chapter on the qi of place. To read a face, a hand, or a hillside is, in this tradition, one skill turned upon different forms.

Mountain, Medicine, Destiny, Divination, and Physiognomy are not five trades but five windows, each opening on the same room.

What makes these five into one study is the common grammar this book is built to display: yin and yang, the five phases, the stems and branches, and the eight trigrams. The cultivator refining his breath, the physician feeling a pulse, the diviner reading a life or a moment, and the geomancer reading a slope are all reading the movement of *qi* through a particular form, by the same logic. The great physician Sun Simiao, as the closing chapter records, made exactly this range the mark of mastery. He asked the true healer for a command of the reckoning of fate, the divination of the *Yi* , and the movements of the heavens, alongside the medicine itself. This book follows his measure. It places the *Inner Classic* at the centre because the medicine is the most fully worked-out of the five and the nearest to the body we all inhabit; but it reads the classic always as one art among five, and the five as one knowledge, so that what is offered here is not a translation only but a map of the whole field, and an argument that the field is one.

A NOTE ON METHOD

On Translation, Names, and Sounds

Every translation in this book was prepared for this volume. The aim throughout was faithfulness first: to carry every element of the source across, to drop nothing quietly, and to let each phrase land with the weight the original intends. The English is meant to be plain and precise at once, never a dictionary-literal word swap, and never loosened into paraphrase. Technical terms are kept accurate and intact, with the Chinese given so that a reader who knows the language can check the rendering against the original.

Classical passages appear in a consistent three-part form. First the Chinese, in traditional characters. Then a romanisation in *pinyin* , the standard modern spelling of Mandarin, to give the sound. Then the English. The reader who wants only the meaning can rest in the English; the reader who wants the texture of the original has the characters and the sound beside it.

A FEW KEY WORDS KEPT IN THE ORIGINAL

Some terms have no single English equivalent that does not distort them. These are kept in romanised form and explained on first use, then gathered in the Glossary. The most important are *qi* (氣), the vital breath or energy; *jing* (精), the dense, fluid essence that is the body's deep reserve; *shen* (神), the spirit or conscious brightness; *yin* and *yang* (陰陽), the paired phases of all process; and *Dao* (道), the Way. Translating *qi* as "energy" or *shen* as "mind" would not be wrong so much as thin. The original words are richer, and they are kept.

ON ROMANISATION

Modern *pinyin* is used for sounds and titles. A few spellings will be familiar from older books in their earlier forms, such as *chi* for *qi* and *Tao* for *Dao* ; the modern spellings are used here for consistency. The *Inner Classic* is cited by its two parts, the *Su Wen* (素問), the "Basic Questions," and the *Ling Shu* (靈樞), the "Spiritual Pivot," each of eighty-one treatises. The numbering follows the received recension of the Tang editor Wang Bing.

HOW TO SAY THE SOUNDS

For a reader who does not know pinyin, a few letters are not said as an English speaker would guess: *q* sounds like *ch* , *x* like a soft *sh* , and *zh* like *j* . So the words this book uses most are said, roughly, *qi* as "chee," *jing* as "jeeng," *shen* as "shun," and *Dao* as "dow" (*yin* and *yang* are said much as they look). Each syllable also carries one of four tones, a rise or fall in pitch that matters in speech; a reader may set the tones aside and still be understood on the page.

ON THE PASSAGES CHOSEN

This book gives the essential passages of the *Inner Classic* , not the whole of its text from beginning to end. Every one of the one hundred and sixty-two treatises is present, and each is opened through its essential passages: the lines in which a treatise states its core teaching, coins the phrase by which it is remembered, or bears most directly on the theme of its gate. The long technical inventories of the original, the catalogues of point locations and the tables of seasonal correspondence, are represented by their key statements rather than printed in full, with the commentary carrying their substance. The aim was that a reader should meet the living thought of every treatise, and that a scholar should always find, through the concordance at the back, exactly which treatise a passage is drawn from and where its neighbours lie. For the complete text in full philological dress, the scholarly editions named in the Sources remain the place to turn.

ON WHAT THIS BOOK IS

This is a book of understanding, not a clinical handbook. It records what the tradition holds and why, including its practices of diet, breath, stillness, and the conservation of essence. It is offered for study and self-cultivation. Nothing in it is medical advice, and the dietary and bodily practices of the old texts are described for comprehension of the tradition, not as a regimen to follow unguided. For diagnosis and treatment, see a qualified physician.

It is worth being clear about which parts of this book are the classic itself and which are the author's own reading of it. The Chinese text and its translation are the *Inner Classic* itself, the historical document, given as faithfully as the craft allows. The thematic arrangement, the commentary, and above all the gathering of the wider Five Arts around the medicine, the reading of a life in the Eight Characters and the Purple Star, the reading of land in Feng Shui, the inner alchemy, and the old ritual arts, are the author's own interpretation and the cultural tradition the classic grew within. They are offered as a way of seeing and as a map of that tradition, not as clinical medicine and not as claims settled by modern science. The medicine of the classic and the arts that surround it are set down here as one historical body of thought; whether to take up any of their practices is left, with that distinction kept clear, to the reader's own judgement and to qualified guidance.

ORIGINS

A Chronology of the Tradition

源流

The lineage the Prologue opened, from Pangu to the Yellow Emperor, runs on into recorded history. This chronology sets the principal figures and works in their order, from the sages of remote antiquity, through the Han in which the Inner Classic settled into the form it still holds, to the Ming physician whose thematic arrangement this edition follows.

High Antiquity *THE AGE OF THE SAGES*

As the Prologue recounts, the line opens in remote antiquity with Pangu, who parted the formless dark into Heaven and Earth; then Fuxi, who drew the eight trigrams from the patterns of the world; Shennong, the Divine Farmer, who tasted the hundred herbs and gave the first medicine; and the Yellow Emperor, Huangdi, in whose name this classic stands. They belong to the age before the written record, which the tradition keeps as the wellspring of its knowledge; with the Zhou the line enters the count of dated years.

The Zhou and the Warring States *C. 6TH TO 3RD CENTURY BCE*

In the centuries of the late Zhou, the Daoist classics took written form: the Daodejing, ascribed to Laozi, and the writings of Zhuangzi, which set down the vision of the Way, of nature, and of the cultivated life on which so much of this book rests. In the same long period the commentaries of the Book of Change matured, and the currents of yin and yang, of the five phases, of cosmology and of medicine gathered toward the synthesis the Inner Classic would make.

The Han *C. 2ND CENTURY BCE TO 2ND CENTURY CE*

It was around the Han that the Huangdi Neijing reached the form in which it has come down, though its materials reach back much further, so that it is best placed across the long span from the Warring States to the Eastern Han (戰國 to 東漢 , roughly 475 BCE to 220 CE): the Su Wen, the Basic Questions, and the Ling Shu, the Spiritual Pivot, each of eighty-one treatises, gathering centuries of accumulated medicine into the cast of a dialogue between the Yellow Emperor and Qibo. The text was the work of no single hand or year but the settling of a long tradition into a canon.

The Tang *7TH TO 8TH CENTURY CE*

Two figures of the Tang shaped the tradition the book carries. Sun Simiao (581-682), honoured as the King of Medicine, sickly in his youth and a healer by his own recovery, wrote the great formularies known as the Prescriptions Worth a Thousand in Gold, and set down, in his essay on the absolute sincerity of the great physician, the ethics by which a healer should practise. Wang Bing, working around the year 762, edited and reordered the Su Wen, supplied the long treatises on the five movements and six qi, and gave the received text the arrangement and the numbering this edition still follows.

The Ming *16TH TO 17TH CENTURY CE*

In the late Ming, the physician Zhang Jingyue, also called Zhang Jiebin (1563-1640), finding the Inner Classic hard to use and poorly studied in his day, compiled the Leijing, the Classified Classic, completed in 1624. He took the whole of the Su Wen and the Ling Shu apart and set them back together by theme rather than by their received order, holding that medicine and the Book of Change spring from a single source. It is his thematic model, four centuries on, that the present edition takes up and carries further.

This Edition *THE PRESENT*

The book stands in that line. Following Zhang Jingyue's example, it gathers the treatises of the Inner Classic by theme into eleven gates, sets the original Chinese beside a fresh English rendering, and joins to the medicine the wider arts of the same tradition, so that a reader today may meet the whole as one body of knowledge rather than as scattered parts.

A NOTE TO THE READER

How This Book Is Arranged

The Inner Classic was never meant to be read from the first page to the last. It came down to us as two collections, the Basic Questions and the Spiritual Pivot, eighty-one chapters each, assembled over centuries by many hands. A single subject lies scattered across a dozen chapters, and a single chapter may turn without warning from the pulse to the stars to the dressing of a wound. For two thousand years this has kept the classic a closed mountain, climbed by physicians and by almost no one else.

In the seventeenth century a physician of the Ming, Zhang Jingyue, did something audacious with it. He took the entire text apart and built it back together by subject, gathering all that the classic says of yin and yang into one place, all that it says of the channels into another, and so on through twelve great categories. He called the result the Classified Classic, the Leijing, and it remains one of the most useful keys ever cut for this lock. This book follows his example, and carries it to the reader of today.

You will therefore not find the chapters here in their ancient order. You will find them gathered into eleven gates, each opening on a single theme: the nurturing of life, yin and yang, the organs and their network, the reading of the body, the channels, the needle, the origins of disease, the art of treatment, the movements of the heavens, the inner work of cultivation, and the wider tradition of the Five Arts in which this medicine has its home. Read the gates in order and each prepares the next; step through any one alone and it stands on its own feet.

Within every gate the shape is the same. Each opens in plain speech, for the reader who simply wants to live well. Then come the words of the classic itself, in a fresh translation, so that you meet the source and not a summary of it. Around those words runs a commentary that asks, of each teaching, the five questions a practitioner must answer: what it is, whom it concerns, when and where it holds, why it is so, and above all how it is to be done, by what method. A teaching one cannot act upon is only half a teaching, and the weight throughout falls on the how. Where a passage opens onto practice, a note sets down what can actually be done; where it touches the inner work, the cultivator will find the thread picked up and carried into the tenth gate.

Every passage keeps its origin. Beneath each one its source is named, whether the Basic Questions or the Spiritual Pivot, and the chapter within, so that a scholar may turn at once to the original and a physician may know exactly where an idea was born. At the back of the book a concordance sets this out in both directions: every original chapter with the gates and pages that draw upon it, and every gate with the full roll of chapters it gathers. Nothing has been moved without leaving a path back to where it stood.

A word on what this book is. The classical passages have been translated afresh from the original Chinese for this volume, and checked against the standard editions and the old commentaries. The fuller scholarly translations are listed in the Sources, and I commend them warmly to anyone who wishes to go further. What this book adds, and what sets it beside those translations rather than among them, is the arrangement and the commentary: the gathering of a scattered classic into eleven clear themes, and the work of carrying each teaching from the page into the clinic and onto the cushion, so that a text of two thousand years becomes not only readable but genuinely usable, by the layperson seeking health, the physician seeking its roots, the cultivator seeking the inner work, and the scholar seeking the source.

Begin, then, where the classic itself begins. Not with disease, but with the art of staying whole.

THE JOURNEY OF THIS BOOK

The Eleven Gates

Eleven doorways into one teaching. Each may be entered alone; together they trace the whole arc, from the keeping of health to the inner work of return.

I

The Hundred Years:

Nurturing Life 養生

Why the people of old lived out their full span while we wear out by half, and the plain discipline that made the difference.

II

The Two That Make the Ten Thousand:

Yin and Yang 陰陽

The single distinction from which the whole of medicine, time, and change unfolds.

III

The Court Within:

The Organs and Their Network 藏象

Your organs as a government of officials, each with a post to keep, a season of its own, and a way of failing.

IV

Reading the Unspoken:

Pulse and Diagnosis 脈色

How a finger laid at the wrist and a glance at the face disclose what the body will not say aloud.

V

The Rivers of the Body:

The Channels and Collaterals 經絡

The hidden network along which qi and blood run, where it surfaces, and where it may be met.

A NOTE TO THE READER

Where to Begin

The gates may be read straight through, first to last, and they are set in an order in which each prepares the next. But the book is also built to be entered at whatever door suits you, and there is more than one good way in. If you are unsure, here are four paths through it.

TO LIVE AND AGE WELL

Begin with the first gate, on nurturing life, and the second, on yin and yang. Read the plain opening of each section and the verses, and let the heavier theory wait. From there the tenth gate, on cultivation, and the closing chapters on stillness will speak most directly to a life lived in health. This is the path that asks the least and gives a great deal.

TO LEARN THE MEDICINE

Read the gates in their order. The body is built up as you go: yin and yang, then the organs, the reading of pulse and colour, the channels, the needle, the course of disease, and the art of treatment. The ninth gate, on the movements and qi of the years, is the steepest climb in the classic and is best kept until the rest is in hand.

TO TAKE UP THE INNER WORK

Begin with the tenth gate, on spirit, essence, and cultivation, and carry on into the closing chapters on the inner elixir and on stillness and return. Then double back to the first gate, on nurturing life, and the second, on yin and yang, which lay the ground the inner work stands on.

TO SEE THE WHOLE TRADITION

Read the front matter on the Five Arts, then the eleventh gate, which sets the medicine among destiny, divination, the reading of forms, and the mountain arts. With that frame in view, the other gates read as so many rooms in one house. The scholar seeking the source will find, beneath every passage, the treatise it came from, and at the back a concordance that leads straight to it.

Wherever you start, one thread runs through all of it. Follow it, and the gates open onto one another.

PART ONE

The Hundred Years

The Art of Nurturing Life

養生

On the nurturing of life. Why the people of high antiquity lived out the full span Heaven gave them, while the people of later ages wear out by half, and the plain discipline that made the difference.

GATE ONE · NURTURING LIFE

The Hundred Years

養生

> *The people of high antiquity who knew the Way patterned themselves on yin and yang and kept in accord with the arts of number.*
>
> Su Wen 1

Ask the book its oldest question first. Why did the people of long ago live out a hundred years with their step still firm, while we are worn and slow at fifty? The classic opens on exactly this, and it does not answer with a herb or a needle. It answers with a way of living. Before there is any talk of disease, there is this gate, and everything that follows rests on it.

Nurturing life, 養生, is the art of keeping the body and the spirit whole so that a life reaches its natural term in good order. It is the least dramatic part of the whole tradition and the most important, for the physician's finest cure only returns a person to where this discipline would have kept them. Zhang Jingyue placed it first among his categories for the same reason the classic does: it is the ground on which medicine, cultivation, and the reading of fate all stand.

Read this gate, then, for five things, the five a practitioner must always settle. What the discipline is: a steady moderation and an attunement to the rhythms outside us. Whom it concerns: everyone, and most of all the person who is not yet ill. When and where it applies: every day, in every season, in the ordinary conduct of waking, eating, working, and rest. Why it works: because body and spirit, kept from waste, stay whole together. And, carrying the most weight, how it is done. The chapters below answer the how in plain and usable terms, and that is where we will linger.

The Question, and the Answer

SU WEN 1

乃問於天師曰：余聞上古之人，春秋皆度百歲，而動作不衰；今時之人，年半百而動作皆衰者，時世異耶？人將失之耶？

nǎi wèn yú tiān shī yuē: yú wén shàng gǔ zhī rén, chūn qiū jiē dù bǎi suì, ér dòng zuò bù shuāi; jīn shí zhī rén, nián bàn bǎi ér dòng zuò jiē shuāi zhě, shí shì yì yé? rén jiāng shī zhī yé?

He asked his Heavenly Teacher: I have heard that the people of high antiquity all passed a hundred years, and their movements did not weaken. The people of today reach but half a hundred, and all their movements have already failed. Is this because the times have changed, or because people have lost the Way?

SU WEN 1

岐伯對曰：上古之人，其知道者，法於陰陽，和於術數，食飲有節，起居有常，不妄作勞，故能形與神俱，而盡終其天年，度百歲乃去。

qí bó duì yuē: shàng gǔ zhī rén, qí zhī dào zhě, fǎ yú yīn yáng, hé yú shù shù, shí yǐn yǒu jié, qǐ jū yǒu cháng, bù wàng zuò láo, gù néng xíng yǔ shén jù, ér jìn zhōng qí tiān nián, dù bǎi suì nǎi qù.

Qibo answered: The people of high antiquity who knew the Way patterned themselves on yin and yang and kept in accord with the arts of number. They ate and drank with measure, rose and rested at regular hours, and did not labour recklessly. So body and spirit stayed whole together, and they lived out the full span Heaven had given, departing only after a hundred years.

The answer is a discipline of four hinges, and not one of them asks you to do more. First, pattern yourself on yin and yang: live by the great alternations of day and night and of the seasons, waking and working with the light, drawing inward with the dark and the cold. Second, keep to the arts of number, which is to say measure and proportion, the right amount and the right timing in all things rather than the most. Third, eat and drink with measure. Fourth, rise and rest at regular hours. And over all four, do not labour recklessly, spending in a day what should be spent across a life.

Set beside the medicine of our own time, this is the original counsel of lifestyle and prevention: regular sleep, moderate food, sustainable effort, a life lived in rhythm rather than in surges. What is easy to miss, and worth saying plainly, is that the prescription is restraint. The body holds a finite store, and long life is less a matter of adding to it than of not squandering it. The people of high antiquity reached their hundred years not because they strove harder, but because they wasted less.

The aim the chapter sets is worth saying plainly, because it is easy to miss: not a long life, but a whole one. Body and spirit are meant to stay sound together to the end, the body still working and the mind still clear, so that a person lives out the full span they were given and only then goes. And nothing in the recipe is hidden. It is the ordinary steadiness of sleep, food, work, and rest, kept up over a lifetime, that the classic is willing to call the Way, which is a high name for very plain habits.

The Stillness That Guards

> SU WEN 1
>
> 夫上古聖人之教下也，皆謂之虛邪賊風，避之有時，恬惔虛無，真氣從之，精神內守，病安從來。
>
> *fū shàng gǔ shèng rén zhī jiào xià yě, jiē wèi zhī xū xié zéi fēng, bì zhī yǒu shí, tián tán xū wú, zhēn qì cóng zhī, jīng shén nèi shǒu, bìng ān cóng lái.*
>
> When the sages of high antiquity taught those below them, they spoke always of the empty evils and robber winds, which are to be avoided each in its season. Be calm and empty, free of striving, and the true qi will follow; keep the essence and spirit guarded within, and from where could illness come?

Here the discipline turns inward, and gives its mechanism. Be calm and empty, free of striving, the classic says, and the true qi follows its proper course; keep the essence and spirit guarded within, and illness has no road by which to come. Calm and emptiness here are not idleness. They name a mind not driven by craving and fear, not scattered outward through the senses and the appetites. When the spirit is not leaking away, the protective qi keeps its post at the surface, and the body is not left open.

The practical reading is direct. Much of what wears a person down is not labour but agitation: the restless wanting, the carried anger, the mind that will not put the day down. To quiet that is itself a medicine, and a way of conserving the very reserve that sickness and age draw upon. This is as close as the ancient text comes to what we would now describe as the long cost of unrelieved stress upon the body's defences and its power to recover.

The line the chapter turns on is that when the mind is calm and asks for little, the true qi follows of itself. This is not only advice for the well. In the clinic it is the quiet half of many treatments, since a heart that will not settle keeps the qi stirred and the sleep broken no matter what else is done, and steadying it is often what finally lets a stubborn case turn. The gate on cultivation, later in the book, returns to this same line and makes a whole practice of it.

This one line is also the seed of the entire inner tradition. To guard the spirit within, to conserve the essence, to still the heart: these are exactly the first steps the later schools of cultivation build upon, turning a counsel of health into a discipline of return. The reader who wishes to follow that road will find it taken up in the tenth gate, where the manuals of inner cultivation, named among the Sources, carry calm and emptiness far beyond the keeping of health. Here it is enough to note where the door is.

The Sun Within the Day

> SU WEN 3
>
> 陽氣者，若天與日，失其所則折壽而不彰，故天運當以日光明。是故陽因而上，衛外者也。
>
> *yáng qì zhě, ruò tiān yǔ rì, shī qí suǒ zé zhé shòu ér bù zhāng, gù tiān yùn dāng yǐ rì guāng míng. shì gù yáng yīn ér shàng, wèi wài zhě yě.*
>
> The yang qi is like Heaven and the sun: lose its proper place, and the lifespan is cut short and never shines out. So as the turning of Heaven takes the sun for its light, in the same way the yang qi rises and guards the outside of the body.

SU WEN 3

故陽氣者，一日而主外，平旦人氣生，日中而陽氣隆，日西而陽氣已虛，氣門乃閉。是故暮而收拒，無擾筋骨，無見霧露，反此三時，形乃困薄。

gù yáng qì zhě, yī rì ér zhǔ wài, píng dàn rén qì shēng, rì zhōng ér yáng qì lóng, rì xī ér yáng qì yǐ xū, qì mén nǎi bì. shì gù mù ér shōu jù, wú rǎo jīn gǔ, wú jiàn wù lù, fǎn cǐ sān shí, xíng nǎi kùn báo.

The yang qi governs the outside of the body across the course of a day: at dawn the human qi is born, at noon the yang qi is at its height, and by sundown the yang qi has emptied and the gate of qi closes. So at dusk one should gather and guard the body, neither straining the sinews and bones nor going out into the mist and dew. To go against these three times of day is to leave the body worn and weak.

The yang qi is the warmth and the activity of the body, and the classic likens it to the sun: it should be bright but contained, and it keeps a daily tide. It is born at dawn, stands highest at noon, and by sundown has emptied, the gate of qi closing for the night. The instruction follows from the image. Live with this tide. Spend the bright hours in activity and outward effort, when the yang is rising and full; at dusk gather inward, and neither strain the sinews and bones nor go out into the cold and the night damp. To go against these three times of the day, the text says without softening it, is to leave the body worn and weak.

It would be hard to state a circadian discipline more exactly. The usable form for a modern life: place demanding work and exertion in the first half of the day; let the evening turn toward winding down rather than winding up; and protect sleep as the hour when the yang withdraws to be restored. The principle is not that late effort is forbidden, but that it is paid for, and the bill is the slow wearing the chapter warns of.

The Balance That Holds

SU WEN 3

凡陰陽之要，陽密乃固，兩者不和，若春無秋，若冬無夏，因而和之，是謂聖度。陰平陽秘，精神乃治；陰陽離決，精氣乃絕。

fán yīn yáng zhī yào, yáng mì nǎi gù, liǎng zhě bù hé, ruò chūn wú qiū, ruò dōng wú xià, yīn ér hé zhī, shì wèi shèng dù. yīn píng yáng mì, jīng shén nǎi zhì; yīn yáng lí jué, jīng qì nǎi jué.

In all that matters between yin and yang, it is the firm sealing of the yang that holds the body sound. When the two fall out of accord, it is as a spring without its autumn, a winter without its summer; to bring them back into accord is what is called the sage's measure. When the yin is even and the yang is sealed, the spirit is kept in order; let yin and yang break apart, and the essence and the qi are cut off.

Here the classic states the whole aim of nurturing life in a single line. Health is not the heaping up of yang nor the hoarding of yin but the even balance of the two, the yin level and the yang held firmly sealed; from that balance the spirit stays whole and in order. Let the two break apart, and essence and qi drain away together. Every discipline in this gate, the seasons, the hours, the guarding stillness, is in the end a way of keeping this one balance.

The word the tradition leaned on hardest is sealed: it is only when the yang is sealed and firm, held and rooted rather than flaring up and scattering, that the two are truly in accord. In the clinic the opposite is a common sight, the flushed, wakeful tiredness of someone whose yang will not settle at night, who runs hot and thin and cannot drop into sleep. Adding more heat is the wrong move; the work is to weigh the yang down and fill the yin beneath it, so the spirit can close and sleep comes back. This is why the later art of quieting the spirit shares a root with the plainest rules of season and hour.

Living by the Four Seasons

SU WEN 2

春三月，此謂發陳，天地俱生，萬物以榮，夜臥早起，廣步於庭，被髮緩形，以使志生，生而勿殺，予而勿奪，賞而勿罰，此春氣之應，養生之道也。逆之則傷肝，夏為寒變，奉長者少。

chūn sān yuè, cǐ wèi fā chén, tiān dì jù shēng, wàn wù yǐ róng, yè wò zǎo qǐ, guǎng bù yú tíng, pī fà huǎn xíng, yǐ shǐ zhì shēng, shēng ér wù shā, yǔ ér wù duó, shǎng ér wù fá, cǐ chūn qì zhī yìng, yǎng shēng zhī dào yě. nì zhī zé shāng gān, xià wèi hán biàn, fèng zhǎng zhě shǎo.

The three months of spring are called the bringing forth of the old. Heaven and Earth are both giving birth, and the ten thousand things flourish. Sleep at night and rise early; walk broadly in the courtyard; loosen the hair and ease the body, so that the will may be born. Give life and do not kill, give and do not take away, reward and do not punish. This is the response to the qi of spring and the way of nourishing life. To go against it harms the liver, and in summer brings a cold-change, so that little is left to supply the season of growth.

What the day is in small, the year is in large. The second chapter takes each season in turn and says when to sleep and to rise, how to carry the will, and what in oneself to nourish, then warns that to live against a season injures the organ that rules it and robs the next season of what it needs. Spring is for bringing the old growth forth; one rises early, walks in the open, and lets plans and intentions begin, favouring gentle growth over force. To live against spring strains the liver, and leaves too little to carry into the heat. The other three seasons keep the same shape, and the practice note below gathers all four into a form you can act on.

SU WEN 2

夫四時陰陽者，萬物之根本也。所以聖人春夏養陽，秋冬養陰，以從其根，故與萬物沉浮於生長之門。逆其根，則伐其本，壞其真矣。故陰陽四時者，萬物之終始也，死生之本也，逆之則災害生，從之則苛疾不起，是謂得道。

fū sì shí yīn yáng zhě, wàn wù zhī gēn běn yě. suǒ yǐ shèng rén chūn xià yǎng yáng, qiū dōng yǎng yīn, yǐ cóng qí gēn, gù yǔ wàn wù chén fú yú shēng zhǎng zhī mén. nì qí gēn, zé fá qí běn, huài qí zhēn yǐ. gù yīn yáng sì shí zhě, wàn wù zhī zhōng shǐ yě, sǐ shēng zhī běn yě, nì zhī zé zāi hài shēng, cóng zhī zé kē jí bù qǐ, shì wèi dé dào.

The four seasons, with their yin and yang, are the root and foundation of the ten thousand things. And so the sage nourishes the yang through spring and summer and the yin through autumn and winter, following this root, and so rises and sinks with the ten thousand things at the gate of birth and growth. To turn against the root is to hack at one's own foundation and to ruin what is true within. Yin and yang and the four seasons are the end and the beginning of all things, the root of death and life: go against them and disaster is born; follow them and no grave illness arises. This is what it means to hold the Way.

This is the root principle beneath the four regimens, and the classic states it here as plainly as it states anything. The seasons are not a setting for health but its very ground: yin and yang across the year are the beginning and the end of all living things, and to keep step with them is what the chapter calls holding the Way. To work against them is not merely to risk discomfort but to strike at one's own foundation, and from that, the text warns, calamity follows of itself.

Two of the most quoted lines in all of Chinese medicine sit in this same short chapter. The first is its counsel to build the yang through spring and summer and the yin through autumn and winter, laying in the store that each half of the year will draw on. The second is the physician's founding rule, to tend the illness before it arrives and settle the disorder before it forms; to reach for medicine only after disease is full, the chapter says, is to dig a well when you are already thirsty. The plain, day-by-day version of this counsel returns in the closing pages on living well.

LIVING WITH THE FOUR SEASONS

Spring (wood, the liver). Sleep at night and rise early; walk in the open air; loosen the body and let intentions and plans take shape. Encourage, do not force. Living against it strains the liver.

Summer (fire, the heart). Sleep at night and rise early; do not resent the long bright days; let the spirit open and express itself outward, and keep the temper from flaring. Living against it strains the heart.

Autumn (metal, the lung). Sleep and rise early, with the fowl; draw the will inward and keep it calm as the air turns keen; gather rather than scatter. Living against it strains the lung.

Winter (water, the kidney). Sleep early and rise after first light; keep the will quiet and held close, as though guarding something of your own; stay warm, and do not throw the pores open in sweat. Living against it strains the kidney.

The single rule beneath the four: in the growing half of the year nourish the yang, staying active and outward; in the gathering half nourish the yin, growing quiet and inward. Spend with the season that is spending, and conserve with the season that conserves.

Treating What Is Not Yet Ill

SU WEN 2

是故聖人不治已病治未病，不治已亂治未亂，此之謂也。夫病已成而後藥之，亂已成而後治之，譬猶渴而穿井，鬥而鑄錐，不亦晚乎！

shì gù shèng rén bù zhì yǐ bìng zhì wèi bìng, bù zhì yǐ luàn zhì wèi luàn, cǐ zhī wèi yě. fū bìng yǐ chéng ér hòu yào zhī, luàn yǐ chéng ér hòu zhì zhī, pì yóu kě ér chuān jǐng, dòu ér zhù zhuī, bù yì wǎn hū!

And so the sage does not treat what is already ill but treats what is not yet ill; he does not bring order to what is already in turmoil but to what is not yet in turmoil. This is the meaning of it. To reach for medicine only after the disease has formed, to impose order only after the turmoil has broken out, is like digging a well after the thirst has come, or forging a weapon after the battle has begun. Is it not already too late?

From the discipline of nurturing life comes the maxim that the whole tradition holds as its summit. The sage does not treat what is already ill but what is not yet ill; he brings order not to the turmoil that has broken out but to the turmoil not yet formed. To reach for medicine only after the disease has taken shape, the classic says, is like digging a well after the thirst has come, or forging a weapon after the battle has begun.

This is the practical reason the nurturing of life stands first, for physician and layperson alike. The work that matters most is done on the not-yet-ill: the faint imbalance, the early sign, the season in which a given organ is exposed. To act there, by the plain disciplines of this gate, is medicine at its height and its cheapest; to wait is to pay later, and dearer. Everything in the gates that follow, the channels, the needle, the formulas, the reading of the years, is in the end in service of this one turn of mind, from cure toward care.

The Span of Years

LING SHU 54

黃帝問於岐伯曰：願聞人之始生，何氣築為基，何立而為楯，何失而死，何得而生？岐伯曰：以母為基，以父為楯。血氣已和，營衛已通，五藏已成，神氣舍心，魂魄畢具，乃成為人。

huáng dì wèn yú qí bó yuē: yuàn wén rén zhī shǐ shēng, hé qì zhù wèi jī, hé lì ér wèi dùn, hé shī ér sǐ, hé dé ér shēng? qí bó yuē: yǐ mǔ wèi jī, yǐ fù wèi dùn. xuè qì yǐ hé, yíng wèi yǐ tōng, wǔ zàng yǐ chéng, shén qì shě xīn, hún pò bì jù, nǎi chéng wèi rén.

The Yellow Emperor asked Qibo: I wish to hear, when a person first comes to be, what qi is built as the foundation, what is set up as the shield, what when lost brings death, and what when kept gives life. Qibo said: The mother is the foundation, the father the shield. When the blood and qi are in harmony and the nutritive and defensive qi run through, when the five organs are complete, the spirit-qi lodges in the heart, and the ethereal and bodily souls are all present, then a person is made.

The Spiritual Pivot asks the plainest question of all, what a person is made from and what a life rests upon, and answers it in a single breath. The mother gives the foundation and the father the shield; and when the blood and qi are in harmony, the nutritive and defensive qi run their courses, the organs are whole, and the spirit settles in the heart with both souls present, then, and only then, is there a person. A human being, in this account, is not a machine assembled but a harmony achieved, and the keeping of that harmony is the whole work of this gate.

LING SHU 54

人生十歲，五藏始定，血氣已通，其氣在下，故好走。二十歲，血氣始盛，肌肉方長，故好趨。三十歲，五藏大定，肌肉堅固，血脈盛滿，故好步。四十歲，五藏六府十二經脈皆大盛以平定，腠理始疏，榮華頹落，髮頗斑白，故好坐。五十歲，肝氣始衰，目始不明。六十歲，心氣始衰，血氣懈惰，故好臥。七十歲，脾氣虛，皮膚枯。八十歲，肺氣衰，魄離，故言善誤。九十歲，腎氣焦，經脈空虛。百歲，五藏皆虛，神氣皆去，形骸獨居而終矣。

rén shēng shí suì, wǔ zàng shǐ dìng, xuè qì yǐ tōng, qí qì zài xià, gù hǎo zǒu. èr shí suì, xuè qì shǐ shèng, jī ròu fāng zhǎng, gù hǎo qū. sān shí suì, wǔ zàng dà dìng, jī ròu jiān gù, xuè mài shèng mǎn, gù hǎo bù. sì shí suì, wǔ zàng liù fǔ shí èr jīng mài jiē dà shèng yǐ píng dìng, còu lǐ shǐ shū, róng huá tuí luò, fà pō bān bái, gù hǎo zuò. wǔ shí suì, gān qì shǐ shuāi, mù shǐ bù míng. liù shí suì, xīn qì shǐ shuāi, xuè qì xiè duò, gù hǎo wò. qī shí suì, pí qì xū, pí fū kū. bā shí suì, fèi qì shuāi, pò lí, gù yán shàn wù. jiǔ shí suì, shèn qì jiāo, jīng mài kōng xū. bǎi suì, wǔ zàng jiē xū, shén qì jiē qù, xíng hái dú jū ér zhōng yǐ.

At ten years the five organs are first settled, the blood and qi are through, and the qi sits in the lower body, so the child loves to run. At twenty the blood and qi begin to flourish and the flesh is growing, so one loves to hurry. At thirty the organs are firmly settled, the flesh solid, the vessels full, so one loves to walk. At forty the organs, the palaces, and the twelve channels are all at their full and steady height; the pores begin to loosen, the bloom begins to fall, the hair turns flecked with grey, so one loves to sit. At fifty the liver-qi begins to wane and the eyes begin to dim. At sixty the heart-qi begins to wane, the blood and qi grow slack, so one loves to lie down. At seventy the spleen-qi is empty and the skin grows dry. At eighty the lung-qi wanes and the bodily soul

> departs, so the speech often errs. At ninety the kidney-qi is parched and the channels stand empty. At a hundred the five organs are all empty and the spirit-qi has gone; the frame remains alone, and the end has come.

The classic then walks the length of a life, ten years at a time, and the picture is unsentimental and exact. The qi rises and gathers through the early decades, so that a child runs, a youth hurries, a grown person walks; it crests near forty, when the hair first greys and one comes to love sitting; and from fifty it withdraws organ by organ, the liver and the eyes first, then the heart and the wish to lie down, the spleen and the skin, the lung and the clarity of speech, the kidney last of all, until at a hundred the organs stand empty, the spirit has gone, and the frame is left alone. To know this curve is not to despair of it. It is to know which way the tide runs at each age, and so to spend the rising years without waste and to guard the falling ones with care.

> LING SHU 6
>
> 黃帝問於伯高曰：余聞形有緩急，氣有盛衰，骨有大小，肉有堅脆，皮有厚薄，其以立壽夭奈何？伯高答曰：形與氣相任則壽，不相任則夭。皮與肉相果則壽，不相果則夭。血氣經絡，勝形則壽，不勝形則夭。
>
> *huáng dì wèn yú bó gāo yuē: yú wén xíng yǒu huǎn jí, qì yǒu shèng shuāi, gǔ yǒu dà xiǎo, ròu yǒu jiān cuì, pí yǒu hòu bó, qí yǐ lì shòu yāo nài hé? bó gāo dá yuē: xíng yǔ qì xiāng rèn zé shòu, bù xiāng rèn zé yāo. pí yǔ ròu xiāng guǒ zé shòu, bù xiāng guǒ zé yāo. xuè qì jīng luò, shèng xíng zé shòu, bù shèng xíng zé yāo.*
>
> The Yellow Emperor asked Bo Gao: I have heard that the form may be loose or tight, the qi flourishing or waning, the bones large or small, the flesh firm or frail, the skin thick or thin; how do these set a person's long life or early death? Bo Gao answered: When the form and the qi are equal to each other, there is long life; when they are not, an early death. When the skin and the flesh hold to each other, there is long life; when they do not, an early death. When the blood, the qi, the channels, and the collaterals are a match for the form, there is long life; when they cannot match the form, an early death.

Why, then, do two people born in the same year not reach the same age? Because the span has a baseline set by the build. Where the form and the qi are matched, where skin and flesh hold firm together, where the blood and the vessels are equal to the body they must supply, a life runs long; where these are mismatched, it runs short. The constitution deals the hand. But it does not play it: the disciplines of this gate, measure and regularity and the quieting of the spirit, are how a modest endowment is made to last, and how a strong one is kept from being thrown away.

FROM THE AUTHOR

I did not come to this gate as a scholar. I came to it as a patient. For years a deep disorder of the spleen and the stomach was read as something it was not, and the more it was met as an acute thing to be suppressed, the longer it kept its hold. What turned it in the end was not a heroic remedy. It was the slow work this chapter describes: measure in food, regularity in sleep, the quieting of a driven mind, the keeping of warmth, and the refusal to spend what I did not have. The classic calls this nurturing life. I have come to call it the ground I stand on, and the first thing I teach.

恬惔虛無，真氣從之。

Be calm and empty, free of striving, and the true qi will follow.

WHERE THIS GATE LEADS

The seasonal discipline rests on a single distinction, taken up in *Gate Two, The Two That Make the Ten Thousand*. The inner side of stillness, the guarding of the spirit, is carried into a full practice in *Gate Ten, The Work of Return*. And the cycle of the seasons opens onto the great cycle of the years in *Gate Nine, The Weather of the Years*.

PART TWO

The Two That Make the Ten Thousand

Yin and Yang

陰陽

On yin and yang. The single distinction from which the whole of medicine, time, change, and the body unfolds, and to which, in the end, all of it returns.

GATE TWO · YIN AND YANG

The Two That Make the Ten Thousand

陰陽

> *Yin and yang are the Way of Heaven and Earth, the cord and net of the ten thousand things.*
>
> Su Wen 5

If the first gate gave the discipline of a whole life, this one gives the idea beneath it, and beneath all the rest. Nearly every page that follows, the organs, the channels, the pulse, the needle, the calendar of the years, is in some way the working out of a single distinction. Learn it well here, and the remainder of the book becomes legible. Yin and yang are not two things. They are not two substances or two forces standing side by side. They are a way of dividing any one whole into its two aspects: the active and the quiet, the warming and the cooling, the outer and the inner, the function and the form. Nothing is yin or yang in itself; each is named only in relation to the other. The outside of the body is yang to its inside; yet within the outside, the back is yang and the front is yin; and within any single organ there is again a yang aspect and a yin aspect. This relativity is the whole of the subtlety, and the place where a beginner most often slips, mistaking yin and yang for fixed labels rather than for a question one asks afresh at every scale.

Read this gate, then, for the same five things. What yin and yang are: the two aspects of any whole. Whom they concern: every patient and every well person, since the body is read this way from the skin to the marrow. When and where they apply: everywhere, at every scale, from the turning of the heavens to a single beat at the wrist. Why they matter: because health is their balance and disease their imbalance. And how they are used: to find, in any complaint, which side has grown too full or too empty, and to restore the mean between them. That last sentence is the physician's whole art in miniature, and we will follow it to the end of the gate.

The Root of All Things

SU WEN 5

陰陽者，天地之道也，萬物之綱紀，變化之父母，生殺之本始，神明之府也。治病必求於本。

yīn yáng zhě, tiān dì zhī dào yě, wàn wù zhī gāng jì, biàn huà zhī fù mǔ, shēng shā zhī běn shǐ, shén míng zhī fǔ yě. zhì bìng bì qiú yú běn.

Yin and yang are the Way of Heaven and Earth, the cord and net of the ten thousand things, the father and mother of all change, the root and beginning of life and death, the dwelling-place of spirit-brightness. In treating illness, one must always seek the root.

SU WEN 6

岐伯對曰：陰陽者，數之可十，推之可百，數之可千，推之可萬，萬之大，不可勝數，然其要一也。

qí bó duì yuē: yīn yáng zhě, shǔ zhī kě shí, tuī zhī kě bǎi, shǔ zhī kě qiān, tuī zhī kě wàn, wàn zhī dà, bù kě shèng shǔ, rán qí yào yī yě.

Qibo answered: Yin and yang may be counted to ten, drawn out to a hundred, counted to a thousand, drawn out to ten thousand; and beyond ten thousand they cannot be numbered, yet their essential is one.

The classic does not introduce yin and yang modestly. It calls them the Way of Heaven and Earth, the cord that binds the ten thousand things, the parent of all change, the root of living and dying, and then gives the healer a command that the whole tradition has obeyed ever since: in treating disease, one must seek the root. A symptom is a surface. Behind it lies a disturbance of the balance, and it is that disturbance, not only its outward sign, that the physician is charged to find and to right.

The second passage answers the obvious worry, that a single pair could not possibly account for so vast a medicine. Yin and yang, it says, may be counted to ten, drawn out to a hundred, to a thousand, to ten thousand, past all counting, and yet their essence is one. The three yin and three yang, the twelve channels, the five phases, the endless tables of correspondence in the pages ahead are all elaborations of this one distinction. Master the one, and the many cease to be a burden to memory and become instead a single idea, seen from many sides. This is also, quietly, the cultivator's discovery, the return of the ten thousand to the one, and the tenth gate takes it up in earnest.

The chapter's answer is that the pair never stops dividing. There is yin within yin and yang within yang: the day is yang, but its morning is the yang within yang and its afternoon the yin within yang, and the same split runs on without end. This is why so simple a scheme can hold so much. Yin and yang are not two fixed boxes but a way of cutting any whole, at any scale, as finely as a case needs. Much of the confusion a beginner feels falls away once this one point is held: the terms are always relative, never absolute.

How the One Divides

SU WEN 5

故積陽為天，積陰為地。陰靜陽躁，陽生陰長，陽殺陰藏。陽化氣，陰成形。寒極生熱，熱極生寒。

gù jī yáng wèi tiān, jī yīn wèi dì. yīn jìng yáng zào, yáng shēng yīn zhǎng, yáng shā yīn cáng. yáng huà qì, yīn chéng xíng. hán jí shēng rè, rè jí shēng hán.

So the massing of yang made Heaven, and the massing of yin made Earth. Yin is still and yang is stirring; yang gives birth and yin brings to growth, yang slays and yin stores away. Yang transforms into qi, and yin completes into form. Cold at its extreme gives birth to heat, and heat at its extreme to cold.

SU WEN 5

故曰：天地者，萬物之上下也；陰陽者，血氣之男女也；水火者，陰陽之徵兆也；陰陽者，萬物之能始也。

gù yuē: tiān dì zhě, wàn wù zhī shàng xià yě; yīn yáng zhě, xuè qì zhī nán nǚ yě; shuǐ huǒ zhě, yīn yáng zhī zhēng zhào yě; yīn yáng zhě, wàn wù zhī néng shǐ yě.

So it is said: Heaven and Earth are the above and below of the ten thousand things; yin and yang are the male and female of blood and qi; water and fire are the emblems of yin

> and yang; and yin and yang are the very capacity from which the ten thousand things begin.

One line here is worth more than a page of definition. Yang transforms into qi, and yin completes into form. Yang is the functional, dispersing, warming, quickening side of anything; yin is the material, condensing, cooling, structuring side. A living body is the two at once: the form that yin builds, kept warm and moving by the qi that yang supplies. And because cold at its extreme gives birth to heat, and heat at its extreme to cold, the two are not fixed enemies but a turning, each passing into the other when pressed to its limit, as midnight begins the return toward noon.

If you want a single image to hold all of this, the classic gives it: water and fire are the emblems of yin and yang. Fire rises, is hot, bright, and restless; water sinks, is cold, dark, and still. Everything else in the table below is only this pair seen in another guise. Read it, but read it remembering the rule of relativity: each term is yang or yin only beside its neighbour.

There is a working rule hidden in this pair. Because yang turns into qi and yin settles into form, a shortage of yang tends to show as things going cold and slack and failing to move, while a shortage of yin shows as things drying, heating, and wearing thin. In the clinic that one line often points the way before any name is reached: is the trouble a loss of the warming, moving side, or of the cooling, building side. The rest of this gate is really only that single question, asked in finer and finer detail.

THE TWO ASPECTS, IN THEIR COMMON CORRESPONDENCES

Yang 陽	Yin 陰
Heaven	Earth
Fire	Water
The sun, the day	The moon, the night
Movement, activity	Stillness, rest
Rising, dispersing	Descending, gathering
The exterior, the surface	The interior, the depths
Function and qi	Substance and form
Warmth, heat	Coolness, cold
Brightness	Shadow
The back, above	The front, below

When the Balance Tips

SU WEN 5

陰勝則陽病，陽勝則陰病。陽勝則熱，陰勝則寒。重寒則熱，重熱則寒。

yīn shèng zé yáng bìng, yáng shèng zé yīn bìng. yáng shèng zé rè, yīn shèng zé hán. chóng hán zé rè, chóng rè zé hán.

When yin prevails, yang sickens; when yang prevails, yin sickens. Yang in excess makes heat, yin in excess makes cold. Cold upon cold turns to heat, and heat upon heat turns to cold.

Here is the whole theory of disease in two lines. Illness is not, in this view, an invader to be named and killed so much as a balance gone wrong: one side grown too full at the other's expense, or one side fallen too empty to hold its place. When yang is in excess there is heat; when yin is in excess there is cold; and either, pushed far enough, flips into its opposite, which is why a high fever can end in a deathly chill.

The method that follows is the physician's first move in every case, before any formula or needle is chosen. Ask which side is in excess and which in want, for everything after turns on the answer. Heat signs, a flushed face, thirst for cold drink, restlessness, a rapid forceful pulse, point toward yang in excess or yin too weak to restrain it. Cold signs, pallor, a craving for warmth, weariness, loose stool, a slow faint pulse, point toward yin in excess or yang too weak to warm. To read the case wrongly here, to warm what is already hot or cool what is already cold, is the gravest of errors, and the rest of the book exists to keep you from it.

First, Yin and Yang

SU WEN 5

善診者，察色按脈，先別陰陽；審清濁，而知部分；視喘息，聽音聲，而知所苦；觀權衡規矩，而知病所主；按尺寸，觀浮沉滑濇，而知病所生。以治無過，以診則不失矣。

shàn zhěn zhě, chá sè àn mài, xiān bié yīn yáng; shěn qīng zhuó, ér zhī bù fèn; shì chuǎn xī, tīng yīn shēng, ér zhī suǒ kǔ; guān quán héng guī jǔ, ér zhī bìng suǒ zhǔ; àn chǐ cùn, guān fú chén huá sè, ér zhī bìng suǒ shēng. yǐ zhì wú guò, yǐ zhěn zé bù shī yǐ.

The skilled diagnostician examines the colour and palpates the pulse, and first of all distinguishes yin from yang. He weighs the clear against the turbid, and so knows which region is affected; he watches the breathing and listens to the voice, and so knows where the suffering lies; he observes the patient against the standards of measure, and so knows what governs the disease; he presses the inch and the cubit and observes the floating, the sinking, the slippery, and the rough, and so knows where the disease arose. Treating in this way he makes no error, and in diagnosis he does not fail.

Before colour, breath, voice, or pulse is weighed, one distinction comes first, and the whole of the reading turns on it: is the pattern a yin one or a yang one? The chapter sets out the full method of examination, looking, listening, and palpating, but it places this single judgement at the head of them all. The later gates fill in the colours of the face and the qualities of the pulse; here the classic fixes the order in which they are to be read, yin and yang before all else.

Reading Yin and Yang at the Wrist

> SU WEN 7
>
> 所謂陰陽者，去者為陰，至者為陽；靜者為陰，動者為陽；遲者為陰，數者為陽。謹熟陰陽，無與眾謀。
>
> *suǒ wèi yīn yáng zhě, qù zhě wèi yīn, zhì zhě wèi yáng; jìng zhě wèi yīn, dòng zhě wèi yáng; chí zhě wèi yīn, shù zhě wèi yáng. jǐn shú yīn yáng, wú yǔ zhòng móu.*
>
> As for yin and yang: what departs is yin, what arrives is yang; the still is yin, the moving is yang; the slow is yin, the rapid is yang. Know yin and yang thoroughly, and you need take counsel of no crowd.

The distinction is not left in the heavens; it is brought down to the fingertips. At the wrist, a pulse is read first of all as yin or yang: what recedes under the finger is yin, what rises to meet it yang; the quiet beat is yin, the lively yang; the slow is yin, the rapid yang. From this first sorting the finer diagnosis unfolds, and the gate on reading the body carries it much further. The classic adds a promise that doubles as a standard: know yin and yang thoroughly, and you need consult no one, for the foundation of judgement is already in your hand.

Restoring the Mean

SU WEN 5

形不足者，溫之以氣；精不足者，補之以味。其高者，因而越之；其下者，引而竭之。

xíng bù zú zhě, wēn zhī yǐ qì; jīng bù zú zhě, bǔ zhī yǐ wèi. qí gāo zhě, yīn ér yuè zhī; qí xià zhě, yǐn ér jié zhī.

Where the form is insufficient, warm it with qi; where the essence is insufficient, supplement it with flavour. What is high, lift and release; what is low, draw downward and drain.

Treatment falls out of all this as plainly as a conclusion from its premises. Where the form is depleted, warm and raise it with qi; where the essence is thin, replenish it with the rich flavours that build substance. The governing principle is the principle of opposites: cool the hot, warm the cold, fill the empty, drain the full, lift what has sunk, settle what has risen. Every herb in the cabinet and every point along the channels serves this one end, the restoration of a mean that has been lost. The eighth gate sets it out as a full art; here it is enough to see that the whole of treatment is already implied by yin and yang.

Yin Within Yin

SU WEN 4

故曰：陰中有陰，陽中有陽。平旦至日中，天之陽，陽中之陽也；日中至黃昏，天之陽，陽中之陰也；合夜至雞鳴，天之陰，陰中之陰也；雞鳴至平旦，天之陰，陰中之陽也。故人亦應之。

gù yuē: yīn zhōng yǒu yīn, yáng zhōng yǒu yáng. píng dàn zhì rì zhōng, tiān zhī yáng, yáng zhōng zhī yáng yě; rì zhōng zhì huáng hūn, tiān zhī yáng, yáng zhōng zhī yīn yě; hé yè zhì jī míng, tiān zhī yīn, yīn zhōng zhī yīn yě; jī míng zhì píng dàn, tiān zhī yīn, yīn zhōng zhī yáng yě. gù rén yì yīng zhī.

So it is said: within the yin there is yin, and within the yang there is yang. From dawn to noon is the yang of Heaven, the yang within the yang; from noon to dusk is the yang of Heaven, the yin within the yang; from nightfall to cockcrow is the yin of Heaven, the yin within the yin; from cockcrow to dawn is the yin of Heaven, the yang within the yin. And the human being answers to this as well.

SU WEN 4

故背為陽，陽中之陽，心也；背為陽，陽中之陰，肺也；腹為陰，陰中之陰，腎也；腹為陰，陰中之陽，肝也；腹為陰，陰中之至陰，脾也。

gù bèi wèi yáng, yáng zhōng zhī yáng, xīn yě; bèi wèi yáng, yáng zhōng zhī yīn, fèi yě; fù wèi yīn, yīn zhōng zhī yīn, shèn yě; fù wèi yīn, yīn zhōng zhī yáng, gān yě; fù wèi yīn, yīn zhōng zhī zhì yīn, pí yě.

So the back is yang, and within that yang the yang is the heart and the yin the lung; the belly is yin, and within that yin the yin is the kidney, the yang the liver, and the most yin of all the spleen.

Here the relativity promised at the opening of this gate is made exact. There is yin within yin and yang within yang, and the same hour or organ may be either, according to what it is set beside. The morning, though it belongs to the day's yang, is the yang within the yang; the afternoon is the yin within the yang; deep night is the yin within the yin, and the hours before dawn the yang within the yin. The body divides the same way: the back is yang and the belly yin, and within each the organs sort again, the heart as the yang within the yang, the kidney as the yin within the yin. Nothing here is fixed. Each thing is named only by its neighbour, and a physician who forgets it will take a relative yang for an absolute one and treat the wrong thing.

The Reaches of the Pair

The one distinction does not stop at the body's halves. Chapter after chapter draws it out into every domain the medicine touches. The classic ranks even the channels by it, calling the greater-yang the warp of the system, the bright-yang its binding cord, the lesser-yang its roving part, and the three grades of yin the outer, the inner, and the extreme.

> SU WEN 79
>
> 三陽為經，二陽為維，一陽為游部；三陰為表，二陰為裏，一陰至絕。
>
> *sān yáng wèi jīng, èr yáng wèi wéi, yī yáng wèi yóu bù; sān yīn wèi biǎo, èr yīn wèi lǐ, yī yīn zhì jué.*
>
> The greater-yang is the warp, the bright-yang the binding cord, the lesser-yang the roving part; the greater-yin is the outer, the lesser-yin the inner, and the reverting-yin reaches to the very end.

It divides the very qi of the body. What the body draws from food is turbid and inclines to yin; what it draws from the air is clear and inclines to yang; the clear pours into the yin tracts and the turbid into the yang, and where the two interfere a disorder of qi follows.

LING SHU 40

黃帝曰：願聞人氣之清濁。岐伯曰：受穀者濁，受氣者清。清者注陰，濁者注陽。清濁相干，命曰亂氣。

huáng dì yuē: yuàn wén rén qì zhī qīng zhuó. qí bó yuē: shòu gǔ zhě zhuó, shòu qì zhě qīng. qīng zhě zhù yīn, zhuó zhě zhù yáng. qīng zhuó xiāng gān, mìng yuē luàn qì.

The Yellow Emperor said: I wish to hear of the clear and the turbid in a person's qi. Qibo said: That which receives the grain is turbid; that which receives the breath is clear. The clear pours into the yin, the turbid into the yang; and when the clear and the turbid interfere with each other, it is called a chaos of qi.

It binds the body to the calendar and the sky. Above the waist is Heaven and below it Earth; the twelve channels of the legs answer to the twelve months and the ten fingers to the ten days, so that the turning seasons and the standing body keep one yin-yang reckoning between them.

LING SHU 41

黃帝曰：余聞天為陽，地為陰，日為陽，月為陰，其合之於人奈何？岐伯曰：腰以上為天，腰以下為地，故天為陽，地為陰。足之十二經脈以應十二月，手之十指以應十日。

huáng dì yuē: yú wén tiān wèi yáng, dì wèi yīn, rì wèi yáng, yuè wèi yīn, qí hé zhī yú rén nài hé? qí bó yuē: yāo yǐ shàng wèi tiān, yāo yǐ xià wèi dì, gù tiān wèi yáng, dì wèi yīn. zú zhī shí èr jīng mài yǐ yīng shí èr yuè, shǒu zhī shí zhǐ yǐ yīng shí rì.

The Yellow Emperor said: I have heard that Heaven is yang and Earth is yin, the sun yang and the moon yin; how are these matched in a person? Qibo said: Above the waist is Heaven, below the waist is Earth; so Heaven is yang and Earth is yin. The twelve channels of the feet answer to the twelve months, and the ten fingers of the hands answer to the ten days.

And it reaches all the way into build and temperament. From the five phases the classic derives twenty-five constitutional types, five within each phase, told apart by colour and form.

> LING SHU 64
>
> 天地之間，六合之內，不離於五，人亦應之。先立五形，金木水火土，別其五色，異其五形之人，而二十五人具矣。
>
> *tiān dì zhī jiān, liù hé zhī nèi, bù lí yú wǔ, rén yì yīng zhī. xiān lì wǔ xíng, jīn mù shuǐ huǒ tǔ, bié qí wǔ sè, yì qí wǔ xíng zhī rén, ér èr shí wǔ rén jù yǐ.*
>
> Between Heaven and Earth, within the six directions, nothing departs from the five, and a person too answers to them. First set down the five forms, metal, wood, water, fire, and earth, distinguish their five colours, and tell apart the people of the five forms; and so the twenty-five types are complete.

A companion chapter extends the same five-fold scheme to the tones and the flavours that suit each type, and then turns it to a question as concrete as why a woman grows no beard. The answer it gives runs straight back to yin and yang.

LING SHU 65

黃帝曰：婦人無鬚者，無血氣乎？岐伯曰：衝脈、任脈，皆起於胞中，上循背裏，為經絡之海。其浮而外者，循腹上行，會於咽喉，別而絡脣口。血氣盛則充膚熱肉，血獨盛則澹滲皮膚，生毫毛。婦人之生，有餘於氣，不足於血，以其數脫血也，衝任之脈不榮脣口，故鬚不生。

huáng dì yuē: fù rén wú xū zhě, wú xuè qì hū? qí bó yuē: chōng mài, rèn mài, jiē qǐ yú bāo zhōng, shàng xún bèi lǐ, wèi jīng luò zhī hǎi. qí fú ér wài zhě, xún fù shàng háng, huì yú yān hóu, bié ér luò chún kǒu. xuè qì shèng zé chōng fū rè ròu, xuè dú shèng zé dàn shèn pí fū, shēng háo máo. fù rén zhī shēng, yǒu yú yú qì, bù zú yú xuè, yǐ qí shuò tuō xuè yě, chōng rèn zhī mài bù róng chún kǒu, gù xū bù shēng.

The Yellow Emperor asked: Women grow no beard; is it that they lack blood and qi? Qibo said: The penetrating vessel and the controlling vessel both rise from within the womb and run up along the inside of the spine, the sea of the channels and collaterals. The part that floats outward runs up the belly, meets at the throat, and branches to net the lips and mouth. When blood and qi are abundant they fill the skin and warm the flesh; when the blood alone is abundant it seeps to the skin and grows the fine hair. A woman, by her nature, has a surplus of qi and a want of blood, because she loses blood again and again; so her penetrating and controlling vessels do not flourish at the lips and mouth, and no beard grows there.

The reasoning is the method of the whole gate in miniature, and worth following step by step. A plain visible fact, the absence of a beard, is referred first to two vessels, the penetrating and the controlling, which rise from the womb and branch to the lips; the vessels are referred in turn to the blood and qi they carry, and that balance to the standing difference between the sexes. A woman, losing blood by her months, runs richer in qi and shorter in blood, so the vessels that would feed the lip fall short, and no beard grows. This is the how of it: one never stops at the sign, but follows it inward, vessel by substance, until it rests on yin and yang. A shorter scheme, last of all, sorts every person into five kinds by that same balance.

LING SHU 72

蓋有太陰之人，少陰之人，太陽之人，少陽之人，陰陽和平之人。凡五人者，其態不同，其筋骨氣血各不等。

gài yǒu tài yīn zhī rén, shào yīn zhī rén, tài yáng zhī rén, shào yáng zhī rén, yīn yáng hé píng zhī rén. fán wǔ rén zhě, qí tài bù tóng, qí jīn gǔ qì xuè gè bù děng.

There are the greater-yin person, the lesser-yin person, the greater-yang person, the lesser-yang person, and the person in whom yin and yang are in balance. These five differ in their bearing, and their sinews, bones, qi, and blood are each unlike.

These last deserve a clinician's notice. The greater-yang person is bold and outward and quick to spend; the greater-yin person is guarded and inward and slow to give; the balanced person keeps to the mean. To know which kind of person sits before you is to know in advance how their qi is likely to run, and how to weigh whatever you then find in them.

TELLING YIN FROM YANG IN YOURSELF

A **yang pattern** leans toward heat, activity, and excess: feeling warm or flushed, thirst for cold drinks, restlessness, a loud and hurried manner, dryness or constipation, a fast and forceful pulse, a red tongue.

A **yin pattern** leans toward cold, quiet, and depletion: feeling cold, pallor, a wish for warmth and rest, tiredness, loose stool, a slow and faint pulse, a pale tongue.

The aim is never to maximise one side. It is to restore the balance: warm what is cold, cool what is hot, rouse what is sluggish, settle what is agitated. A healthy body, like a good year, is one whose two aspects turn smoothly into each other, neither holding the field too long.

YIN AND YANG

Essential Verses

These are among the gate's most quoted lines in the classic, gathered here for study.

> SU WEN 4
>
> 夫精者，身之本也。故藏於精者，春不病溫。夫上古聖人之教下也，皆謂之虛邪賊風，避之有時。
>
> *fū jīng zhě, shēn zhī běn yě. gù cáng yú jīng zhě, chūn bù bìng wēn. fū shàng gǔ shèng rén zhī jiào xià yě, jiē wèi zhī xū xié zéi fēng, bì zhī yǒu shí.*
>
> The essence is the root of the body. Thus one who stores essence well will not fall to warm disease in spring. When the sages of high antiquity taught those below them, they spoke always of the depleting evils and robber winds, and of avoiding them in their season.

Everything the body can muster against a seasonal illness is drawn from one reserve, the stored essence, and the yin held within is the ground the active yang stands upon. Spend that reserve through a hard winter and the spring opening is left undefended, so the warm disease that arrives in the third month is really the previous winter's depletion coming due. The discipline the line asks for is seasonal husbandry: guard the essence through the cold months with rest, warmth, and restraint, so the store is full when spring's heat tests it, and let summer's sweat issue freely rather than trapping it, since sweat held in becomes autumn's fever. Read this way, the doctrine of yin and yang turns into a plain ledger of saving and spending kept across the year, in which each season collects on the one before.

SU WEN 7

凡陽有五，五五二十五陽。所謂陰者，真藏也，見則為敗，敗必死也；所謂陽者，胃脘之陽也。別於陽者，知病處也；別於陰者，知死生之期。

fán yáng yǒu wǔ, wǔ wǔ èr shí wǔ yáng. suǒ wèi yīn zhě, zhēn zàng yě, jiàn zé wèi bài, bài bì sǐ yě; suǒ wèi yáng zhě, wèi wǎn zhī yáng yě. bié yú yáng zhě, zhī bìng chù yě; bié yú yīn zhě, zhī sǐ shēng zhī qī.

There are five yangs, and five times five makes twenty-five yangs. What is called the yin is the true-organ pulse: when it appears the organ is failing, and failing it must die. What is called the yang is the yang of the stomach cavity. One who can distinguish the yang knows where the disease lies; one who can distinguish the yin knows the term of death or life.

Beneath every pulse the chapter asks the physician to find two things at once. One is the living stomach-qi, felt as a soft, rounded fullness within the beat, the yang of the pulse; the other is the bare true-organ stroke that surfaces only when that fullness is gone, the yin. The distinction settles a case, because the presence of stomach-qi is the presence of a reserve and its absence is a body laid open. So the hand works in two passes: feel first for the rounded stomach quality, which tells where the trouble sits, and then for whether the underlying organ stroke has come up hard and naked, which tells how much time remains. Prognosis here is nothing more than separating two qualities in a single touch of the finger.

SU WEN 79

三陽為父，三陰為母；二陽為衛，二陰為雌；一陽為紀，一陰為獨使。三陽一陰，太陽脈勝，一陰不得止，內亂五藏，外為驚駭。

sān yáng wèi fù, sān yīn wèi mǔ; èr yáng wèi wèi, èr yīn wèi cí; yī yáng wèi jì, yī yīn wèi dú shǐ. sān yáng yī yīn, tài yáng mài shèng, yī yīn bù dé zhǐ, nèi luàn wǔ zàng, wài wèi jīng hài.

The three-yang is father, the three-yin is mother; the two-yang is guard, the two-yin is consort; the one-yang is the cord, the one-yin the solitary envoy. When three-yang

> meets one-yin and the greater-yang pulse prevails, the one-yin cannot hold; within it throws the five organs into disorder, and without it shows as fright and alarm.

The chapter hands the physician a kind of kinship chart for the six channel-divisions, ranking them as father and mother, guard and consort, cord and lone envoy. Naming relations rather than listing parts is the whole point, because a relation tells you how two divisions will behave when they meet, which one leads and which must give way. The reading then runs straight: see which yang and which yin are joined in the patient, judge from the pulse which is prevailing, and trace the result from their fixed bond. Here the greater-yang overpowers the one-yin, which cannot restrain it, so the disorder turns inward to throw the five organs into confusion and outward as startle and fear. It is yin-yang doctrine sharpened into a working calculus of the channels.

FROM THE AUTHOR

The same distinction I read in a client's pulse I read in a chart of birth and in the lie of a piece of land. Where is the warmth here, and where the cold; what is rising, and what has sunk; which aspect rules, and which is starved. The Five Arts are not five subjects but one eye, trained on different objects. Learn to see yin and yang truly in any one of them, and you have begun to see it in all.

數之可十，推之可萬，然其要一也。

Counted to ten, drawn out to ten thousand, yet its essence is one.

WHERE THIS GATE LEADS

The seasonal discipline of *Gate One* is simply yin and yang applied to the year. The officials of *Gate Three, The Court Within* divide at once into yin organs and yang organs. Diagnosis in *Gate Four, Reading the Unspoken* begins, as we have seen, by telling yin from yang. Treatment in *Gate Eight, The Physician's Hand* is the restoring of their balance. And the return of the ten thousand to the one is the inner work of *Gate Ten, The Work of Return*.

PART THREE

The Court Within

The Organs and Their Network

藏象

On the visceral systems. The organs read not as parts laid upon a table but as a court of officials, each with an office to keep, a tissue and a season of its own, and a spirit in its care.

GATE THREE · THE ORGANS AND THEIR NETWORK

The Court Within

藏象

> *The heart is the office of the sovereign, and from it the brightness of spirit issues.*
>
> Su Wen 8

Open a modern anatomy and the organs appear as a catalogue of parts, each to be named, weighed, and set aside. Open this gate and they appear as a court. The heart is the sovereign, the lung its chancellor, the liver its general, the gallbladder its judge, and health is the good order of the whole government, not the soundness of any single piece taken alone.

The name of this gate, cang xiang, says what is meant: the organs within, cang, and their manifestations without, xiang. For the classic an organ is not only the flesh beneath the rib. It is a sphere of function, known by what it governs and by how it shows itself, in a tissue, a colour, an opening of the senses, an emotion, a season. The heart is read in the face, the liver in the eyes and the nails, the kidney in the bones and the hair of the head. The hidden interior is written upon the visible surface, and learning to read that surface is half of diagnosis. This is why the gate matters even to a reader who will never lift a needle: your own face and nails and sleep are already telling you which office is strained.

As in every gate, five questions shape the reading, though here the fifth carries the most weight. The organs, to begin with, are not lumps of tissue but a network of offices, each one announcing itself somewhere on the surface. They concern everyone, sick or well, since any body can be read this way, and the reading is done everywhere: in the consulting room, certainly, but also in the quiet daily noticing of one's own face, nails, and sleep. All of this matters because the body is a single interdependent government in which no office falls alone. The method, though, is the heart of the gate. Trace a complaint back to the office behind it; confirm that office by its outward signs; then treat it together with the organs it leans upon, never as a part lifted out of the whole. To treat an office within its web of dependence, rather than in isolation, is the whole distance between this medicine and a catalogue of parts.

The Twelve Officials

SU WEN 8

心者，君主之官也，神明出焉。肺者，相傅之官，治節出焉。肝者，將軍之官，謀慮出焉。膽者，中正之官，決斷出焉。膻中者，臣使之官，喜樂出焉。

xīn zhě, jūn zhǔ zhī guān yě, shén míng chū yān. fèi zhě, xiàng fù zhī guān, zhì jié chū yān. gān zhě, jiāng jūn zhī guān, móu lǜ chū yān. dǎn zhě, zhōng zhèng zhī guān, jué duàn chū yān. dàn zhōng zhě, chén shǐ zhī guān, xǐ lè chū yān.

The heart is the office of the sovereign, and from it the brightness of spirit issues. The lung is the office of the chancellor and tutor, and from it the ordering of the rhythms issues. The liver is the office of the general, and from it planning and deliberation issue. The gallbladder is the office of the upright judge, and from it decisions issue. The centre of the chest is the office of the envoy, and from it joy and gladness issue.

SU WEN 8

脾胃者，倉廩之官，五味出焉。大腸者，傳道之官，變化出焉。小腸者，受盛之官，化物出焉。腎者，作強之官，伎巧出焉。三焦者，決瀆之官，水道出焉。膀胱者，州都之官，津液藏焉，氣化則能出矣。

pí wèi zhě, cāng lǐn zhī guān, wǔ wèi chū yān. dà cháng zhě, chuán dào zhī guān, biàn huà chū yān. xiǎo cháng zhě, shòu shèng zhī guān, huà wù chū yān. shèn zhě, zuò qiáng zhī guān, jì qiǎo chū yān. sān jiāo zhě, jué dú zhī guān, shuǐ dào chū yān. páng guāng zhě, zhōu dōu zhī guān, jīn yè cáng yān, qì huà zé néng chū yǐ.

The spleen and stomach are the office of the granary, and from them the five flavours issue. The large intestine is the office of conveyance, and from it the transformation of waste issues. The small intestine is the office that receives the full, and from it the transforming of matter issues. The kidney is the office of toil and strength, and from it skill and ingenuity issue. The triple burner is the office that clears the channels, and from it the waterways issue. The bladder is the office of the regional capital, where the fluids are stored, and when the qi transforms them, they can be sent out.

SU WEN 8

凡此十二官者，不得相失也。故主明則下安，以此養生則壽，歿世不殆，以為天下則大昌。主不明則十二官危，使道閉塞而不通，形乃大傷，以此養生則殃，以為天下者，其宗大危，戒之戒之。

fán cǐ shí èr guān zhě, bù dé xiāng shī yě. gù zhǔ míng zé xià ān, yǐ cǐ yǎng shēng zé shòu, mò shì bù dài, yǐ wèi tiān xià zé dà chāng. zhǔ bù míng zé shí èr guān wēi, shǐ dào bì sāi ér bù tōng, xíng nǎi dà shāng, yǐ cǐ yǎng shēng zé yāng, yǐ wèi tiān xià zhě, qí zōng dà wēi, jiè zhī jiè zhī.

These twelve offices must never lose their bond with one another. So when the sovereign is clear, all below are at peace; live by this, and life is long and ends without peril; rule a realm by this, and it flourishes greatly. But when the sovereign is not clear, the twelve offices fall into danger, the roads between them close and no longer pass, and the body is gravely harmed; live by this, and life meets calamity; rule a realm by this, and its line stands in grave danger. Guard against it, guard against it.

The court is not decoration; it is a way of thinking. Each office holds a charge. The heart rules and houses the spirit, so a clear mind is a sound heart. The lung, as chancellor, sets the rhythms, the breath and the pace of the qi. The liver, as general, plans and moves, and turns wrathful when it is thwarted. The gallbladder decides; the granary of spleen and stomach feeds the realm; the intestines carry and sort; the kidney does the hard labour and keeps the deep reserve; the triple burner holds the waterways open; the bladder stores and releases. Name the failing office by its charge, and the disorder half explains itself.

Then comes the law that governs the whole court. The twelve offices must never lose their bond, and everything turns upon the ruler. When the sovereign is clear, all below are at peace, life is long, and a realm prospers; when the sovereign is darkened, the roads between the offices close, and the body is gravely harmed. The teaching for the physician, and for anyone who would keep their own health, is double. Treat the network and not the lone symptom. And above all keep the heart, the seat of the mind and the spirit, clear, for when it is troubled the entire government suffers under it. Here medicine and cultivation meet, and the tenth gate takes up the thread.

The image the chapter is best remembered for stands at its head: the heart is the office of the sovereign, and from it the spirit and its clarity come forth. The rest are ranked below it, the lung as chancellor, the liver as general, and so on, each a post in a single court. The point is not decoration. If the sovereign is bright, the chapter says, the whole realm is steady; if the sovereign is troubled, the twelve posts are all put in danger. That is the classic's way of setting the settled spirit at the centre of health rather than at its edge.

The Roots of Life

SU WEN 9

帝曰：藏象何如？岐伯曰：心者，生之本，神之變也，其華在面，其充在血脈，為陽中之太陽，通於夏氣。肺者，氣之本，魄之處也，其華在毛，其充在皮，為陽中之太陰，通於秋氣。腎者，主蟄，封藏之本，精之處也，其華在髮，其充在骨，為陰中之少陰，通於冬氣。

dì yuē: zàng xiàng hé rú? qí bó yuē: xīn zhě, shēng zhī běn, shén zhī biàn yě, qí huá zài miàn, qí chōng zài xuè mài, wèi yáng zhōng zhī tài yáng, tōng yú xià qì. fèi zhě, qì zhī běn, pò zhī chù yě, qí huá zài máo, qí chōng zài pí, wèi yáng zhōng zhī tài yīn, tōng yú qiū qì. shèn zhě, zhǔ zhé, fēng cáng zhī běn, jīng zhī chù yě, qí huá zài fà, qí chōng zài gǔ, wèi yīn zhōng zhī shào yīn, tōng yú dōng qì.

The Emperor asked: What are the manifestations of the organs? Qibo said: The heart is the root of life and the seat of the spirit's changes; its flowering shows in the face, its fullness in the blood vessels; it is the greater yang within the yang, and joins with the qi of summer. The lung is the root of the qi and the dwelling of the bodily soul; its flowering shows in the body hair, its fullness in the skin; it is the greater yin within the yang, and joins with the qi of autumn. The kidney governs the storing-away, the root of sealing and hoarding and the dwelling of the essence; its flowering shows in the hair of the head, its fullness in the bones; it is the lesser yin within the yin, and joins with the qi of winter.

SU WEN 9

肝者，罷極之本，魂之居也，其華在爪，其充在筋，以生血氣，其味酸，其色蒼，為陽中之少陽，通於春氣。脾、胃、大腸、小腸、三焦、膀胱者，倉廩之本，營之居也，名曰器，能化糟粕，轉味而入出者也，其華在脣四白，其充在肌，其味甘，其色黃，此至陰之類，通於土氣。凡十一臟，取決於膽也。

gān zhě, bà jí zhī běn, hún zhī jū yě, qí huá zài zhǎo, qí chōng zài jīn, yǐ shēng xuè qì, qí wèi suān, qí sè cāng, wèi yáng zhōng zhī shào yáng, tōng yú chūn qì. pí, wèi, dà cháng, xiǎo cháng, sān jiāo, páng guāng zhě, cāng lǐn zhī běn, yíng zhī jū yě, míng yuē qì, néng huà zāo pò, zhuǎn wèi ér rù chū zhě yě, qí huá zài chún sì bái, qí chōng zài jī, qí wèi gān, qí sè huáng, cǐ zhì yīn zhī lèi, tōng yú tǔ qì. fán shí yī zàng, qǔ jué yú dǎn yě.

The liver is the root of endurance and the home of the ethereal soul; its flowering shows in the nails, its fullness in the sinews; it brings forth the blood and qi, its flavour sour and its colour green; it is the lesser yang within the yang, and joins with the qi of spring. The spleen, stomach, large intestine, small intestine, triple burner, and bladder are the root of the granary and the dwelling of the nutritive qi; they are named the vessels, for they can transform the dregs and turn the flavours, taking in and sending out; their flowering shows in the white rim of the lips, their fullness in the flesh, their flavour sweet and their colour yellow; they are of the kind of the utmost yin, and join with the qi of earth. Of all the eleven organs, the decision rests with the gallbladder.

Asked outright what the organs show, the classic answers one by one, and the pattern is exact. Each organ is the root of something, houses one of the spirits, flowers in a tissue you can see, fills a tissue you can feel, and joins with a season of the year. The heart is the root of life and flowers in the face. The lung is the root of the qi and flowers in the skin and its fine hair. The kidney is the root of sealing and storing, holds the essence and the will, and flowers in the bones and the hair of the head. The liver is the root of endurance and flowers in the nails and the sinews. The spleen, with its fellow vessels, is the root of the granary and flowers in the lips and the flesh.

This is what makes the hidden legible. A dull and lifeless complexion speaks of the heart; brittle nails and failing eyes of the liver; thinning hair and aching bones of the kidney; dry skin and a weak voice of the lung; pale slack lips of the spleen. The senses keep the same rule: the eyes open to the liver, the ears to the kidney, the tongue to the heart, the nose to the lung, the mouth to the spleen. The table below gathers the five organs into a single view.

THE FIVE ORGANS AND HOW THEY SHOW THEMSELVES

ORGAN	ITS OFFICE	SPIRIT IT HOUSES	SHOWS ITSELF IN	SEASON
Heart 心	The sovereign	The spirit, shen	The face; the vessels; the tongue	Summer
Lung 肺	The chancellor	The bodily soul, po	The skin and body hair; the nose	Autumn
Liver 肝	The general	The ethereal soul, hun	The nails and sinews; the eyes	Spring
Spleen 脾	The granary	The intent, yi	The lips and flesh; the mouth	Late summer
Kidney 腎	The worker of power	The will, zhi	The head hair and bones; the ears	Winter

What Stores and What Transmits

SU WEN 11

所謂五藏者，藏精氣而不瀉也，故滿而不能實。六腑者，傳化物而不藏，故實而不能滿也。所以然者，水穀入口，則胃實而腸虛；食下，則腸實而胃虛。故曰實而不滿，滿而不實也。

suǒ wèi wǔ zàng zhě, cáng jīng qì ér bù xiè yě, gù mǎn ér bù néng shí. liù fǔ zhě, chuán huà wù ér bù cáng, gù shí ér bù néng mǎn yě. suǒ yǐ rán zhě, shuǐ gǔ rù kǒu, zé wèi shí ér cháng xū; shí xià, zé cháng shí ér wèi xū. gù yuē shí ér bù mǎn, mǎn ér bù shí yě.

What are called the five organs store the essential qi and do not drain it, so they are filled but never replete. The six palaces convey and transform what passes through and do not store it, so they are replete but never filled. The reason is this: when food and drink enter the mouth, the stomach is replete while the intestines are empty; when the food goes down, the intestines are replete while the stomach is empty. So it is said: replete but not filled, filled but not replete.

SU WEN 11

黃帝問曰：余聞方士，或以腦髓為藏，或以腸胃為藏，或以為腑，敢問更相反，皆自謂是，不知其道，願聞其說。岐伯對曰：腦、髓、骨、脈、膽、女子胞，此六者，地氣之所生也，皆藏於陰而象於地，故藏而不瀉，名曰奇恆之府。

huáng dì wèn yuē: yú wén fāng shì, huò yǐ nǎo suǐ wèi zàng, huò yǐ cháng wèi wèi zàng, huò yǐ wèi fǔ, gǎn wèn gèng xiāng fǎn, jiē zì wèi shì, bù zhī qí dào, yuàn wén qí shuō. qí bó duì yuē: nǎo, suǐ, gǔ, mài, dǎn, nǚ zǐ bāo, cǐ liù zhě, dì qì zhī suǒ shēng yě, jiē cáng yú yīn ér xiàng yú dì, gù cáng ér bù xiè, míng yuē qí héng zhī fǔ.

The Yellow Emperor asked: I have heard the practitioners; some take the brain and marrow for organs, some take the bowels and stomach for organs, and some take them for palaces. They contradict one another, each calling himself right, and I do not know

> the principle of it; I wish to hear the explanation. Qibo answered: The brain, the marrow, the bones, the vessels, the gallbladder, and the womb, these six are born of the qi of Earth; all of them store within the yin and take Earth for their image, so they store and do not drain, and are named the curious and constant palaces.

The court divides into two kinds of office, and the difference is one of function, not merely of where each sits. The five organs, the zang, store the essential qi and do not pour it out; they are filled, yet never stuffed. The six palaces, the fu, the stomach and intestines and their fellows, pass food and waste through and transform it; they are stuffed, yet never filled, for as one fills the next empties. The treasure is kept in the zang; the traffic is kept moving by the fu. They sicken in different ways and are treated in different ways, and to confuse the two is to mistake the storehouse for the road.

The classic then names a third kind, the curious and constant palaces: the brain, the marrow, the bones, the vessels, the gallbladder, and the womb. Shaped like the hollow fu yet storing like the solid zang, they keep what is most precious, the marrow and the deep essence, and they sit cleanly in neither column. It is here, at the brain and the marrow and the womb, that the medicine of the organs reaches toward the inner work of essence and spirit, the subject of the tenth gate.

The Substances the Organs Make

The court does more than govern; it manufactures. The organs are the body's makers and keepers of its vital substances, and the classic distinguishes those substances with care, refusing to let them blur into a single word.

> LING SHU 30
>
> 兩神相搏，合而成形，常先身生，是謂精。上焦開發，宣五穀味，熏膚充身澤毛，若霧露之溉，是謂氣。腠理發泄，汗出溱溱，是謂津。穀入氣滿，淖澤注於骨，補益腦髓，是謂液。中焦受氣取汁，變化而赤，是謂血。壅遏營氣，令無所避，是謂脈。
>
> *liǎng shén xiāng bó, hé ér chéng xíng, cháng xiān shēn shēng, shì wèi jīng. shàng jiāo kāi fā, xuān wǔ gǔ wèi, xūn fū chōng shēn zé máo, ruò wù lù zhī gài, shì wèi qì. còu lǐ fā xiè, hàn chū qín qín, shì wèi jīn. gǔ rù qì mǎn, nào zé zhù yú gǔ, bǔ yì nǎo suí, shì wèi yè. zhōng jiāo shòu qì qǔ zhī, biàn huà ér chì, shì wèi xuè. yōng è yíng qì, lìng wú suǒ bì, shì wèi mài.*
>
> When the two spirits grapple and join to form the body, that which is always born before the body is called the essence. When the upper burner opens and spreads the flavours of the five grains, warming the skin, filling the body, and moistening the hair like the watering of mist and dew, that is called the qi. When the pores open and the sweat comes streaming, that is called the jin fluid. When grain enters and the qi is full, and the rich moisture pours into the bones and replenishes the brain and marrow, that is called the ye fluid. When the middle burner receives the qi and takes its juice, transforming it to red, that is called the blood. When the nutritive qi is hemmed in and given nowhere to stray, that is called the vessel.

Six are named, and each has its origin. The essence is what forms before the body itself, the deep reserve drawn from both parents. The qi is what the upper burner spreads from the grain, warming the skin and moistening the hair like mist. The thin jin fluid is what comes out as sweat; the thick ye fluid is what pours into the bones and feeds the brain and marrow. The blood is the grain's juice transformed to red in the middle burner; and the vessel is what hems the nutritive qi and gives it nowhere to stray. The use of the list is exact: to read a depletion, the physician names which of the six is short, and from there which organ that makes or stores it has failed.

SU WEN 23

五味所入：酸入肝，辛入肺，苦入心，鹹入腎，甘入脾，是謂五入。五氣所病：心為噫，肺為咳，肝為語，脾為吞，腎為欠為嚏，胃為氣逆為噦為恐，大腸小腸為泄，下焦溢為水，膀胱不利為癃，不約為遺溺，膽為怒，是謂五病。

wǔ wèi suǒ rù: suān rù gān, xīn rù fèi, kǔ rù xīn, xián rù shèn, gān rù pí, shì wèi wǔ rù. wǔ qì suǒ bìng: xīn wèi yī, fèi wèi ké, gān wèi yǔ, pí wèi tūn, shèn wèi qiàn wèi tì, wèi wèi qì nì wèi yuě wèi kǒng, dà cháng xiǎo cháng wèi xiè, xià jiāo yì wèi shuǐ, páng guāng bù lì wèi lóng, bù yuē wèi yí nì, dǎn wèi nù, shì wèi wǔ bìng.

Where the five flavours enter: the sour enters the liver, the pungent the lung, the bitter the heart, the salty the kidney, and the sweet the spleen; these are called the five entries. The diseases of the five kinds of qi: the heart makes belching, the lung cough, the liver talkativeness, the spleen swallowing, and the kidney yawning and sneezing; the stomach makes counterflowing qi, hiccough, and fear; the large and small intestines make diarrhoea; the lower burner overflowing makes water; the bladder, when it does not run freely, makes dribbling stoppage, and when it does not hold, makes incontinence; the gallbladder makes anger. These are called the five diseases.

The correspondences run both ways, into the organs and out of them. Each flavour enters its own organ, the sour to the liver, the pungent to the lung, the bitter to the heart, the salty to the kidney, the sweet to the spleen; and each organ, when its qi is disturbed, has its own signature complaint, the heart belching, the lung coughing, the kidney yawning and sneezing, the stomach turning its qi back as hiccup. This is a diagnostic shorthand: a craving or a reflex is read back to the office it speaks for.

SU WEN 10

心之合脈也，其榮色也，其主腎也。肺之合皮也，其榮毛也，其主心也。肝之合筋也，其榮爪也，其主肺也。脾之合肉也，其榮脣也，其主肝也。腎之合骨也，其榮髮也，其主脾也。

xīn zhī hé mài yě, qí róng sè yě, qí zhǔ shèn yě. fèi zhī hé pí yě, qí róng máo yě, qí zhǔ xīn yě. gān zhī hé jīn yě, qí róng zhǎo yě, qí zhǔ fèi yě. pí zhī hé ròu yě, qí róng chún yě, qí zhǔ gān yě. shèn zhī hé gǔ yě, qí róng fà yě, qí zhǔ pí yě.

The heart pairs with the vessels; it blossoms in the complexion, and what governs it is the kidney. The lung pairs with the skin; it blossoms in the body hair, and what governs it is the heart. The liver pairs with the sinews; it blossoms in the nails, and what governs it is the lung. The spleen pairs with the flesh; it blossoms in the lips, and what governs it is the liver. The kidney pairs with the bones; it blossoms in the hair of the head, and what governs it is the spleen.

The same chapter ties each organ to a tissue it pairs with, a sign it flowers in, and another organ that holds it in check. The heart pairs with the vessels and shows in the face; the lung with the skin and shows in the body hair; the liver with the sinews and shows in the nails; the spleen with the flesh and shows in the lips; the kidney with the bones and shows in the hair of the head. And each is governed by another along the round of the five phases, so that a trouble that looks to be the liver's may in truth be a weak lung failing to restrain it. To read the surface well is therefore never to read one organ alone, but the ring of five that check and feed each other.

FIGURE · THE FIVE PHASES

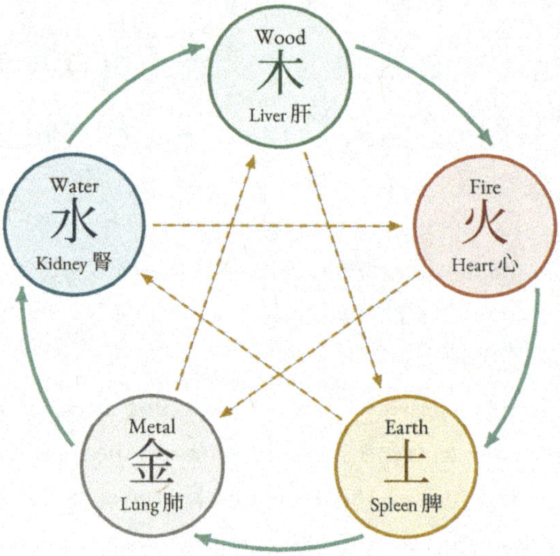

The five phases in their generating cycle (相生, the outer ring) and their controlling cycle (相剋, the inner star), each phase paired with the organ it governs.

Each phase governs far more than a single organ. A season, a direction, a colour, a taste, an emotion, and a voice all belong to the same five, so that one pattern runs from the turning of the seasons all the way to the sound of a person's voice.

THE FIVE PHASES AND THEIR CORRESPONDENCES

PHASE	SEASON	DIRECTION	COLOUR	TASTE	EMOTION	SOUND
Wood 木	Spring	East	Green	Sour	Anger	Shouting
Fire 火	Summer	South	Red	Bitter	Joy	Laughter
Earth 土	Late summer	Centre	Yellow	Sweet	Pensiveness	Singing
Metal 金	Autumn	West	White	Pungent	Grief	Weeping
Water 水	Winter	North	Black	Salty	Fear	Groaning

LING SHU 36

水穀皆入於口，其味有五，各注其海，津液各走其道。天暑衣厚則腠理開，故汗出；天寒則腠理閉，氣濕不行，水下留於膀胱，則為溺與氣。悲哀氣並則為泣，中熱胃緩則為唾。邪氣內逆，則氣為之閉塞而不行，不行則為水脹。

shuǐ gǔ jiē rù yú kǒu, qí wèi yǒu wǔ, gè zhù qí hǎi, jīn yè gè zǒu qí dào. tiān shǔ yī hòu zé còu lǐ kāi, gù hàn chū; tiān hán zé còu lǐ bì, qì shī bù xíng, shuǐ xià liú yú páng guāng, zé wèi nì yǔ qì. bēi āi qì bìng zé wèi qì, zhōng rè wèi huǎn zé wèi tuò. xié qì nèi nì, zé qì wèi zhī bì sāi ér bù xíng, bù xíng zé wèi shuǐ zhàng.

Water and grain all enter the mouth; their flavours are five, each pouring into its own sea, and the fluids each run their own road. When the weather is hot and the clothing thick, the pores open and so there is sweat; when the weather is cold, the pores close, the moist qi does not move, the water settles down into the bladder, and there becomes urine and breath-vapour. When grief gathers the qi, there are tears; when there is heat within and the stomach is slack, there is spittle; and when an evil qi turns back inside, the qi is thereby blocked from moving, and what does not move becomes water-swelling.

Even the body's fluids sort by the five, and by the conditions that call them out: sweat in heat, urine and vapour in cold, tears in grief, spittle when the stomach slackens with heat, and water-swelling when an errant qi blocks the flow. An abnormal fluid is thus a message like any other sign, and is read back to the organ and the state behind it.

The Body Within, and the Shape of Health

The classic did not only reason about the organs; it measured them, and asked plainly why some bodies fall ill and others do not.

> LING SHU 47
>
> 五藏者，所以藏精神血氣魂魄者也；六府者，所以化水穀而行津液者也。此人之所以具受於天也。五藏皆堅者無病，五藏皆脆者不離於病。
>
> *wǔ zàng zhě, suǒ yǐ cáng jīng shén xuè qì hún pò zhě yě; liù fǔ zhě, suǒ yǐ huà shuǐ gǔ ér xíng jīn yè zhě yě. cǐ rén zhī suǒ yǐ jù shòu yú tiān yě. wǔ zàng jiē jiān zhě wú bìng, wǔ zàng jiē cuì zhě bù lí yú bìng.*
>
> The five organs are that which stores the essence and the spirit, the blood and the qi, the ethereal and the bodily souls; the six palaces are that which transforms water and grain and moves the fluids. This is what every person receives complete from Heaven. When the five organs are all firm, there is no illness; when they are all frail, one is never free of illness.

Here is the division of labour in one line, and a verdict on constitution besides. The five organs store what is precious, the essence and spirit, the blood and qi and the two souls; the six palaces transform food and move the fluids. And the firmness of the organs is itself a kind of health: where they are all firm there is no illness, where they are all frail one is never quite free of it. The teaching for the physician is to weigh the build before the complaint, guarding the frail-organ body and trusting the firm one to bear more.

LING SHU 31

黃帝問於伯高曰：余願聞六府傳穀者，腸胃之小大長短，受穀之多少奈何？伯高曰：胃紆曲屈，伸之長二尺六寸，大一尺五寸，徑五寸，大容三斗五升。小腸後附脊，左環迴周疊積，長三丈二尺。迴腸當臍左環，長二丈一尺。廣腸傅脊，長二尺八寸。

huáng dì wèn yú bó gāo yuē: yú yuàn wén liù fǔ chuán gǔ zhě, cháng wèi zhī xiǎo dà cháng duǎn, shòu gǔ zhī duō shǎo nài hé? bó gāo yuē: wèi yū qū qū, shēn zhī cháng èr chǐ liù cùn, dà yī chǐ wǔ cùn, jìng wǔ cùn, dà róng sān dòu wǔ shēng. xiǎo cháng hòu fù jí, zuǒ huán huí zhōu dié jī, cháng sān zhàng èr chǐ. huí cháng dāng qí zuǒ huán, cháng èr zhàng yī chǐ. guǎng cháng fù jí, cháng èr chǐ bā cùn.

The Yellow Emperor asked Bo Gao: I should like to hear, of the six palaces that pass the grain along, the size and length of the intestines and stomach, and how much grain each receives. Bo Gao said: The stomach, coiled and bent, when drawn out straight is two chi six cun long, a chi and a half around, five cun across, and holds at most three dou five sheng. The small intestine, attached behind to the spine, circling leftward in folded coils, is three zhang two chi long. The looping intestine, turning leftward at the navel, is two zhang one chi. The broad intestine, laid against the spine, is two chi eight cun.

LING SHU 32

黃帝曰：願聞人之不食，七日而死，何也？伯高曰：胃大一尺五寸，徑五寸，長二尺六寸，橫屈受水穀三斗五升，其中之穀常留二斗，水一斗五升而滿。故平人日再後，後二升半，一日中五升，七日五七三斗五升，而留水穀盡矣。故平人不食飲七日而死者，水穀精氣津液皆盡故也。

huáng dì yuē: yuàn wén rén zhī bù shí, qī rì ér sǐ, hé yě? bó gāo yuē: wèi dà yī chǐ wǔ cùn, jìng wǔ cùn, cháng èr chǐ liù cùn, héng qū shòu shuǐ gǔ sān dòu wǔ shēng, qí zhōng zhī gǔ cháng liú èr dòu, shuǐ yī dòu wǔ shēng ér mǎn. gù píng rén rì zài hòu, hòu èr shēng bàn, yī rì zhōng wǔ shēng, qī rì wǔ qī sān dòu wǔ shēng, ér liú shuǐ gǔ jìn yǐ. gù píng rén bù shí yǐn qī rì ér sǐ zhě, shuǐ gǔ jīng qì jīn yè jiē jìn gù yě.

The Yellow Emperor said: I should like to know why a person who does not eat dies in seven days. Bo Gao said: The stomach is a chi and a half around, five cun across, two chi six cun long, and bent crosswise it receives three dou five sheng of water and grain; of this, two dou of grain remain within and a dou and a half of water fill it. Now an ordinary person voids twice a day, two and a half sheng each time, five sheng in a day; in seven days, seven times five, that is three dou five sheng, and the stored water and grain are spent. So when an ordinary person neither eats nor drinks for seven days and dies, it is because the essence-qi and the fluids of water and grain are all used up.

The tradition is often thought purely speculative, yet here it measures: the coil of the stomach drawn straight, the length of the intestines in zhang and chi, the dou and sheng each will hold, and from these the reasoning that a person without food dies in about seven days, when the stored grain and its fluids are spent. This is the empirical floor beneath a famous insistence, that the qi made from food is the root of life, and that a pulse or a body without that stomach-made qi is in grave danger.

SU WEN 29

帝曰：脾不主時何也？岐伯曰：脾者土也，治中央，常以四時長四藏，各十八日寄治，不得獨主於時也。脾藏者常著胃土之精也，土者生萬物而法天地，故上下至頭足，不得主時也。

dì yuē: pí bù zhǔ shí hé yě? qí bó yuē: pí zhě tǔ yě, zhì zhōng yāng, cháng yǐ sì shí cháng sì zàng, gè shí bā rì jì zhì, bù dé dú zhǔ yú shí yě. pí zàng zhě cháng zhù wèi tǔ zhī jīng yě, tǔ zhě shēng wàn wù ér fǎ tiān dì, gù shàng xià zhì tóu zú, bù dé zhǔ shí yě.

The Emperor asked: Why does the spleen not govern a season of its own? Qibo said: The spleen is earth, and it governs the centre; it constantly nourishes the four other organs through the four seasons, lodged in each for eighteen days, and so cannot govern a season of its own. The spleen forever holds fast the essence of the stomach-earth; and earth, which gives birth to the ten thousand things and takes its law from Heaven and Earth, reaches above and below from head to foot, and so cannot be confined to one season.

One office holds the centre of this economy. The spleen, as earth, rules no single season of its own but lends its qi to the other four organs through the whole year, and carries the stomach's essence out to the four limbs; when it fails, the limbs lose their nourishment and grow useless. This is why the spleen and stomach are treated as the pivot of the body, and why so much of therapy, then and now, begins by mending them.

SU WEN 24

形樂志苦，病生於脈，治之以灸刺。形樂志樂，病生於肉，治之以鍼石。形苦志樂，病生於筋，治之以熨引。形苦志苦，病生於咽嗌，治之以甘藥。形數驚恐，經絡不通，病生於不仁，治之以按摩醪藥。是謂五形志也。

xíng lè zhì kǔ, bìng shēng yú mài, zhì zhī yǐ jiǔ cì. xíng lè zhì lè, bìng shēng yú ròu, zhì zhī yǐ zhēn shí. xíng kǔ zhì lè, bìng shēng yú jīn, zhì zhī yǐ yùn yǐn. xíng kǔ zhì kǔ, bìng shēng yú yàn ài, zhì zhī yǐ gān yào. xíng shuò jīng kǒng, jīng luò bù tōng, bìng shēng yú bù rén, zhì zhī yǐ àn mó láo yào. shì wèi wǔ xíng zhì yě.

When the body is at ease but the disposition troubled, the disease arises in the vessels, and is treated with moxa and needle. When both body and disposition are at ease, the disease arises in the flesh, and is treated with needle and stone. When the body is hard-pressed but the disposition at ease, the disease arises in the sinews, and is treated with hot compress and stretching. When both body and disposition are hard-pressed, the disease arises in the throat, and is treated with sweet medicines. When the body is often startled and afraid and the channels and collaterals are blocked, the disease arises as numbness, and is treated with massage and medicinal wine. These are called the five conditions of body and disposition.

Last, the classic sorts illness by the meeting of body and mind, ease or hardship in the one, ease or trouble in the other, and matches each pairing to where disease settles and how to meet it: moxa and needle, the stone, warming and stretching, sweet herbs, or massage. The method is to read not the organ only but the life around it. A comfortable body carrying a troubled mind tends to ail in the vessels and asks for one hand; a hard-worked body with an easy mind ails in the sinews and asks for another. The court within is answerable, always, to the conditions without.

READING THE COURT FROM OUTSIDE

The face and the tongue, the heart. A dull, grey, or bluish complexion, or a tongue too pale or too red, points to the sovereign and the blood it moves.

The eyes and the nails, the liver. Tired or dry eyes, brittle or ridged nails, point to the general, and often to a life under strain.

The head hair, the bones and teeth, the hearing, the kidney. Early greying or thinning, a weak low back and knees, fading hearing, point to the deep reserve.

The skin, the voice, the nose, the lung. Dry skin, frequent colds, a faint voice, point to the chancellor of the qi.

The lips, the appetite, the limbs, the spleen. Pale slack lips, a heavy tiredness in the limbs, a poor appetite, point to the granary. A change at the surface is a message from an office within, and the fourth gate teaches how to read it closely.

THE ORGANS AND THEIR NETWORK

Essential Verses

These are among the gate's most quoted lines in the classic, gathered here for study.

SU WEN 29

陽道實，陰道虛。故犯賊風虛邪者，陽受之；食飲不節，起居不時者，陰受之。陽受之則入六府，陰受之則入五藏。

yáng dào shí, yīn dào xū. gù fàn zéi fēng xū xié zhě, yáng shòu zhī; shí yǐn bù jié, qǐ jū bù shí zhě, yīn shòu zhī. yáng shòu zhī zé rù liù fǔ, yīn shòu zhī zé rù wǔ zàng.

The way of yang tends to repletion, the way of yin to depletion. Thus one who is struck by robber wind and depleting evil, the yang receives it; one whose food and drink are intemperate, whose rising and resting keep no hour, the yin receives it. What the yang receives enters the six bowels; what the yin receives enters the five organs.

Two doors lead into the body, and the chapter is careful to keep them apart. An outside assault, a robber wind or depleting cold, enters by the yang and strikes the six bowels; an inside fault, irregular food or broken hours, enters by the yin and lodges in the five organs. How an illness began therefore predicts how deep it has gone, since the yang takes its blows at the surface where repletion shows and the yin takes its abuses in the interior where depletion settles. The physician reads the cause first: a wind turns attention to the bowels and the exterior, intemperate living to the organs and the interior, and the disease is met at the level its origin has reached rather than at the symptom on view. The bare formula, yang full and yin empty, becomes a map from how a disease started to where it has come to rest.

> LING SHU 32
>
> 胃滿則腸虛，腸滿則胃虛，更虛更滿，故氣得上下。五藏安定，血脈和利，精神乃居。
>
> *wèi mǎn zé cháng xū, cháng mǎn zé wèi xū, gèng xū gèng mǎn, gù qì dé shàng xià. wǔ zàng ān dìng, xuè mài hé lì, jīng shén nǎi jū.*
>
> When the stomach is full the intestine is empty; when the intestine is full the stomach is empty; emptying and filling by turns, and so the qi is able to move up and down. When the five organs are settled, when blood and vessels run smooth and free, then essence and spirit take up their dwelling.

The gut works like a pump that is never full at both ends at once: when the stomach fills the intestine has emptied, when the intestine fills the stomach stands empty, and it is this emptiness by turns that keeps a space open ahead for the qi to descend into. On that steady up-and-down traffic two larger things rest, the settling of the organs and the housing of essence and spirit, so the line ties the most ordinary fact of digestion to the dwelling of the spirit itself. What it asks of the physician is to support the alternation rather than overrun it: not to pile food on an unemptied stomach, to keep the downward passage clear so the rhythm holds, and to remember that a spirit which cannot rest often traces back to a tract that has lost its beat.

LING SHU 47

人之血氣精神者，所以奉生而周於性命者也。五藏者，所以藏精神血氣魂魄者也。視其外應，以知其內藏，則知所病矣。

rén zhī xuè qì jīng shén zhě, suǒ yǐ fèng shēng ér zhōu yú xìng mìng zhě yě. wǔ zàng zhě, suǒ yǐ cáng jīng shén xuè qì hún pò zhě yě. shì qí wài yīng, yǐ zhī qí nèi cáng, zé zhī suǒ bìng yǐ.

A person's blood, qi, essence, and spirit are what serve life and complete the round of one's allotted span. The five organs are what store the essence and spirit, the blood and qi, the ethereal and bodily souls. Observe the outward correspondences, and so know the inner organs, and you will know where the disease lies.

An organ, in this reading, is a storehouse, and what it stores is the body's life: the blood and qi, the essence and spirit, the ethereal and bodily souls. Life itself is the keeping of these stores intact, and because each organ throws its condition onto a fixed outer sign, that inner state can be read at the surface without opening the body. The method follows from this directly. Gather the outward signs, the colour and lustre, the state of the tissue and the opening of the senses that belong to an organ, and reason back to the organ that owns them, letting the visible stand witness for the hidden. It is the warrant beneath the whole of diagnosis by correspondence, the reason a face or a fingernail can name a trouble seated deep in the trunk.

FROM THE AUTHOR

Of all the offices, watch the sovereign. A heart that cannot rest, a mind crowded and driven, will disorder a body more surely than any single weak organ; settle the heart, and the whole court settles with it. This is why the keeping of health and the work of cultivation are not two roads but one, and why a quiet mind belongs at the head of any treatment, in this gate and in the last.

主明則下安。

When the sovereign is clear, all below are at peace.

WHERE THIS GATE LEADS

The organs sort at once into the yin and yang of *Gate Two*, the storing zang being yin and the transmitting fu yang. Their outward signs are read at the wrist and the face in *Gate Four, Reading the Unspoken*. How each office falls ill is the matter of *Gate Seven, How Illness Begins*. And the spirits the organs house, the shen and the hun and the rest, are the inward concern of *Gate Ten, The Work of Return*.

PART FOUR

Reading the Unspoken

Pulse and Diagnosis

脈色

On diagnosis. How the physician, with a finger laid at the wrist and a steady eye upon the face, hears what the body itself cannot put into words.

GATE FOUR · PULSE AND DIAGNOSIS

Reading the Unspoken

脈色

> *The pulse is the storehouse of the blood.*
>
> Su Wen 17

A patient tells you what they have noticed. The body tells you what they have not. Long before a complaint has a name, it has a colour in the face, a weight in the voice, a rhythm at the wrist; and the physician's first art is to read these signs that lie below speech. This gate is about that reading.

The tradition gathers diagnosis under four heads: looking, listening and smelling, asking, and feeling the pulse. This gate dwells on the two the classic trusts above the rest and returns to again and again, the pulse and the complexion, mai and se. The pulse, taken at the wrist, is the clearest single window onto the state of the qi and the blood; the face, the eyes, and the tongue confirm it and refine it. Together they let a skilled hand know not only that something is wrong but where it sits and which way it is moving.

Read this gate for the same five things. What it reads are the body's silent signs, the pulse above all and the colour beside it; whom it serves is every patient, and anyone who would learn to notice the early turn of their own health. It belongs to the opening of a consultation, and best to the stillness of early morning, and its purpose is to find a disturbance and judge where it is heading before a single remedy is chosen. The method, though, is the refrain of the whole gate: never trust one sign alone, but read several together, each checked against the others, against the stomach-qi, and against the season.

The Art of Examination

SU WEN 17

黃帝問曰：診法何如？岐伯對曰：診法常以平旦，陰氣未動，陽氣未散，飲食未進，經脈未盛，絡脈調勻，氣血未亂，故乃可診有過之脈。切脈動靜而視精明，察五色，觀五臟有餘不足，六腑強弱，形之盛衰，以此參伍，決死生之分。

huáng dì wèn yuē: zhěn fǎ hé rú? qí bó duì yuē: zhěn fǎ cháng yǐ píng dàn, yīn qì wèi dòng, yáng qì wèi sàn, yǐn shí wèi jìn, jīng mài wèi shèng, luò mài diào yún, qì xuè wèi luàn, gù nǎi kě zhěn yǒu guò zhī mài. qiè mài dòng jìng ér shì jīng míng, chá wǔ sè, guān wǔ zàng yǒu yú bù zú, liù fǔ qiáng ruò, xíng zhī shèng shuāi, yǐ cǐ cān wǔ, jué sǐ shēng zhī fēn.

The Yellow Emperor asked: How is diagnosis to be done? Qibo answered: Diagnosis is best done at dawn, when the yin qi has not yet stirred and the yang qi has not yet scattered, when food and drink have not yet been taken, the channels are not yet full and the collaterals are even, and the qi and blood are not yet thrown into disorder; only then can a pulse at fault be read. Feel the movement and stillness of the pulse and look into the clear light of the eyes; examine the five colours, observe where the five organs have too much or too little and where the six palaces are strong or weak, and weigh the flourishing or decline of the body; cross-check these against one another, and decide the division between life and death.

SU WEN 17

夫脈者，血之府也。長則氣治，短則氣病，數則煩心，大則病進，上盛則氣高，下盛則氣脹，代則氣衰，細則氣少，濇則心痛。渾渾革至如湧泉，病進而色弊；綿綿其去如弦絕，死。

fū mài zhě, xuè zhī fǔ yě. cháng zé qì zhì, duǎn zé qì bìng, shuò zé fán xīn, dà zé bìng jìn, shàng shèng zé qì gāo, xià shèng zé qì zhàng, dài zé qì shuāi, xì zé qì shǎo, sè zé xīn tòng. hún hún gé zhì rú yǒng quán, bìng jìn ér sè bì; mián mián qí qù rú xián jué, sǐ.

The pulse is the storehouse of the blood. A long pulse means the qi is in order; a short one, that the qi is ill; a rapid one, a vexed heart; a large one, that the disease is advancing. Full above, the qi is raised high; full below, the qi is distended; when it skips a beat, the qi is waning; when fine, the qi is scant; when rough, there is pain in the heart. When it arrives turbid and surging like a gushing spring, the disease is advancing and the colour failing; when it departs faint and trailing like a snapping bowstring, the patient dies.

The method has both a setting and a procedure. The setting is calm: the classic asks for the quiet of dawn, before food and exertion have stirred the qi, when the channels are even and a fault shows plainly. Few of us will examine literally at first light, but the principle holds, that one reads a body at rest, not one just hurried in from the street, and gives it a few quiet breaths first. The procedure is to gather many things at once: feel the movement of the pulse, look into the clear light of the eyes, read the five colours, judge where each organ is full or empty, weigh the vigour of the body, and then cross-check them, the classic's word is to weigh them five by five, before deciding. This is the heart of the art and its safeguard against error: a single sign can mislead, but agreement among several can be trusted.

How much one finger can gather, the second passage shows. A long, ample pulse tells of qi in good order; a short one, of qi already ill; a rapid one, of a heart vexed with heat; a large and swelling one, of a disease still advancing. Full under the fingers toward the wrist, the qi is driven upward; full toward the elbow, it is distended below; a pulse that skips is a waning qi, a thready one a scant qi, a rough dragging one the sign of pain at the heart. None of these is read in isolation; each is one reading among the several the examiner is weighing at once.

The Stomach-Qi in the Pulse

SU WEN 18

黃帝問曰：平人何如？岐伯對曰：人一呼脈再動，一吸脈亦再動，呼吸定息脈五動，閏以太息，命曰平人。平人者，不病也。常以不病調病人，醫不病，故為病人平息以調之為法。

huáng dì wèn yuē: píng rén hé rú? qí bó duì yuē: rén yī hū mài zài dòng, yī xī mài yì zài dòng, hū xī dìng xī mài wǔ dòng, rùn yǐ tài xī, mìng yuē píng rén. píng rén zhě, bù bìng yě. cháng yǐ bù bìng diào bìng rén, yī bù bìng, gù wèi bìng rén píng xī yǐ diào zhī wèi fǎ.

The Yellow Emperor asked: What is the pulse of a normal person? Qibo answered: In one exhalation the pulse beats twice, and in one inhalation it beats twice again; across a settled breath the pulse beats five times, with an added beat at a longer breath. Such a one is called a normal person, and a normal person is one who is not ill. The physician, being himself not ill, uses his own unhurried breath as the measure by which he adjusts and reads the breathing of the sick. This is the method.

SU WEN 18

平人之常氣稟於胃，胃者平人之常氣也，人無胃氣曰逆，逆者死。

píng rén zhī cháng qì bǐng yú wèi, wèi zhě píng rén zhī cháng qì yě, rén wú wèi qì yuē nì, nì zhě sǐ.

The constant qi of a normal person is received from the stomach; the stomach is the source of that constant qi. A person without stomach qi is in counterflow, and counterflow means death.

Before any subtle reading come two plain measures. The first is rate. In a healthy person the pulse beats about five times to one full, easy breath; far fewer beats speak of cold or a scant qi, far more of heat or distress. And the physician takes his own unhurried breath as the ruler against which he counts, which is why his own steadiness is itself part of the instrument, and why a flustered examiner reads badly.

The second measure is the one the whole tradition prizes most: the stomach-qi. Whatever its season or shape, a healthy pulse has a soft, rooted, unforced quality, the living sign that the stomach is still making qi and blood out of food. A pulse that has lost this, gone hard and bare and rootless, is the gravest finding in the book, for as the classic says without softening it, a person without stomach-qi is in counterflow, and counterflow is death. Before you name the pulse fast or slow, floating or deep, feel first for that soft rootedness; its presence is the difference between a disorder and a danger.

The rule the chapter draws from this is as blunt as any in the book: where there is stomach-qi there is life, and where it is gone there is death. In practice it means a pulse is read not only for its rate or shape but for a certain soft, rounded, unforced quality underneath, the sign that the body is still feeding and renewing itself. A pulse that has lost that quality, however strong it seems, is the graver finding. It is one of the oldest and steadiest of all the bedside judgements this medicine makes.

The Pulse of the Seasons

SU WEN 19

黃帝問曰：春脈如弦，何如而弦？岐伯對曰：春脈者肝也，東方木也，萬物之所以始生也，故其氣來軟弱輕虛而滑，端直以長，故曰弦，反此者病。帝曰：何如而反？岐伯曰：其氣來實而強，此謂太過，病在外；其氣來不實而微，此謂不及，病在中。帝曰：春脈太過與不及，其病皆何如？岐伯曰：太過則令人善忘，忽忽眩冒而巔疾；其不及則令人胸痛引背，下則兩脅胠滿。

huáng dì wèn yuē: chūn mài rú xián, hé rú ér xián? qí bó duì yuē: chūn mài zhě gān yě, dōng fāng mù yě, wàn wù zhī suǒ yǐ shǐ shēng yě, gù qí qì lái ruǎn ruò qīng xū ér huá, duān zhí yǐ zhǎng, gù yuē xián, fǎn cǐ zhě bìng. dì yuē: hé rú ér fǎn? qí bó yuē: qí qì lái shí ér qiáng, cǐ wèi tài guò, bìng zài wài; qí qì lái bù shí ér wēi, cǐ wèi bù jí, bìng zài zhōng. dì yuē: chūn mài tài guò yǔ bù jí, qí bìng jiē hé rú? qí bó yuē: tài guò zé lìng rén shàn wàng, hū hū xuàn mào ér diān jí; qí bù jí zé lìng rén xiōng tòng yǐn bèi, xià zé liǎng xié qū mǎn.

The Yellow Emperor asked: The spring pulse is like a bowstring; how is it bowstring-like? Qibo answered: The spring pulse is the liver, the wood of the east, by which the ten thousand things begin to be born; so its qi comes soft, weak, light, and smooth, straight and long, and is therefore called bowstring. A pulse contrary to this is ill. The Emperor asked: How is it contrary? Qibo said: When its qi comes full and strong, this is excess, and the disease is on the outside; when it comes not full but faint, this is deficiency, and the disease is within. The Emperor asked about the illnesses of each. Qibo said: In excess it makes a person forgetful, dizzy and clouded, with disorder at the crown; in deficiency it brings pain in the chest drawing through to the back, and below, a fullness in both flanks.

The pulse is not the same all year, and it ought not to be. As the yang rises through spring and summer, the pulse rises toward the surface and grows full; as the yang withdraws through autumn and winter, the pulse sinks and firms. So the healthy spring pulse is faintly taut, like a string just drawn; the summer pulse comes full and falls away, like a hook; the autumn pulse floats light at the surface; the winter pulse lies deep and firm as a stone. A pulse that matches its season is well; one wearing the wrong season's character is a warning. And when the season's softness has wholly gone, leaving only the bare, hard, so-called true-organ pulse, the classic counts it fatal, for the stomach-qi that softened it is spent. The table gathers the five.

SEASON	ORGAN	PULSE	HOW IT FEELS
Spring 春	Liver	Taut, wiry	Soft and light, straight and long, like a string just drawn
Summer 夏	Heart	Full, hook-like	Comes full and strong, departs faint, rising and falling away
Autumn 秋	Lung	Floating	Light and near the surface, easily met by a gentle touch
Winter 冬	Kidney	Sinking, stony	Deep and firm, found only with a pressing finger
Late summer 長夏	Spleen	Moderate	Even and soft, rich in stomach-qi, the temperate mean of all

The Three Regions and Nine Indicators

SU WEN 20

帝曰：何謂三部？岐伯曰：有下部，有中部，有上部，部各有三候，三候者，有天有地有人也。上部天，兩額之動脈；上部地，兩頰之動脈；上部人，耳前之動脈。中部天，手太陰也；中部地，手陽明也；中部人，手少陰也。下部天，足厥陰也；下部地，足少陰也；下部人，足太陰也。

dì yuē: hé wèi sān bù? qí bó yuē: yǒu xià bù, yǒu zhōng bù, yǒu shàng bù, bù gè yǒu sān hòu, sān hòu zhě, yǒu tiān yǒu dì yǒu rén yě. shàng bù tiān, liǎng é zhī dòng mài; shàng bù dì, liǎng jiá zhī dòng mài; shàng bù rén, ěr qián zhī dòng mài. zhōng bù tiān, shǒu tài yīn yě; zhōng bù dì, shǒu yáng míng yě; zhōng bù rén, shǒu shào yīn yě. xià bù tiān, zú jué yīn yě; xià bù dì, zú shào yīn yě; xià bù rén, zú tài yīn yě.

The Emperor asked: What are the three regions? Qibo said: There is a lower region, a middle, and an upper, and each region has three indicators, the three being a Heaven, an Earth, and a Human. In the upper region, the Heaven is the throbbing vessel at the two temples, the Earth the throbbing vessel at the two cheeks, the Human the throbbing vessel before the ears. In the middle region, the Heaven is the hand greater-yin, the Earth the hand bright-yang, the Human the hand lesser-yin. In the lower region, the Heaven is the foot reverting-yin, the Earth the foot lesser-yin, the Human the foot greater-yin.

SU WEN 20

中部之候雖獨調，與眾藏相失者死。中部之候相減者死。目內陷者死。帝曰：何以知病之所在？岐伯曰：察九候，獨小者病，獨大者病，獨疾者病，獨遲者病，獨熱者病，獨寒者病，獨陷下者病。

zhōng bù zhī hòu suī dú diào, yǔ zhòng zàng xiāng shī zhě sǐ. zhōng bù zhī hòu xiāng jiǎn zhě sǐ. mù nèi xiàn zhě sǐ. dì yuē: hé yǐ zhī bìng zhī suǒ zài? qí bó yuē: chá jiǔ hòu, dú xiǎo zhě bìng, dú dà zhě bìng, dú jí zhě bìng, dú chí zhě bìng, dú rè zhě bìng, dú hán zhě bìng, dú xiàn xià zhě bìng.

Even if the indicators of the middle region alone are in tune, when they have lost concord with the other organs, it means death; when the middle indicators dwindle away, it means death; when the eyes are sunken, it means death. The Emperor asked: How does one know where the disease lies? Qibo said: Examine the nine indicators. The one that alone is small marks disease; the one that alone is large marks disease; the one alone hurried, the one alone slow, the one alone hot, the one alone cold, the one alone sunken, each marks disease.

The classic also keeps a whole-body method, older and broader than the wrist alone. It divides the body into three regions, upper, middle, and lower, each with three pulsing points, nine in all, and reads a particular organ or region at each. In the lower region it takes the liver, the kidney, and the spleen and stomach; in the middle, the lung, the chest, and the heart; in the upper, the head, the mouth and teeth, and the ears and eyes. Later practice would concentrate this whole map into the three positions of the wrist, but the principle never changed.

And the principle is comparison. Health is concord among the nine, all in step, none standing apart. To find where a disease lies, the examiner looks for the one indicator that breaks from its fellows: the one that alone is small, or alone large, alone hurried or alone slow, alone hot or alone cold. That single point out of step names the region in trouble. Here again the method is not to trust one reading but to weigh each against the rest, and to let the odd one out point the way.

What the chapter asks for is a whole survey rather than a single reading. The hand goes to three regions, each with three indicators, at the head, the hands, and the feet, and life and death are judged by how their fullness and emptiness stand against one another. A pulse means nothing on its own; it means something only measured against the others, and against what an even, healthy pulse feels like. So the first skill to build is that feel for the even pulse, because without it the abnormal cannot be seen. This is diagnosis as a reading of the whole field of qi, not a guess drawn from one corner of it.

The Colours of the Face

Before the wrist, there is the face. The classic reads the complexion as closely as the pulse, and gives each region of the face and each shade of colour a settled meaning.

> LING SHU 49
>
> 五色各見其部，察其浮沈以知淺深，察其澤夭以觀成敗，察其散摶以知遠近，視色上下以知病處。青黑為痛，黃赤為熱，白為寒，是謂五官。
>
> *wǔ sè gè jiàn qí bù, chá qí fú shěn yǐ zhī qiǎn shēn, chá qí zé yāo yǐ guān chéng bài, chá qí sàn tuán yǐ zhī yuǎn jìn, shì sè shàng xià yǐ zhī bìng chù. qīng hēi wèi tòng, huáng chì wèi rè, bái wèi hán, shì wèi wǔ guān.*
>
> Each of the five colours shows in its own region of the face. Observe whether it floats or sinks, to know whether the trouble is shallow or deep; observe whether it is moist or withered, to see whether it tends toward recovery or toward ruin; observe whether it is scattered or gathered, to know whether the disease is far off or near; and read the colour high or low upon the face, to know where the disease sits. Green and black mean pain, yellow and red mean heat, and white means cold.

The method is exact and worth learning as a sequence. Each colour appears in its own region; whether it floats near the surface or sinks tells how shallow or deep the trouble lies; whether it is moist or withered tells whether the case tends to recovery or to ruin; whether it is scattered or gathered tells whether the disease is near or far; and the height of the colour on the face tells where it sits. The shades themselves are read plainly: green and black for pain, yellow and red for heat, white for cold. None of this asks a single instrument, only a trained and unhurried eye.

LING SHU 37

黃帝曰：願聞五官。岐伯曰：鼻者，肺之官也；目者，肝之官也；口脣者，脾之官也；舌者，心之官也；耳者，腎之官也。故肺病者喘息鼻張，肝病者眥青，脾病者脣黃，心病者舌卷短、顴赤，腎病者顴與顏黑。

huáng dì yuē: yuàn wén wǔ guān. qí bó yuē: bí zhě, fèi zhī guān yě; mù zhě, gān zhī guān yě; kǒu chún zhě, pí zhī guān yě; shé zhě, xīn zhī guān yě; ěr zhě, shèn zhī guān yě. gù fèi bìng zhě chuǎn xī bí zhāng, gān bìng zhě zì qīng, pí bìng zhě chún huáng, xīn bìng zhě shé juǎn duǎn, quán chì, shèn bìng zhě quán yǔ yán hēi.

The Yellow Emperor said: I wish to hear of the five offices. Qibo said: The nose is the office of the lung; the eyes, the office of the liver; the mouth and lips, the office of the spleen; the tongue, the office of the heart; the ears, the office of the kidney. So in disease of the lung the breath pants and the nostrils flare; in disease of the liver the corners of the eyes turn green; in disease of the spleen the lips turn yellow; in disease of the heart the tongue curls and shortens and the cheekbones redden; and in disease of the kidney the cheekbones and the brow are dark.

The face speaks organ by organ as well as colour by colour, for the five orifices are the outward offices of the five organs: the nose answers to the lung, the eyes to the liver, the lips to the spleen, the tongue to the heart, the ears to the kidney. So flaring nostrils and panting breath accuse the lung, green at the corners of the eyes the liver, yellow lips the spleen, a curled short tongue and red cheekbones the heart, a darkened brow the kidney. A sign at an orifice is read straight back to the office it serves.

SU WEN 15

黃帝問曰：余聞揆度奇恆，所指不同，用之奈何？岐伯對曰：揆度者，度病之淺深也；奇恆者，言奇病也。請言道之至數，五色脈變，揆度奇恆，道在於一。

huáng dì wèn yuē: yú wén kuí dù qí héng, suǒ zhǐ bù tóng, yòng zhī nài hé? qí bó duì yuē: kuí dù zhě, dù bìng zhī qiǎn shēn yě; qí héng zhě, yán qí bìng yě. qǐng yán dào zhī zhì shù, wǔ sè mài biàn, kuí dù qí héng, dào zài yú yī.

The Yellow Emperor asked: I have heard of gauging-and-measuring and of the curious-and-constant, which point to different things; how are they used? Qibo answered: Gauging-and-measuring is the measuring of how shallow or deep a disease lies; the curious-and-constant speaks of the unusual diseases. Let me tell of the utmost number of the Way: the five colours and the changes of the pulse, the gauging-and-measuring and the curious-and-constant, their Way lies in being one.

All of this the classic gathers under two arts. Gauging measures how deep a disease has travelled; the curious and the constant tell an unusual illness from an ordinary one. And it insists that the Way lies in the One: colour and pulse are not two separate skills but a single coherent reading, in which depth and ordinariness are the two questions always being asked.

Reading the Inside from the Outside

Beneath the whole of diagnosis lies one principle: the hidden interior can be read from the visible exterior. The classic states it almost as a law of nature.

> LING SHU 45
>
> 日與月焉，水與鏡焉，鼓與響焉。夫日月之明，不失其影；水鏡之察，不失其形；鼓響之應，不後其聲。故遠者司外揣內，近者司內揣外，是謂陰陽之極，天地之蓋。
>
> *rì yǔ yuè yān, shuǐ yǔ jìng yān, gǔ yǔ xiǎng yān. fū rì yuè zhī míng, bù shī qí yǐng; shuǐ jìng zhī chá, bù shī qí xíng; gǔ xiǎng zhī yīng, bù hòu qí shēng. gù yuǎn zhě sī wài chuāi nèi, jìn zhě sī nèi chuāi wài, shì wèi yīn yáng zhī jí, tiān dì zhī gài.*
>
> It is like the sun and the moon, like water and a mirror, like a drum and its echo. The brightness of the sun and moon never loses the shadow it casts; the clear surface of water and mirror never loses the form set before it; the answering of the drum's echo never lags behind the sound. So from afar one reads the outside to gauge the inside, and close at hand one reads the inside to gauge the outside; this is the very limit of yin and yang, the canopy of Heaven and Earth.

As the sun casts a shadow that never lies, as a mirror holds the form set before it, as a drum returns its echo without delay, so the inner state answers faithfully in the outer sign. This is the licence beneath the entire art: from afar one reads the outside to gauge the inside, and the reverse close at hand. Every visible mark, rightly read, is a true report from within.

SU WEN 76

夫脈之大小滑濇浮沈，可以指別；五藏之象，可以類推；五藏相音，可以意識；五色微診，可以目察。能合脈色，可以萬全。

fū mài zhī dà xiǎo huá sè fú shěn, kě yǐ zhǐ bié; wǔ zàng zhī xiàng, kě yǐ lèi tuī; wǔ zàng xiāng yīn, kě yǐ yì shí; wǔ sè wēi zhěn, kě yǐ mù chá. néng hé mài sè, kě yǐ wàn quán.

The largeness or smallness, the slipperiness or roughness, the floating or sinking of a pulse can be told apart by the finger; the images of the five organs can be reasoned out by their kind; the resonances of the five organs can be grasped by the understanding; and the faint signs of the five colours can be examined by the eye. One who can join the pulse and the colour together will be whole in ten thousand cases.

But the outer signs must be read together, never one alone. The pulse is told by the finger, the images of the organs by reasoning, the colours by the eye; and the one who joins pulse and colour into a single judgement will not err in ten thousand cases. This cross-checking, one channel of evidence against another, is the method the gate returns to again and again.

SU WEN 80

診有大方，坐起有常，出入有行，以轉神明。必清必淨，上觀下觀，按脈動靜，循尺滑濇寒溫之意，視其大小，合之病能，逆從以得，復知病名，診可十全。

zhěn yǒu dà fāng, zuò qǐ yǒu cháng, chū rù yǒu xíng, yǐ zhuǎn shén míng. bì qīng bì jìng, shàng guān xià guān, àn mài dòng jìng, xún chǐ huá sè hán wēn zhī yì, shì qí dà xiǎo, hé zhī bìng néng, nì cóng yǐ dé, fù zhī bìng míng, zhěn kě shí quán.

There is a great method in diagnosis: a settled bearing in sitting and rising, an order in coming and going, so as to keep the spirit-brightness turning clear and pure. Look above and look below; press the pulse in its movement and its stillness; run the finger along the forearm for the sense of its slipperiness or roughness, its cold or warmth; observe whether the signs are large or small; match all of this to what the disease is able

> to do; grasp what runs against and what runs with it; and then the name of the disease is known, and the diagnosis is whole ten times in ten.

The examination itself has a discipline. The classic asks for a settled bearing and a clear mind, then a fixed order: look above and below, press the pulse in movement and stillness, run the finger along the forearm for its texture and warmth, weigh whether the signs are large or small, and match all of it to what the disease can do. Done so, the reading is whole ten times in ten; done carelessly, it misleads.

> LING SHU 74
>
> 黃帝問於岐伯曰：余欲無視色持脈，獨調其尺，以言其病，從外知內，為之奈何？岐伯曰：審其尺之緩急、大小、滑濇，肉之堅脆，而病形定矣。尺膚熱甚，脈盛躁者，病溫也；尺膚寒，其脈小者，泄、少氣。
>
> *huáng dì wèn yú qí bó yuē: yú yù wú shì sè chí mài, dú diào qí chǐ, yǐ yán qí bìng, cóng wài zhī nèi, wèi zhī nài hé? qí bó yuē: shěn qí chǐ zhī huǎn jí, dà xiǎo, huá sè, ròu zhī jiān cuì, ér bìng xíng dìng yǐ. chǐ fū rè shèn, mài shèng zào zhě, bìng wēn yě; chǐ fū hán, qí mài xiǎo zhě, xiè, shǎo qì.*
>
> The Yellow Emperor asked Qibo: I should like, without looking at the colour or taking the pulse, to judge a disease from the skin of the forearm alone, knowing the inside from the outside; how is it done? Qibo said: Examine the forearm skin for its looseness or tightness, its largeness or smallness, its slipperiness or roughness, and the firmness or softness of its flesh, and the form of the disease is settled. When the forearm skin is very hot and the pulse full and agitated, the disease is a febrile warmth; when the forearm skin is cold and the pulse small, there is diarrhoea and a scantness of qi.

The principle is concrete enough that a disease can be judged from the forearm skin alone, knowing the inside from the outside: its looseness or tightness, its warmth, the firmness of its flesh. A forearm hot to the touch over a full, agitated pulse marks a febrile heat; a cold forearm over a small pulse marks diarrhoea and a scantness of qi. Even a patch of skin is a readable surface.

Signs of Warning, and Signs in Sleep and Tears

Some readings serve prognosis, the honest judging of danger; and some reach the hidden states that no ordinary sign betrays.

SU WEN 48

脈至而搏，血衄身熱者死。脈至如喘，名曰暴厥，暴厥者不知與人言。脈至如數，使人暴驚，三四日自已。脈至如火薪然，是心精之予奪也，草乾而死。脈至如散葉，是肝氣予虛也，木葉落而死。

mài zhì ér bó, xuè nǜ shēn rè zhě sǐ. mài zhì rú chuǎn, míng yuē bào jué, bào jué zhě bù zhī yǔ rén yán. mài zhì rú shuò, shǐ rén bào jīng, sān sì rì zì yǐ. mài zhì rú huǒ xīn rán, shì xīn jīng zhī yǔ duó yě, cǎo qián ér sǐ. mài zhì rú sàn yè, shì gān qì yǔ xū yě, mù yè luò ér sǐ.

When the pulse arrives throbbing, with nosebleed and a hot body, death follows. When the pulse arrives like panting, it is named sudden reversal, and the one in sudden reversal cannot speak with others. When the pulse arrives as if rapid, it brings a sudden fright that heals of itself in three or four days. When the pulse arrives like kindled brushwood, the heart's essence is being robbed, and the patient dies when the grasses wither. When the pulse arrives like scattered leaves, the liver-qi is failing, and he dies when the leaves fall.

The classic catalogues the ominous pulses without flinching. A throbbing pulse with nosebleed and a hot body foretells death; a pulse like panting names a sudden collapse in which the person cannot speak; a pulse flaring like a kindled flame says the heart's essence is being given up, and names even the season of the end. These are not symptoms to be eased but verdicts to be known, and the physician who cannot read them cannot speak truthfully of what is coming.

LING SHU 43

陰氣盛則夢涉大水而恐懼，陽氣盛則夢大火而燔焫，陰陽俱盛則夢相殺。上盛則夢飛，下盛則夢墮。甚飢則夢取，甚飽則夢予。肝氣盛則夢怒，肺氣盛則夢恐懼哭泣，心氣盛則夢善笑恐畏。

yīn qì shèng zé mèng shè dà shuǐ ér kǒng jù, yáng qì shèng zé mèng dà huǒ ér fán ruò, yīn yáng jù shèng zé mèng xiāng shā. shàng shèng zé mèng fēi, xià shèng zé mèng duò. shèn jī zé mèng qǔ, shèn bǎo zé mèng yǔ. gān qì shèng zé mèng nù, fèi qì shèng zé mèng kǒng jù kū qì, xīn qì shèng zé mèng shàn xiào kǒng wèi.

When the yin qi is in excess, one dreams of wading great waters in fear; when the yang qi is in excess, one dreams of great fires that scorch and burn; when both are in excess, one dreams of killing and being killed. When the upper body is over-full, one dreams of flying; when the lower is over-full, one dreams of falling. In great hunger one dreams of taking; in great fullness, of giving. When the liver-qi is in excess one dreams of anger; when the lung-qi is in excess, of fear and weeping; when the heart-qi is in excess, of laughing and of dread.

Even sleep reports the body's state. When an evil lodges and unsettles the souls, it surfaces as a dream cast in the body's own imbalance: an excess of yin as wading deep cold water in fear, an excess of yang as great fires; an over-full upper body as flying, an over-full lower as falling; the liver in excess as anger, the lung as weeping. A patient's dreams, asked after gently, can confirm where the disturbance lies.

SU WEN 81

夫心者，五藏之專精也；目者，其竅也；華色者，其榮也。是以人有德也，則氣和於目；有亡，憂知於色。水之精為志，火之精為神，水火相感，神志俱悲，是以目之水生也。

fū xīn zhě, wǔ zàng zhī zhuān jīng yě; mù zhě, qí qiào yě; huá sè zhě, qí róng yě. shì yǐ rén yǒu dé yě, zé qì hé yú mù; yǒu wáng, yōu zhī yú sè. shuǐ zhī jīng wèi zhì, huǒ zhī jīng wèi shén, shuǐ huǒ xiāng gǎn, shén zhì jù bēi, shì yǐ mù zhī shuǐ shēng yě.

The heart is the gathered essence of the five organs; the eye is its opening; and the bloom of the complexion is its flowering. So when a person is at peace, the qi runs harmonious in the eyes; and when something is lost, the grief of it is known in the colour. The essence of water is the will, the essence of fire is the spirit; when water and fire move upon each other and the spirit and the will both grieve, the water of the eye is born, and this is weeping.

And the subtlest sign of all is the eye. The heart is the gathered essence of the organs, the eye its opening, the complexion its flowering; so peace runs harmonious in the eyes and loss shows in the colour. When water and fire, the will and the spirit, grieve together, the water of the eye is born, and we weep. To read a face well is, in the end, to read the spirit behind it.

WHAT THE PULSE TELLS, AND WHERE

Rate. About four or five beats to one calm breath. Much slower suggests cold or a weak qi; much faster suggests heat or distress. Steady your own breathing first, and use it as the measure.

Depth. A pulse met by a light touch (floating) points to the surface, or to a yang that is not anchored; one found only by pressing deep (sinking) points to the interior, or to cold.

The stomach-qi. Above all, feel whether the pulse is soft and rooted, which is good, or hard and rootless, which is grave. This single quality matters more than rate or depth.

The positions. At each wrist the pulse is read in three places: the inch nearest the hand, the bar behind it, and the cubit further still. By long tradition the left wrist reads the heart, the liver, and the kidney from inch to cubit; the right reads the lung, the spleen and stomach, and the deep kidney-yang. A change at one position points to its organ. The fuller art of reading these is the work of years; this is enough to begin.

FIGURE · THE THREE POSITIONS

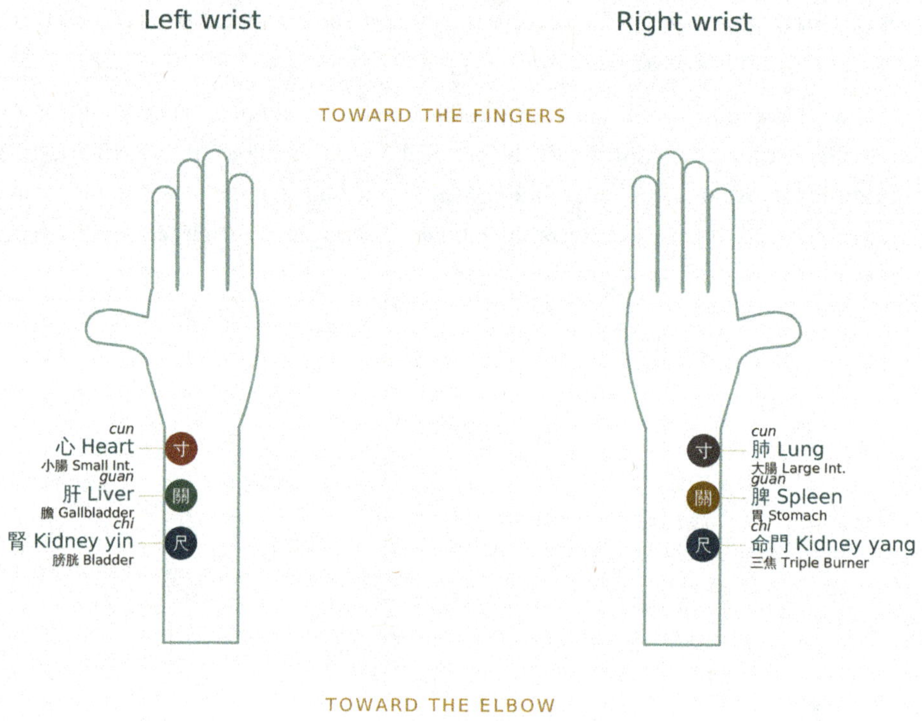

The radial pulse is read at three positions on each wrist, the inch (cun/寸), the bar (guan/關), and the cubit (chi/尺), the inch toward the fingers and the cubit toward the elbow, and at two depths beneath each finger. In one arrangement the deep level is taken for the yin organ and the surface for its paired yang organ, so that twelve channels are felt at six points: heart, liver, and kidney on the left, lung, spleen, and the gate of life on the right. Schools differ: others read the same depth as the yin and yang aspect of one organ rather than a change of organ.

PULSE AND DIAGNOSIS

Essential Verses

These are among the gate's most quoted lines in the classic, gathered here for study.

SU WEN 19

五藏受氣於其所生，傳之於其所勝，氣舍於其所生，死於其所不勝。病之且死，必先傳行，至其所不勝，病乃死。真藏脈見者，死。

wǔ zàng shòu qì yú qí suǒ shēng, chuán zhī yú qí suǒ shèng, qì shě yú qí suǒ shēng, sǐ yú qí suǒ bù shèng. bìng zhī qiě sǐ, bì xiān chuán xíng, zhì qí suǒ bù shèng, bìng nǎi sǐ. zhēn zàng mài jiàn zhě, sǐ.

Each of the five organs receives qi from the one it engenders, transmits it to the one it overcomes, lodges in the one that engenders it, and dies at the one that overcomes it. When a disease is about to prove fatal, it first passes along this course, and only when it reaches the organ that overcomes it does the patient die. When the true-organ pulse appears, death follows.

A disease does not wander at random through the organs; it travels the fixed lines of engendering and overcoming, lodging harmlessly in a mother-organ but turning deadly when it arrives at the organ that conquers its own. Because the path runs by rule, it can be forecast and the end foreseen. The physician traces where the illness now sits within the five phases, projects its next step along the conquest sequence, and watches whether it is moving toward the organ that overcomes the patient's weakest. The bared true-organ pulse, the stroke with no stomach-qi to soften it, is the final confirmation that the reserve standing between the patient and that conquest has run out. The five phases here are less a diagram than a clock for the course of grave illness.

> SU WEN 20
>
> 三部九候，所以決死生之要會也。必先知經脈，然後知病脈。必審捫循三部九候之盛虛，而調之，無問其病，以平為期。
>
> *sān bù jiǔ hòu, suǒ yǐ jué sǐ shēng zhī yào huì yě. bì xiān zhī jīng mài, rán hòu zhī bìng mài. bì shěn mén xún sān bù jiǔ hòu zhī shèng xū, ér diào zhī, wú wèn qí bìng, yǐ píng wèi qī.*
>
> The three regions and nine indicators are the essential meeting-ground for deciding death and life. One must first know the normal channel pulse, and only then can one know the diseased pulse. One must carefully feel and trace the fullness and emptiness across the three regions and nine indicators, and regulate accordingly, not asking after the named disease, taking the return to evenness as the goal.

Rather than reading a single wrist, this chapter sends the hand across the whole body, three regions each with three indicators, and judges life and death by how their fullness and emptiness stand against one another. A diseased pulse means nothing except against a known healthy one, so the work begins by fixing in the hand what an even channel feels like; only then are the nine sites palpated in turn and weighed together to locate excess and deficiency. From there the physician regulates toward balance, treating the imbalance the fingers actually find rather than the name the patient offers, with evenness as the only target. Diagnosis becomes a survey of the entire field of qi, not an inference drawn from one corner of it.

SU WEN 76

別於陽者，知病從來；別於陰者，知死生之期。知陽者知陰，知陰者知陽。夫聖人之治病，循法守度，援物比類，化之冥冥。

bié yú yáng zhě, zhī bìng cóng lái; bié yú yīn zhě, zhī sǐ shēng zhī qī. zhī yáng zhě zhī yīn, zhī yīn zhě zhī yáng. fū shèng rén zhī zhì bìng, xún fǎ shǒu dù, yuán wù bǐ lèi, huà zhī míng míng.

One who distinguishes the yang knows whence the disease came; one who distinguishes the yin knows the term of death and life. To know the yang is to know the yin, and to know the yin is to know the yang. When the sage treats illness, he follows the method and keeps the measure, draws on things by likeness and class, and works his changes in the unseen.

Every case carries two readings, and a physician who takes only one is half-blind: the yang aspect tells where the disease came from, the yin aspect what is likely to become of it, and each implies the other, since cause and outcome are two faces of one pattern. The sage who treats this way does not improvise. He keeps to a settled method and a fixed measure, reasons from the known to the unknown by likeness and class, comparing the case before him to its kind, and so brings about cures whose working is too fine to point at. The line binds disciplined technique to the trained intuition that lets a practitioner see at once where a disease began and where it is going.

SU WEN 81

夫心者，五藏之專精也，目者其竅也，華色者其榮也。是以人有德也，則氣和於目；有亡，憂知於色。泣涕者，腦也，腦者陰也。

fū xīn zhě, wǔ zàng zhī zhuān jīng yě, mù zhě qí qiào yě, huá sè zhě qí róng yě. shì yǐ rén yǒu dé yě, zé qì hé yú mù; yǒu wáng, yōu zhī yú sè. qì tì zhě, nǎo yě, nǎo zhě yīn yě.

The heart is the concentrated essence of the five organs; the eyes are its portal, and the bloom of the complexion its flowering. Thus when a person is whole, the qi is harmonious in the eyes; when something is lost, grief is known in the colour. Tears come from the brain, and the brain is yin.

The heart gathers the concentrated essence of all five organs, and it shows that gathering through two windows, the light of the eyes and the colour of the face, so that an inner condition surfaces before a word is spoken. A whole person looks out with a clear, harmonious eye; one who has lost something wears the loss as a shadow in the complexion, which is why the face cannot lie about feeling or depletion. The physician therefore watches the steadiness and lustre of the gaze and the bloom of the colour as a direct reading of the heart-spirit and the body's reserve, and takes even tears as rising from the yin depths rather than the surface. It is the ground of inspecting the spirit, the first of the four examinations, set down as a plain account of why the heart is legible in the face.

LING SHU 37

五官者，五藏之閱也。五色各見其部，察其浮沉，以知淺深；察其澤夭，以觀成敗；察其散摶，以知遠近；視色上下，以知病處。

wǔ guān zhě, wǔ zàng zhī yuè yě. wǔ sè gè jiàn qí bù, chá qí fú chén, yǐ zhī qiǎn shēn; chá qí zé yāo, yǐ guān chéng bài; chá qí sàn tuán, yǐ zhī yuǎn jìn; shì sè shàng xià, yǐ zhī bìng chù.

The five offices are the outward viewing-windows of the five organs. The five colours each appear in their proper region; observe whether the colour floats or sinks, to know whether the disease is shallow or deep; observe whether it is moist or withered, to see whether it is mending or failing; observe whether it is scattered or gathered, to know whether it is recent or long-standing; note where on the face the colour lies, high or low, to know the seat of the disease.

A colour on the face answers four different questions at once, and the chapter teaches the physician to ask them one at a time. Whether it floats or sinks tells the depth of the disease; whether it is moist or withered tells whether the condition is mending or failing; whether it is gathered or scattered tells whether it is recent or long-standing; and where it sits on the face tells which organ is involved. Because the same hue means different things along each of these axes, reading a complexion is never a matter of naming a colour but of weighing it in four dimensions. Worked through in order, the art turns into something a practitioner can actually follow, with the five offices serving as fixed windows onto the five organs behind them.

FROM THE AUTHOR

Of everything in this gate, the stomach-qi is the hardest to learn, because it is not a number but a texture, the difference between a pulse that is alive under the finger and one that is merely strong. No book conveys it; only many wrists, felt slowly, in a quiet hour, with the breath settled. Once it can be felt, a passing trouble can be told from a real danger, and that one judgement is worth more than a hundred named pulses.

以此參伍，決死生之分。

Cross-check these against one another, and decide the division between life and death.

WHERE THIS GATE LEADS

Every pulse is read first as the yin or yang of *Gate Two*, what recedes and what rises, the slow and the rapid. The colours and signs at the surface belong to the organs of *Gate Three, The Court Within*. The particular pulses and signs of named illnesses are gathered in *Gate Seven, How Illness Begins*. And the treatment a reading calls for is the work of *Gate Eight, The Physician's Hand*.

PART FIVE

The Rivers of the Body

The Channels and Collaterals

經絡

On the channels. The hidden network of rivers along which qi and blood run, binding every organ to the surface and to one another, and the ground on which the needle does its work.

GATE FIVE · THE CHANNELS AND COLLATERALS

The Rivers of the Body

經絡

> *The channels are that by which life and death are decided.*
>
> Ling Shu 10

Beneath the skin runs a map that no dissection lays out as the classic draws it: a network of rivers along which the qi and the blood travel, joining every organ to the surface and to one another. Open the body and you will not find the channels labelled there; yet press the right place on the forearm and a sensation runs toward the chest, and the network announces itself. This gate is the chart of those rivers.

The word for the network is jingluo, and it names two things. The jing, the channels, are the twelve great rivers, deep and longitudinal, each tied to one of the organs. The luo, the collaterals, are their branching, surfacing tributaries, the smaller vessels that web outward toward the skin. Together they are the conduits through which qi and blood reach every corner of the body, and they are the ground beneath two whole arts: the placing of the needle, and the understanding of how a disease travels inward from the surface or outward from within.

Read this gate for the same five things. What it is, to begin with, is the conduit network of channels and collaterals, the hidden rivers along which qi and blood run. It concerns everyone, and most directly anyone who would understand acupuncture, for this is the map the needle works from. It applies throughout the body, at the particular places where the channels surface and can be reached. It matters because qi and blood must flow freely, and a blocked channel is a sick one. And it is used by knowing each channel's course, the organ it serves, its partner within, and the points at which it may be met.

Why the Channels Matter

LING SHU 10

黃帝曰：人始生，先成精，精成而腦髓生，骨為幹，脈為營，筋為剛，肉為牆，皮膚堅而毛髮長。穀入於胃，脈道以通，血氣乃行。

huáng dì yuē: rén shǐ shēng, xiān chéng jīng, jīng chéng ér nǎo suǐ shēng, gǔ wèi gàn, mài wèi yíng, jīn wèi gāng, ròu wèi qiáng, pí fū jiān ér máo fà zhǎng. gǔ rù yú wèi, mài dào yǐ tōng, xuè qì nǎi xíng.

The Yellow Emperor said: When a person first comes to be, the essence forms before all else; once the essence is formed, the brain and the marrow are born. The bones make the framework, the vessels the channels of nourishment, the sinews the bindings, the flesh the walls; the skin hardens, and the hair grows long. When grain enters the stomach, the paths of the vessels open, and the blood and qi begin to move.

LING SHU 10

經脈者，所以能決死生，處百病，調虛實，不可不通。

jīng mài zhě, suǒ yǐ néng jué sǐ shēng, chù bǎi bìng, diào xū shí, bù kě bù tōng.

The channels are that by which life and death are decided, the hundred diseases are settled, and vacuity and repletion are set right. They must not go unmastered, and must never be left blocked.

The classic places the channels among the first things made in a body. Once the essence has formed and the brain and marrow have arisen, the bones frame it, the sinews bind it, the flesh walls it, and the vessels are laid down as its channels of nourishment; and only when grain enters the stomach and opens those paths do the blood and qi begin to move. The channels are not an afterthought drawn upon the flesh. They are part of how the body is built, and how it is fed.

From this follows the plainest statement in the whole literature of why the channels are studied at all. By them life and death are decided, the hundred diseases settled, and vacuity and repletion set right; they must not go unmastered, and must never be left blocked. The sentence is worth weighing slowly, because it makes flow itself the measure of health. Where the qi and blood move freely the body thrives; where a channel is obstructed, disease gathers at the block. Almost everything the needle does, in the gate that follows, is the freeing of a flow that has stalled.

Deep Rivers, Surfacing Streams

> LING SHU 10
>
> 經脈十二者，伏行分肉之間，深而不見。諸脈之浮而常見者，皆絡脈也。
>
> *jīng mài shí èr zhě, fú xíng fēn ròu zhī jiān, shēn ér bù jiàn. zhū mài zhī fú ér cháng jiàn zhě, jiē luò mài yě.*
>
> The twelve channels run hidden between the partings of the flesh, deep and out of sight. The vessels that float at the surface and are always to be seen are, every one of them, the collaterals.

It is worth being clear about what can and cannot be seen. The twelve great channels run hidden deep between the partings of the flesh; they are not the blue vessels visible at the surface. Those surface vessels, the ones you can see on the back of a hand, are collaterals, the branching tributaries of the system. The channels proper are inferred from their effects and their points, not observed directly, which is why the tradition maps them with such care: they are the deep structure, and the visible collaterals are only where that structure breaks the surface.

FIGURE · THE TWELVE CHANNELS AND THE TWO VESSELS

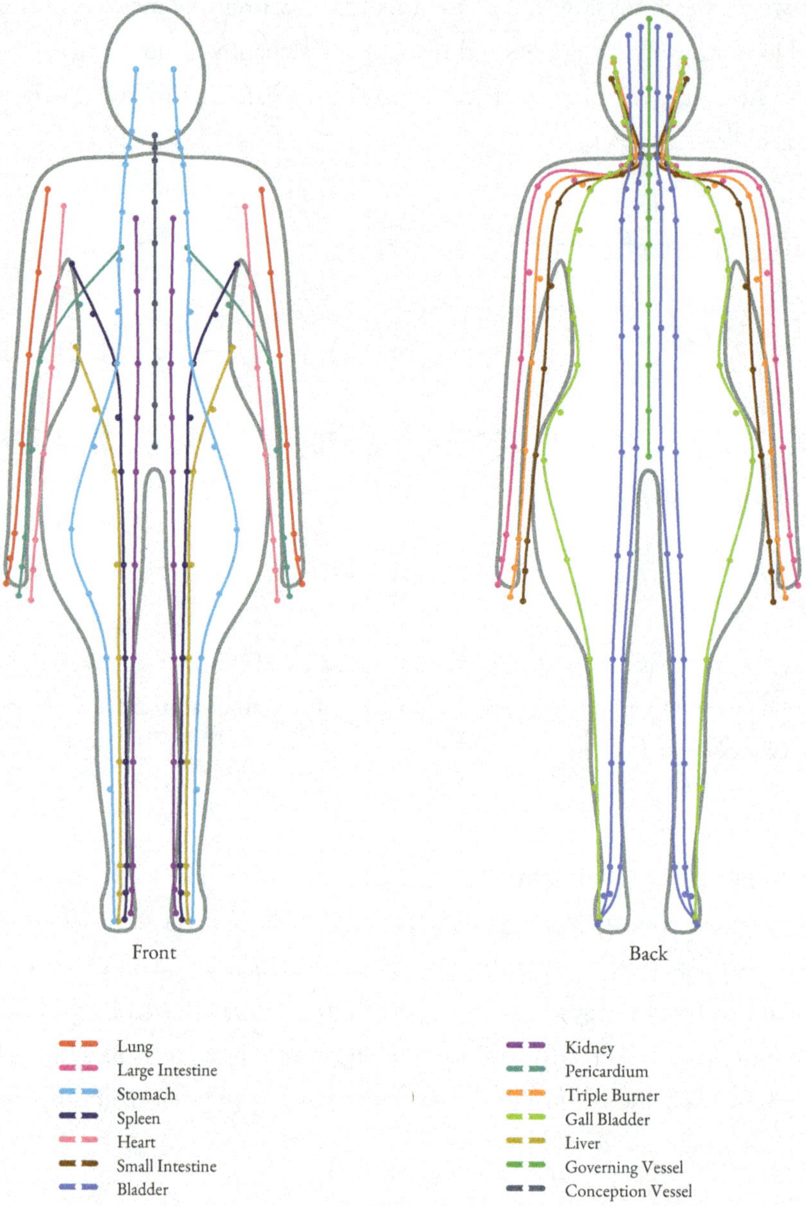

The twelve channels and the two great vessels, each in its own colour with its points marked. The front carries the inner-arm and medial-leg channels, the Stomach, and the Conception Vessel up the midline; the back carries the outer-arm channels, the Bladder in its two lines down the back, the Gallbladder along the flanks, and the Governing Vessel up the spine and over the head. Together they form one circuit, the path the qi travels round the body in a day.

The Twelve Channels

LING SHU 10

肺手太陰之脈，起於中焦，下絡大腸，還循胃口，上膈屬肺，從肺系橫出腋下，下循臑內，行少陰心主之前，下肘中，循臂內上骨下廉，入寸口，上魚，循魚際，出大指之端。是動則病肺脹滿，膨膨而喘咳，缺盆中痛。是主肺所生病者，咳，上氣喘渴，煩心胸滿，臑臂內前廉痛厥，掌中熱。氣盛有餘，則肩背痛，汗出中風，小便數而欠；氣虛則肩背痛寒，少氣不足以息。

fèi shǒu tài yīn zhī mài, qǐ yú zhōng jiāo, xià luò dà cháng, hái xún wèi kǒu, shàng gé shǔ fèi, cóng fèi xì héng chū yè xià, xià xún nào nèi, xíng shào yīn xīn zhǔ zhī qián, xià zhǒu zhōng, xún bì nèi shàng gǔ xià lián, rù cùn kǒu, shàng yú, xún yú jì, chū dà zhǐ zhī duān. shì dòng zé bìng fèi zhàng mǎn, péng péng ér chuǎn ké, quē pén zhōng tòng. shì zhǔ fèi suǒ shēng bìng zhě, ké, shàng qì chuǎn kě, fán xīn xiōng mǎn, nào bì nèi qián lián tòng jué, zhǎng zhōng rè. qì shèng yǒu yú, zé jiān bèi tòng, hàn chū zhōng fēng, xiǎo biàn shuò ér qiàn; qì xū zé jiān bèi tòng hán, shǎo qì bù zú yǐ xī.

The lung channel of the hand greater-yin rises in the middle burner, descends to net the large intestine, turns back along the mouth of the stomach, climbs through the diaphragm to belong to the lung, then crosses out from the lung system below the armpit, runs down the inner arm in front of the heart-governor channel, passes through the middle of the elbow, follows the inner forearm along the lower edge of the bone, enters the inch-mouth at the wrist, rises to the mound of the thumb, follows its border, and comes out at the tip of the thumb. When this channel is disturbed, there is a fullness and distension of the lung, a laboured panting and cough, and pain in the hollow above the collarbone. As the channel governing what the lung gives rise to, its illnesses are coughing, the qi rising with panting and thirst, a vexed heart and a full chest, pain and reversal along the front of the inner arm, and heat in the centre of the palm. When its qi is replete and in excess, there is pain in the shoulder and back, sweating, and frequent scant urination; when its qi is vacuous, there is cold pain in the shoulder and back, and a breath too slight to draw.

The lung channel, given here in full, is the model for how the classic describes all twelve. Each entry traces a course, naming where the channel rises, the organ it belongs to and the partner organ it nets along the way, and where it ends at the fingers or toes. Then it gives two sets of disorders: the illnesses that appear when the channel itself is disturbed, and the illnesses of what its organ gives rise to, divided again by whether the qi is in excess or in want. Learn one entry well and the other eleven fall into the same shape.

The twelve are six matched pairs. Each runs either along the arm or along the leg, each is either yin or yang, and each is tied to one organ and coupled with that organ's partner. Set in the order in which the qi flows through them, they form a single circuit, which the table below lays out.

CHANNEL	ORGAN	ASPECT	PAIRED WITH
Hand greater-yin 手太陰	Lung	yin	Large Intestine
Hand bright-yang 手陽明	Large Intestine	yang	Lung
Foot bright-yang 足陽明	Stomach	yang	Spleen
Foot greater-yin 足太陰	Spleen	yin	Stomach
Hand lesser-yin 手少陰	Heart	yin	Small Intestine
Hand greater-yang 手太陽	Small Intestine	yang	Heart
Foot greater-yang 足太陽	Bladder	yang	Kidney
Foot lesser-yin 足少陰	Kidney	yin	Bladder
Hand reverting-yin 手厥陰	Pericardium	yin	Triple Burner
Hand lesser-yang 手少陽	Triple Burner	yang	Pericardium
Foot lesser-yang 足少陽	Gallbladder	yang	Liver
Foot reverting-yin 足厥陰	Liver	yin	Gallbladder

The Forms of the Channel System

The twelve channels are the trunk of the system, but not the whole of it. Around them and beneath them the classic maps several further networks, each with its own use and its own kind of disorder.

LING SHU 11

足太陽之正，別入於膕中，其一道下尻五寸，別入於肛，屬於膀胱，散之腎，循膂當心入散；直者，從膂上出於項，復屬於太陽。此為一經也。

zú tài yáng zhī zhèng, bié rù yú guó zhōng, qí yī dào xià kāo wǔ cùn, bié rù yú gāng, shǔ yú páng guāng, sàn zhī shèn, xún lǚ dāng xīn rù sàn; zhí zhě, cóng lǚ shàng chū yú xiàng, fù shǔ yú tài yáng. cǐ wèi yī jīng yě.

The divergence of the foot greater-yang separates and enters the hollow behind the knee. One branch descends five cun below the sacrum and enters the anus, joins the bladder, spreads to the kidney, then follows the spine to the level of the heart and disperses there; the straight branch rises along the spine, emerges at the nape, and rejoins the greater-yang. This is one channel and its divergence.

Deepest are the divergences: inner branches that leave a main channel, dive to the organ it pairs with, and later rejoin the surface. They are how a yin channel and its yang partner are knit together within, and how an organ can be reached from a point on the limb. To needle a channel, then, is sometimes to touch an organ it never seems to pass near.

LING SHU 13

足太陽之筋，起於足小指，上結於踝，邪上結於膝，其下循足外側，結於踵，上循跟，結於膕。其病小指支跟腫痛，膕攣，脊反折，項筋急。

zú tài yáng zhī jīn, qǐ yú zú xiǎo zhǐ, shàng jié yú huái, xié shàng jié yú xī, qí xià xún zú wài cè, jié yú zhǒng, shàng xún gēn, jié yú guó. qí bìng xiǎo zhǐ zhī gēn zhǒng tòng, guó luán, jí fǎn zhé, xiàng jīn jí.

The sinew of the foot greater-yang begins at the little toe, rises and binds at the ankle, slants upward and binds at the knee, runs below along the outer side of the foot and binds at the heel, then climbs the heel-cord and binds at the back of the knee. Its disorders are pain and swelling from the little toe to the heel, cramp behind the knee, the spine bent stiffly back, and the sinews of the nape drawn tight.

Alongside the channels run the sinew channels, the musculotendinous lines that begin at the toes and fingers and bind fast at the joints. Their disorders are not of the organs but of movement: pain, cramp, stiffness, and spasm along the line. A complaint of a locked knee or a drawn nape is read on the sinew channel and treated along its course, not as an illness of the inner organs.

SU WEN 56

凡十二經絡脈者，皮之部也。是故百病之始生也，必先於皮毛，邪中之則腠理開，開則入客於絡脈，留而不去，傳入於經，留而不去，傳入於府，廩於腸胃。其入於絡也，則絡脈盛色變。

fán shí èr jīng luò mài zhě, pí zhī bù yě. shì gù bǎi bìng zhī shǐ shēng yě, bì xiān yú pí máo, xié zhōng zhī zé còu lǐ kāi, kāi zé rù kè yú luò mài, liú ér bù qù, chuán rù yú jīng, liú ér bù qù, chuán rù yú fǔ, lǐn yú cháng wèi. qí rù yú luò yě, zé luò mài shèng sè biàn.

All twelve channels and their collaterals are the regions of the skin. So when the hundred diseases first arise, they begin always in the skin and hair; when an evil strikes there, the pores open, and opening, it enters and lodges in the collaterals; staying and not leaving, it passes into the channels; staying and not leaving, it passes into the palaces, to be stored in the bowels and stomach. When it enters the collaterals, they grow full and their colour changes.

Outermost lie the cutaneous regions, the patches of skin that belong to each channel. Disease entering from without follows a fixed road inward: skin, then collateral, then channel, then palace. This is the whole reason an illness caught at the skin is slight and the same illness, left to travel inward, grows grave; and it is how the depth of a case is judged, by how far along that road it has already gone.

SU WEN 57

帝曰：絡之陰陽，亦應其經乎？岐伯曰：陰絡之色應其經，陽絡之色變無常，隨四時而行也。寒多則凝泣，凝泣則青黑；熱多則淖澤，淖澤則黃赤，此皆常色，謂之無病。五色具見者，謂之寒熱。

dì yuē: luò zhī yīn yáng, yì yīng qí jīng hū? qí bó yuē: yīn luò zhī sè yīng qí jīng, yáng luò zhī sè biàn wú cháng, suí sì shí ér xíng yě. hán duō zé níng qì, níng qì zé qīng hēi; rè duō zé nào zé, nào zé zé huáng chì, cǐ jiē cháng sè, wèi zhī wú bìng. wǔ sè jù jiàn zhě, wèi zhī hán rè.

The Emperor asked: Do the yin and yang of the collaterals also answer to their channels? Qibo said: The colour of a yin collateral answers to its channel, but the colour of a yang collateral changes without constancy, shifting with the four seasons. Where cold is much, the blood congeals, and congealed it is green-black; where heat is much, it runs moist, and moist it is yellow-red. All of these are constant colours and are called no-disease; but when all five colours appear together, that is called cold-and-heat.

Even the small surface collaterals declare themselves by colour, cold congealing them to blue and black, heat flushing them yellow and red. The visible vessels under the skin are thus a plain gauge of cold and heat, read with nothing but the eye.

LING SHU 5

太陽根於至陰，結於命門。命門者，目也。陽明根於厲兌，結於顙大。顙大者，鉗耳也。少陽根於竅陰，結於窗籠。窗籠者，耳中也。

tài yáng gēn yú zhì yīn, jié yú mìng mén. mìng mén zhě, mù yě. yáng míng gēn yú lì duì, jié yú sǎng dà. sǎng dà zhě, qián ěr yě. shào yáng gēn yú qiào yīn, jié yú chuāng lóng. chuāng lóng zhě, ěr zhong yě.

The greater-yang roots at the Reaching-Yin point on the little toe and knots at the Gate of Life, which is the eye. The bright-yang roots at the Stern-Toe point and knots at the great brow, which is beside the ear. The lesser-yang roots at the Orifice-Yin point and knots at the Window-Cage, which is within the ear.

And the channels are not an even mesh. They have roots and knots, rooting at the tips of the toes and fingers and knotting at the head and the chest, so that the small points at the ends of the limbs command the whole length of a channel. This is why a point at the end of a toe can move a trouble seated at the eye.

The Channels Measured

The classic did not leave the channels as metaphor. It measured them, as carefully as it measured the organs, and tied every measure to the body itself.

LING SHU 12

黃帝問於岐伯曰：經脈十二者，外合於十二經水，而內屬於五藏六府。夫十二經水者，其有大小、深淺、廣狹、遠近各不同，五藏六府之高下、小大、受穀之多少亦不等。此人之所以參天地而應陰陽也。

huáng dì wèn yú qí bó yuē: jīng mài shí èr zhě, wài hé yú shí èr jīng shuǐ, ér nèi shǔ yú wǔ zàng liù fǔ. fū shí èr jīng shuǐ zhě, qí yǒu dà xiǎo, shēn qiǎn, guǎng xiá, yuǎn jìn gè bù tóng, wǔ zàng liù fǔ zhī gāo xià, xiǎo dà, shòu gǔ zhī duō shǎo yì bù děng. cǐ rén zhī suǒ yǐ cān tiān dì ér yìng yīn yáng yě.

The Yellow Emperor asked Qibo: The twelve channels join, without, to the twelve river-waters, and belong, within, to the five organs and six palaces. The twelve rivers differ each from each in size and depth, in breadth and nearness; and the organs and palaces too are each unlike in their height and size and in how much grain they receive. This is how a person stands in correspondence with Heaven and Earth and answers to yin and yang.

The twelve channels are matched to twelve real rivers, each differing in size and depth and nearness, and the match was not poetry alone: it set how deep a channel could be needled and how much it could bear. A channel likened to a deep, broad river is approached differently from one likened to a shallow stream.

LING SHU 14

黃帝問於伯高曰：脈度言經脈之長短，何以立之？伯高曰：先度其骨節之大小廣狹長短，而脈度定矣。頭之大骨圍二尺六寸，胸圍四尺五寸，腰圍四尺二寸。

huáng dì wèn yú bó gāo yuē: mài dù yán jīng mài zhī cháng duǎn, hé yǐ lì zhī? bó gāo yuē: xiān dù qí gǔ jié zhī dà xiǎo guǎng xiá cháng duǎn, ér mài dù dìng yǐ. tóu zhī dà gǔ wéi èr chǐ liù cùn, xiōng wéi sì chǐ wǔ cùn, yāo wéi sì chǐ èr cùn.

The Yellow Emperor asked Bo Gao: The measure of the vessels speaks of the length of the channels; on what is it founded? Bo Gao said: First measure the bones and joints, their size and breadth and length, and the measure of the vessels is fixed. The great bone of the head is two chi six cun around, the chest four chi five cun, the waist four chi two cun.

To find anything on the body, the body itself is made the ruler. The bones are measured in proportional units, the head so many around, the chest, the waist, the length of each limb, so that a point may be located on any person, tall or short, by proportion rather than by a fixed inch. This bone-measurement is the ground of point-location still.

LING SHU 17

手之六陽，從手至頭，長五尺，五六三丈。手之六陰，從手至胸中，三尺五寸。足之六陽，從足上至頭，八尺，六八四丈八尺。足之六陰，從足至胸中，六尺五寸。凡都合一十六丈二尺，此氣之大經隧也。

shǒu zhī liù yáng, cóng shǒu zhì tóu, cháng wǔ chǐ, wǔ liù sān zhàng. shǒu zhī liù yīn, cóng shǒu zhì xiōng zhōng, sān chǐ wǔ cùn. zú zhī liù yáng, cóng zú shàng zhì tóu, bā chǐ, liù bā sì zhàng bā chǐ. zú zhī liù yīn, cóng zú zhì xiōng zhōng, liù chǐ wǔ cùn. fán dōu hé yī shí liù zhàng èr chǐ, cǐ qì zhī dà jīng suì yě.

The six yang channels of the hands, from hand to head, are five chi each, six fives making three zhang. The six yin of the hands, from hand to chest, are three chi five cun each. The six yang of the feet, from foot to head, are eight chi each, six eights making four zhang eight chi. The six yin of the feet, from foot to chest, are six chi five cun each.

> All together they come to sixteen zhang two chi: these are the great conduits along which the qi runs.

The channels themselves are then given lengths, the arm-yang five chi, the leg-yang eight, and the rest, summing to sixteen zhang and two chi of conduit in all. The qi that fills them has a measured road to run; and once the road has a length, the number of times the qi can travel it in a day becomes a thing one can reckon, which is where the circuit of qi begins.

The Circuit of Qi

> LING SHU 16
>
> 營氣之道，內穀為寶。穀入於胃，乃傳之肺，流溢於中，布散於外，精專者行於經隧，常營無已，終而復始，是謂天地之紀。
>
> *yíng qì zhī dào, nèi gǔ wèi bǎo. gǔ rù yú wèi, nǎi chuán zhī fèi, liú yì yú zhōng, bù sàn yú wài, jīng zhuān zhě xíng yú jīng suì, cháng yíng wú yǐ, zhōng ér fù shǐ, shì wèi tiān dì zhī jì.*
>
> The way of the nutritive qi treasures the grain within. When grain enters the stomach, it is passed on to the lung, brimming over within and spreading abroad without; its pure and concentrated part travels in the channel-tunnels, circulating without end, finishing and beginning again. This is called the cord of Heaven and Earth.

The channels are not twelve separate pipes but one continuous round. The nutritive qi, drawn from the grain in the stomach and sent first to the lung, passes from channel to channel in a fixed order, brimming and spreading, circulating without end, finishing and beginning again, in a rhythm the classic dares to call the cord of Heaven and Earth. The order is the order of the table above, from the lung onward, returning at last from the liver to the lung to begin once more.

Because the round is tied to the day, each channel has its high hour, when its qi is fullest. This is the basis of the daily tide the practice note sets out, and of an old and useful observation: the hour at which a person reliably wakes in the night, or feels a complaint sharpen, often points to the channel then at its flood. To know the circuit is to know not only where to treat but when.

The Tides of Qi

The channels are not still water but a tide. The classic traces where that tide is raised, how it divides, and how often it turns in a day.

SU WEN 21

食氣入胃，散精於肝，淫氣於筋。食氣入胃，濁氣歸心，淫精於脈，脈氣流經，經氣歸於肺，肺朝百脈，輸精於皮毛。毛脈合精，行氣於府，府精神明，留於四藏，氣歸於權衡。權衡以平，氣口成寸，以決死生。

shí qì rù wèi, sàn jīng yú gān, yín qì yú jīn. shí qì rù wèi, zhuó qì guī xīn, yín jīng yú mài, mài qì liú jīng, jīng qì guī yú fèi, fèi cháo bǎi mài, shū jīng yú pí máo. máo mài hé jīng, xíng qì yú fǔ, fǔ jīng shén míng, liú yú sì zàng, qì guī yú quán héng. quán héng yǐ píng, qì kǒu chéng cùn, yǐ jué sǐ shēng.

The qi of food enters the stomach, scatters its essence to the liver, and floods the sinews with qi. The qi of food enters the stomach, and its denser part returns to the heart, flooding the vessels with essence; the qi of the vessels flows into the channels, the channel-qi returns to the lung, and the lung, to which the hundred vessels pay court, sends the essence out to the skin and body hair. The hair and the vessels join their essence, carrying the qi back to the palaces; the essence of the palaces, clear and bright, abides in the four organs, and the qi returns to its balance. When the balance is level, the qi-mouth completes its measure, and by it life and death are decided.

The tide begins at the stomach. The qi of food scatters its essence to the liver and floods the sinews; its denser part goes to the heart and floods the vessels; the vessel-qi runs along the channels and gathers at the lung, which gives audience to the hundred vessels and sends essence out to the skin; and the whole comes to balance at the wrist, where the qi-mouth becomes the inch by which life and death are judged. This one passage joins food, organ, channel, lung, and pulse into a single circuit, and is the reason the wrist can report the whole body.

LING SHU 18

人受氣於穀，穀入於胃，以傳與肺，五藏六府皆以受氣。其清者為營，濁者為衛，營在脈中，衛在脈外，營周不休，五十而復大會，陰陽相貫，如環無端。

rén shòu qì yú gǔ, gǔ rù yú wèi, yǐ chuán yǔ fèi, wǔ zàng liù fǔ jiē yǐ shòu qì. qí qīng zhě wèi yíng, zhuó zhě wèi wèi, yíng zài mài zhōng, wèi zài mài wài, yíng zhōu bù xiū, wǔ shí ér fù dà huì, yīn yáng xiāng guàn, rú huán wú duān.

A person receives qi from grain. The grain enters the stomach and is passed on to the lung, and the five organs and six palaces all receive their qi from it. The clear part becomes the nutritive qi and the turbid the defensive; the nutritive runs within the vessels, the defensive outside them. The nutritive circles without rest, meeting again in a great conjunction after fifty circuits, yin and yang threaded one through the other like a ring that has no end.

The qi so raised divides in two. The clear part becomes the nutritive qi, which runs inside the vessels and feeds; the turbid becomes the defensive qi, which runs outside them and guards. The two circle without rest and meet again in a great conjunction every fifty circuits, yin and yang like a ring without end. A want of the nutritive shows as poor nourishment and a thin pulse; a want of the defensive as easy sweating and a body open to cold.

LING SHU 15

人一呼脈再動，氣行三寸；一吸脈亦再動，氣行三寸；呼吸定息，氣行六寸。一日一夜一萬三千五百息，氣行五十營於身，水下百刻，日行二十八宿。

rén yī hū mài zài dòng, qì xíng sān cùn; yī xī mài yì zài dòng, qì xíng sān cùn; hū xī dìng xī, qì xíng liù cùn. yī rì yī yè yī wàn sān qiān wǔ bǎi xī, qì xíng wǔ shí yíng yú shēn, shuǐ xià bǎi kè, rì xíng èr shí bā xiù.

With one exhalation the pulse beats twice and the qi moves three cun; with one inhalation the pulse beats twice again and the qi moves three cun; in one full breath the qi moves six cun. In a day and a night there are thirteen thousand five hundred breaths,

> and the qi completes fifty circuits of the body, while the water-clock runs down its hundred marks and the sun passes through the twenty-eight lodges of heaven.

The rhythm is exact, and tied to the breath: six cun of travel to a breath, thirteen thousand five hundred breaths to a day and night, fifty circuits of the body while the sun crosses its twenty-eight lodges. The body keeps time with the sky, and the pace of the breath is the pace of the circulation, which is why a settled breath steadies everything downstream of it.

> LING SHU 76
>
> 衛氣之行，一日一夜五十周於身，晝日行於陽二十五周，夜行於陰二十五周，周於五藏。是故平旦陰盡，陽氣出於目，目張則氣上行於頭。
>
> *wèi qì zhī xíng, yī rì yī yè wǔ shí zhōu yú shēn, zhòu rì xíng yú yáng èr shí wǔ zhōu, yè xíng yú yīn èr shí wǔ zhōu, zhōu yú wǔ zàng. shì gù píng dàn yīn jǐn, yáng qì chū yú mù, mù zhāng zé qì shàng xíng yú tóu.*
>
> The course of the defensive qi makes fifty circuits of the body in a day and a night: by day it runs twenty-five circuits through the yang, the outer body, and by night twenty-five through the yin, circling the five organs. So at daybreak, when the yin is spent, the yang qi issues from the eyes; the eyes open, and the qi rises to the head.

The defensive qi keeps a march of its own across the day. By day it runs twenty-five circuits through the outer yang; by night twenty-five through the inner organs. When at dawn it surfaces to the yang and issues from the eyes, we wake; when at dusk it sinks into the yin, we sleep. This is the classic's account of the sleep-and-waking rhythm, and of why a disordered defensive qi keeps a person from rest.

LING SHU 59

黃帝曰：衛氣之留於腹中，蓄積不行，使人支脅中滿，喘呼逆息，何以去之？伯高曰：其氣積於胸中者，上取之；積於腹中者，下取之。

huáng dì yuē: wèi qì zhī liú yú fù zhōng, xù jī bù xíng, shǐ rén zhī xié zhōng mǎn, chuǎn hū nì xī, hé yǐ qù zhī? bó gāo yuē: qí qì jī yú xiōng zhōng zhě, shàng qǔ zhī; jī yú fù zhōng zhě, xià qǔ zhī.

The Yellow Emperor said: When the defensive qi lingers in the belly, gathered and not moving, so that it makes the flanks and the middle full and the breath come panting and against its course, how is it cleared? Bo Gao said: Where the qi is heaped in the chest, draw it off from above; where it is heaped in the belly, draw it off from below.

When the defensive qi stalls and heaps up out of its place, it brings fullness in the flanks and a panting, counter-running breath; and the remedy follows the lodging, drawn off from above when it gathers in the chest, from below when it gathers in the belly. The method is plain: treat the qi where it has actually collected.

LING SHU 52

能知六經標本者，可以無惑於天下。故下虛則厥，下盛則熱；上虛則眩，上盛則熱痛。

néng zhī liù jīng biāo běn zhě, kě yǐ wú huò yú tiān xià. gù xià xū zé jué, xià shèng zé rè; shàng xū zé xuàn, shàng shèng zé rè tòng.

One who knows the root and the branch of the six channels need never be at a loss in the world. Where the lower end is empty there is cold reversal in the limbs, where it is over-full there is heat; where the upper end is empty there is dizziness, where it is over-full there is heat and pain.

And each channel is read at its two ends, the root at the limbs and the branch at the head and trunk. Emptiness at the lower end brings cold reversal in the limbs and fullness brings heat; emptiness above brings dizziness and fullness heat and pain. To know which end of a channel is empty and which is full is to know where the needle should go.

The Four Seas, and the Beat That Never Stops

Beneath the moving tide lie its reservoirs; and at a few places the tide can be felt directly, beating without pause.

> LING SHU 33
>
> 人有髓海，有血海，有氣海，有水穀之海，凡此四者，以應四海也。胃者，水穀之海；衝脈者，為十二經之海；膻中者，為氣之海；腦者，為髓之海。
>
> *rén yǒu suǐ hǎi, yǒu xuè hǎi, yǒu qì hǎi, yǒu shuǐ gǔ zhī hǎi, fán cǐ sì zhě, yǐ yīng sì hǎi yě. wèi zhě, shuǐ gǔ zhī hǎi; chōng mài zhě, wèi shí èr jīng zhī hǎi; dàn zhōng zhě, wèi qì zhī hǎi; nǎo zhě, wèi suǐ zhī hǎi.*
>
> A person has a sea of marrow, a sea of blood, a sea of qi, and a sea of grain and water; these four answer to the four seas of the world. The stomach is the sea of grain and water; the penetrating vessel is the sea of the twelve channels; the chest-centre is the sea of qi; and the brain is the sea of marrow.

The body has four seas that feed the whole: the stomach, the sea of grain and water; the penetrating vessel, the sea of the channels and their blood; the chest, the sea of qi; the brain, the sea of marrow. A want in any one has its own signs, and to fill or drain the right sea is to right the body at its source. A bone-deep weariness and a hollow, ringing head may be an emptiness of the sea of marrow or the sea of qi, met at the points that command those seas, rather than a complaint of any single organ.

LING SHU 62

黃帝曰：經脈十二，而手太陰、足少陰、陽明，獨動不休，何也？岐伯曰：是明胃脈也。胃為五藏六府之海，其清氣上注於肺，肺氣從太陰而行之，故動而不止。

huáng dì yuē: jīng mài shí èr, ér shǒu tài yīn, zú shào yīn, yáng míng, dú dòng bù xiū, hé yě? qí bó yuē: shì míng wèi mài yě. wèi wèi wǔ zàng liù fǔ zhī hǎi, qí qīng qì shàng zhù yú fèi, fèi qì cóng tài yīn ér xíng zhī, gù dòng ér bù zhǐ.

The Yellow Emperor asked: Of the twelve channels, why do the hand greater-yin at the wrist, the foot lesser-yin, and the bright-yang alone pulse without ceasing? Qibo said: This makes the stomach vessel plain. The stomach is the sea of the organs and palaces; its clear qi pours upward to the lung, and the lung-qi runs out along the greater-yin, and so the pulse beats and does not stop.

At a few places the channel can be felt to beat without ceasing, the wrist most of all, and the reason is again the stomach. As the sea of the organs and palaces it sends its clear qi up to the lung; the lung drives it out along the hand greater-yin; and so the wrist pulse beats and does not stop. This closes the circle with the gate of diagnosis, for it is precisely this stomach-made qi, felt at the wrist, that the physician reads, and its presence there that means life. The rivers of the body, fed from four seas, turning by the breath, and legible at the wrist: this is the channel system entire.

THE PAIRS AND THE DAILY TIDE

Each yin organ is coupled with a yang partner, sharing a turn of the circuit, so that treating one can reach the other. The six pairs are lung and large intestine, spleen and stomach, heart and small intestine, kidney and bladder, pericardium and triple burner, liver and gallbladder.

The qi floods each channel in turn across the day. Waking or worsening at the same hour points to the organ then at its height.

FIGURE · THE CIRCULATION OF THE DAY

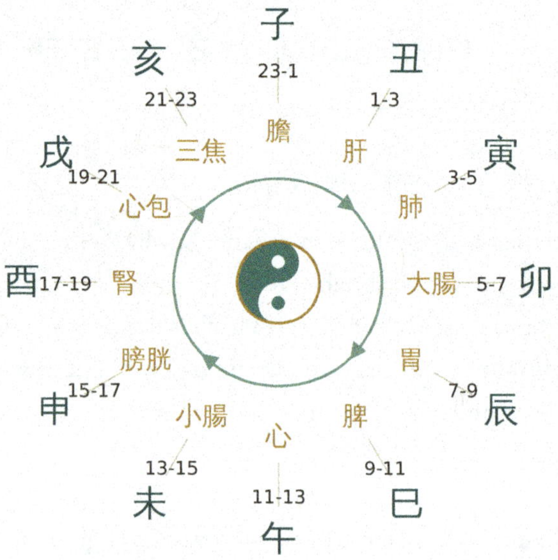

The qi completes one round of the body in a day and a night, cresting in each channel for two hours in turn, marked here by the twelve earthly branches with midnight (子) at the top and noon (午) below. The tide runs Lung, Large Intestine, Stomach, Spleen, Heart, Small Intestine, Bladder, Kidney, Pericardium, Triple Burner, Gallbladder, Liver, and back to the Lung, so that the hour at which an organ is fullest, and the hour it is emptiest twelve hours opposite, became a guide for both diagnosis and the timing of treatment. This daily round of the channels is what later practice came to call the meridian clock (子午流注).

3–5 a.m. : Lung
5–7 a.m. : Large Intestine
7–9 a.m. : Stomach
9–11 a.m. : Spleen
11 a.m.–1 p.m. : Heart
1–3 p.m. : Small Intestine
3–5 p.m. : Bladder
5–7 p.m. : Kidney
7–9 p.m. : Pericardium
9–11 p.m. : Triple Burner
11 p.m.–1 a.m. : Gall Bladder
1–3 a.m. : Liver

THE CHANNELS AND COLLATERALS

Essential Verses

These are among the gate's most quoted lines in the classic, gathered here for study.

SU WEN 56

皮者脈之部也。邪客於皮則腠理開，開則邪入客於絡脈，絡脈滿則注於經脈，經脈滿則入舍於府藏也。故皮者有分部，不與而生大病也。

pí zhě mài zhī bù yě. xié kè yú pí zé còu lǐ kāi, kāi zé xié rù kè yú luò mài, luò mài mǎn zé zhù yú jīng mài, jīng mài mǎn zé rù shě yú fǔ zàng yě. gù pí zhě yǒu fēn bù, bù yǔ ér shēng dà bìng yě.

The skin is the territory of the channels. When an evil settles in the skin the interstices open; opening, the evil enters and lodges in the network vessels; when the network vessels are full it pours into the channel vessels; when the channels are full it enters and lodges in the bowels and organs. Thus the skin is divided into territories, and to neglect them is to let great disease arise.

An evil works inward in stages, and the skin is the first and cheapest place to halt it. Settling there, it opens the interstices and slips into the network vessels; left alone, it pours from the networks into the channels, and from the channels into the bowels and organs, growing graver at every step. Since the skin is parcelled into zones that each report to a channel, the physician can read the zone where trouble shows to name the channel behind it, and act at that outer level, on the interstices and the small vessels, before the evil sinks any further. The line makes the body's outer covering at once the earliest reading-surface and the first line of defence, and turns neglect of the surface into the very means by which a small complaint becomes a great one.

> SU WEN 57
>
> 經有十二，絡有十五，凡二十七氣以上下。所行之處，經之大者，少也。脈之見者，皆絡脈也。諸絡脈皆不能經大節之間，必行絕道而出，入復合於皮中。
>
> *jīng yǒu shí èr, luò yǒu shí wǔ, fán èr shí qī qì yǐ shàng xià. suǒ xíng zhī chù, jīng zhī dà zhě, shǎo yě. mài zhī jiàn zhě, jiē luò mài yě. zhū luò mài jiē bù néng jīng dà jié zhī jiān, bì xíng jué dào ér chū, rù fù hé yú pí zhōng.*
>
> There are twelve channels and fifteen networks, twenty-seven streams of qi in all moving up and down. Of the courses they run, the great trunks of the channels are few; the vessels one can see are all network vessels. None of the network vessels can pass through the spaces of the great joints; they must run by side-roads, emerge, and re-enter to join again within the skin.

What the eye finds at the surface is never the deep channel but the branching network, for the great trunks run hidden and few while every visible vessel is a collateral. The distinction is practical rather than scholarly: the spider veins and surface vessels a needle can reach carry network qi, not the deep current, and the networks themselves detour around the large joints by side-paths, surfacing and re-entering through the skin. Knowing this, the needle-worker treats the accessible superficial courses for what they are, while keeping a clear picture of the great channels running beneath them, out of reach. The verse is a map of which vessels lie within the hand's grasp and which do not.

LING SHU 14

先度其骨節之大小廣狹長短，而脈度定矣。頭之大骨圍二尺六寸，發所覆者顱至項尺二寸，髮以下至頤長一尺，君子終折。

xiān dù qí gǔ jié zhī dà xiǎo guǎng xiá cháng duǎn, ér mài dù dìng yǐ. tóu zhī dà gǔ wéi èr chǐ liù cùn, fā suǒ fù zhě lú zhì xiàng chǐ èr cùn, fà yǐ xià zhì yí cháng yī chǐ, jūn zǐ zhōng zhé.

First measure the size of the bones and joints, their breadth and narrowness, their length, and the measure of the vessels is thereby fixed. The great bone of the head has a circumference of two feet six inches; from the hairline-covered skull to the nape is one foot two inches; from below the hairline to the chin is one foot; and for a well-proportioned person these are taken as the standard divisions.

Before a single point can be found, the bones must be measured, since the lengths of the channels and the seats of the points are not fixed inches but proportional divisions of each person's own frame. The standard segments run between bony landmarks, the skull to the nape, the hairline to the chin, and these are scaled to the body in front of the physician, so that one canon of locations can fit a tall person and a small one alike. This is the quiet metrology beneath all channel and acupuncture work: take the proportional units from the patient's own skeleton, and only then place the points. Without it, a table of locations would fit no one exactly, and the needle would miss by the difference between two bodies.

LING SHU 15

人經脈上下左右前後二十八脈，周身十六丈二尺，以應二十八宿。漏水下百刻，以分晝夜。氣行交通於中，一周於身，下水二刻。

rén jīng mài shàng xià zuǒ yòu qián hòu èr shí bā mài, zhōu shēn shí liù zhàng èr chǐ, yǐ yīng èr shí bā xiù. lòu shuǐ xià bǎi kè, yǐ fēn zhòu yè. qì xíng jiāo tōng yú zhōng, yī zhōu yú shēn, xià shuǐ èr kè.

A person's channel vessels, above and below, left and right, front and back, number twenty-eight, sixteen zhang two chi around the body, answering to the twenty-eight

> lunar lodges. The water-clock drips down one hundred marks to divide day and night; the qi runs and communicates within, and one full circuit of the body corresponds to two marks of the dripping water.

Here the body's inner traffic is set against the clock: twenty-eight vessels of a fixed total length, around which the qi completes fifty circuits in a day and night, timed by the dripping of the water-clock. The reckoning matters because it places the circulation in step with the hours and the heavens, so that where the qi has reached at any moment can be worked out. Knowing that one full circuit takes two of the hundred daily marks lets the physician relate the qi's position to the time of day, which is the seed of needling and treating in accord with the hour when the qi is present at a given place. The circulation, in this telling, is not a vague flow but a measurable, clock-able motion.

> LING SHU 33
>
> 腦為髓之海，其輸上在於其蓋，下在風府。衝脈者，為十二經之海，其輸上在於大杼，下出於巨虛之上下廉。膻中者，為氣之海。胃者，水穀之海。
>
> *nǎo wèi suǐ zhī hǎi, qí shū shàng zài yú qí gài, xià zài fēng fǔ. chōng mài zhě, wèi shí èr jīng zhī hǎi, qí shū shàng zài yú dà zhù, xià chū yú jù xū zhī shàng xià lián. dàn zhōng zhě, wèi qì zhī hǎi. wèi zhě, shuǐ gǔ zhī hǎi.*
>
> The brain is the sea of marrow; its transport points lie above at the crown and below at Wind-Mansion. The thoroughfare vessel is the sea of the twelve channels; its transport points lie above at the Great-Shuttle and below issue at the upper and lower edges of the great-void points. The chest-centre is the sea of qi; the stomach is the sea of water and grain.

The body's largest pools are gathered here into four seas, the marrow, the channel-blood, the qi, and the nourishment, each a reservoir with a fixed upper and lower point of access. The power of the scheme is that a whole class of fullness or emptiness can be met at its reservoir rather than chased vessel by vessel: name the disordered sea from its signs, then needle its upper and lower transport-points to drain a flooded sea or replenish a depleted one. A marrow-sea run dry, for instance, is reached at the crown and at Wind-Mansion. The four seas give treatment a set of master controls over the deepest stores of substance and qi in the body.

LING SHU 52

五藏者，所以藏精神血氣魂魄者也。六府者，所以化水穀而行津液者也。胸氣有街，腹氣有街，頭氣有街，脛氣有街。故氣在頭者，止之於腦。

wǔ zàng zhě, suǒ yǐ cáng jīng shén xuè qì hún pò zhě yě. liù fǔ zhě, suǒ yǐ huà shuǐ gǔ ér xíng jīn yè zhě yě. xiōng qì yǒu jiē, fù qì yǒu jiē, tóu qì yǒu jiē, jìng qì yǒu jiē. gù qì zài tóu zhě, zhǐ zhī yú nǎo.

The five organs are what store the essence and spirit, the blood and qi, the ethereal and bodily souls. The six bowels are what transform water and grain and move the fluids. There is a thoroughfare for the qi of the chest, a thoroughfare for the belly, a thoroughfare for the head, a thoroughfare for the lower leg. Thus qi that is in the head is halted at the brain.

Alongside the named channels run four broad avenues, the qi thoroughfares of the head, chest, belly, and lower leg, where qi travels apart from the channel lines. They matter because they open a direct corridor to a whole region's qi, the shortcut a vessel-by-vessel model lacks: locate the disordered region, enter its thoroughfare at the proper station, head-qi halted at the brain, chest-qi at the back-transports and breastbone, and so move or settle the qi of an entire zone at once. The verse rounds out the precise channels with regional highways the physician can take when a whole area, and not a single line, has gone wrong.

LING SHU 62

足之陽明，何因而動？胃氣上注於肺，其悍氣上衝頭者，循咽，上走空竅，循眼系，入絡腦，出顑，下客主人，循牙車，合陽明，並下人迎，此胃氣別走於陽明者也。

zú zhī yáng míng, hé yīn ér dòng? wèi qì shàng zhù yú fèi, qí hàn qì shàng chōng tóu zhě, xún yàn, shàng zǒu kōng qiào, xún yǎn xì, rù luò nǎo, chū kǎn, xià kè zhǔ rén, xún yá chē, hé yáng míng, bìng xià rén yíng, cǐ wèi qì bié zǒu yú yáng míng zhě yě.

Why does the foot yang-brightness pulse? The stomach-qi pours upward into the lung, and its fierce portion, rushing up to the head, follows the throat, ascends to the orifices, follows the eye-tie, enters to net the brain, emerges at the temple, descends to Guest-

> Host, follows the jaw, joins the yang-brightness, and runs down beside Man's-Welcome, this being the stomach-qi branching off into the yang-brightness.

Certain points visibly throb, and the chapter explains why by tracing the route of that beat at the yang-brightness, following the stomach's vigorous qi up the throat to the brain and back down the face and neck to Man's-Welcome. The anatomy earns its keep at the bedside: it ties the pulse of these points to the strength of the stomach-qi feeding them, so the practitioner can read a throbbing point as a window onto that source-qi and follow the named path to make sense of sensation referred across the face. A curious observation, that some points beat visibly, becomes a traceable map of the stomach-qi's surge through the head, and the force of the beat becomes a gauge of the source's vigour.

> LING SHU 76
>
> 歲有十二月，日有十二辰，子午為經，卯酉為緯。衛氣之行，一日一夜五十周於身，晝日行於陽二十五周，夜行於陰二十五周，周於五藏。
>
> *suì yǒu shí èr yuè, rì yǒu shí èr chén, zi wǔ wèi jīng, mǎo yǒu wèi wěi. wèi qì zhī xíng, yī rì yī yè wǔ shí zhōu yú shēn, zhòu rì xíng yú yáng èr shí wǔ zhōu, yè xíng yú yīn èr shí wǔ zhōu, zhōu yú wǔ zàng.*
>
> The year has twelve months, the day twelve double-hours; the meridian runs from north to south, the parallel from east to west. The course of the defensive qi makes fifty circuits of the body in a day and night, twenty-five through the yang by day and twenty-five through the yin by night, circling the five organs.

The guard-qi keeps a timetable, and the chapter reads it off the clock: by day it patrols the outer yang, by night it withdraws into the yin and the organs, fifty rounds in all. Because the guard is concentrated in different territory at different hours, its strength at any one place rises and falls with the time of day, and treatment is timed to where it then is. Surface and yang complaints are best met while it patrols the exterior by day; disturbances of sleep arise when its nightly passage into the yin is blocked and the guard is left stranded in the yang. The line gives the body's defence a schedule the physician can set against the hour.

FROM THE AUTHOR

Whether the channels are real is a question that tends to dissolve in practice rather than in argument. Where a point is engaged well, a heaviness or a spreading warmth moves along the very line the old charts drew, often reaching somewhere the needle never touched; the classic calls this the arrival of the qi. The map asks for no belief in advance. Followed with care, it asserts itself, river by river.

經脈者，所以能決死生。

The channels are that by which life and death are decided.

WHERE THIS GATE LEADS

Each channel is tied to one of the officials of *Gate Three, The Court Within*, and divides into the yin and yang of *Gate Two*. The state of the channels is read at the wrist in *Gate Four, Reading the Unspoken*. And the points where these rivers surface, and the art of meeting them with the needle, are the whole concern of *Gate Six, The Point of the Needle*.

PART SIX

The Point of the Needle

Acupuncture and the Needle

鍼刺

On the needle. The Inner Classic's central therapy: a fine needle set at points along the channels to move what is stuck and fill what is spent, working not by adding to the body but by regulating the qi it already holds.

GATE SIX · ACUPUNCTURE AND THE NEEDLE

The Point of the Needle

鍼刺

> *Where there is emptiness, fill it; where there is fullness, drain it.*
>
> Ling Shu 1

If the earlier gates describe the body and teach the reading of it, this gate is where the physician's hand at last moves. For the Inner Classic, and above all for the Spiritual Pivot, the needle is the central therapy, and much of that book is in plain fact a manual of it. The chapters gathered here set out what the needle is, how it works, where it is placed and when, and what must never be done with it.

The first thing to grasp is what the needle does, and does not do. It adds no substance to the body. It carries no drug. It works entirely by regulating the qi already present, drawing the full toward the empty, releasing what is pent, recalling what has scattered. A slender piece of metal set briefly at the right point moves the body's own forces, and that is the whole of it, which is why so much of the art lies not in the needle but in the judgement behind it.

The classic is unusually direct about this. It warns that the rules of needling are easy to recite and hard to master, that the crude practitioner watches the body while the superior one watches the qi, and that the single proof of a needle well placed is the arrival of the qi beneath it. Everything in this gate returns, in the end, to that one feeling at the fingertip.

The Nine Needles

The classic does not speak of one needle but of nine, each a different shape made for a different task.

> LING SHU 1
>
> 九鍼之名，各不同形：一曰鑱鍼，二曰員鍼，三曰鍉鍼，四曰鋒鍼，五曰鈹鍼，六曰員利鍼，七曰毫鍼，八曰長鍼，九曰大鍼。
>
> *jiǔ zhēn zhī míng, gè bù tóng xíng: yī yuē chán zhēn, èr yuē yuán zhēn, sān yuē dī zhēn, sì yuē fēng zhēn, wǔ yuē pī zhēn, liù yuē yuán lì zhēn, qī yuē háo zhēn, bā yuē cháng zhēn, jiǔ yuē dà zhēn.*
>
> The nine needles have nine names and nine forms: the first is the arrowhead needle, the second the round needle, the third the blunt needle, the fourth the sharp-edged needle, the fifth the lance needle, the sixth the round-sharp needle, the seventh the fine needle, the eighth the long needle, and the ninth the great needle.

The nine range from the broad arrow-head, for lancing a heat at the skin, through the round-bodied needle that presses without piercing, to the long needle for a deep-seated trouble and the fine hair-needle, the most used of all, for the ordinary regulation of the channels. To choose the needle is already half the treatment, for a shallow heat and a deep cold do not call for the same instrument; and the classic faults the practitioner who reaches for one needle to meet everything.

Under all nine needles lies a single instruction, the one the whole art keeps returning to: where there is emptiness, fill it; where there is fullness, drain it; where the stale and stagnant has settled, clear it out; where an evil prevails, reduce it. Every needle and every technique that follows is only a way of carrying out one of those four moves. It is worth holding onto, because the crowd of points and names can hide how simple the underlying aim stays: to take from where there is too much and give to where there is too little, until the balance comes back.

FIGURE · THE NINE NEEDLES

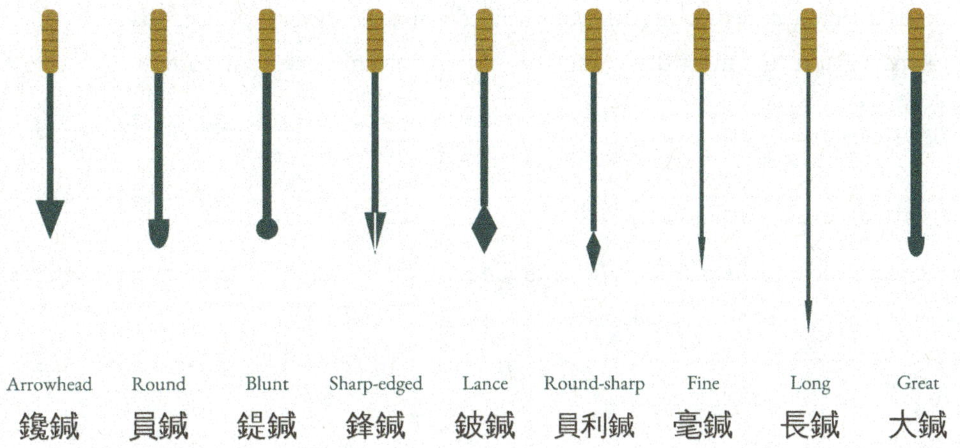

The nine needles of the Numinous Pivot, each shaped to its task. The arrowhead (鑱) for shallow heat in the skin; the round (員) and the blunt (鍉) for stroking and pressing the flesh without piercing; the sharp-edged (鋒) and the lance (鈹) for letting blood and draining abscesses; the round-sharp (員利) for acute pain; the fine (毫), commonest of all, for the ordinary work of regulation; the long (長) for deep-seated disorders; and the great (大) for draining water from a swollen joint.

LING SHU 78

九鍼者，天地之大數也，始於一而終於九。故一以法天，二以法地，三以法人，四以法時，五以法音，六以法律，七以法星，八以法風，九以法野。

jiǔ zhēn zhě, tiān dì zhī dà shù yě, shǐ yú yī ér zhōng yú jiǔ. gù yī yǐ fǎ tiān, èr yǐ fǎ dì, sān yǐ fǎ rén, sì yǐ fǎ shí, wǔ yǐ fǎ yīn, liù yǐ fǎ lǜ, qī yǐ fǎ xīng, bā yǐ fǎ fēng, jiǔ yǐ fǎ yě.

The nine needles answer to the great numbers of Heaven and Earth, beginning at one and ending at nine. So the first takes its pattern from Heaven, the second from Earth, the third from Man, the fourth from the seasons, the fifth from the tones, the sixth from the pitch-pipes, the seventh from the stars, the eighth from the winds, and the ninth from the wild lands. Each needle has its own form and its own work.

The nine were not a random set. The classic matches them to the nine domains of the world, Heaven and Earth and Man, the seasons, the tones, the pitch-pipes, the stars, the winds, and the wild lands, so that the toolkit itself mirrors the cosmos the body belongs to. Behind the scheme is a practical claim: that there is a needle fitted to every kind of disorder, from the most superficial to the most deep, and that the physician's task is to know which one a case asks for.

The Heart of the Method

Beneath the nine instruments lies a single method, which the classic states in a few dense lines that the rest of the tradition spent centuries unfolding.

> LING SHU 1
>
> 小鍼之要，易陳而難入。粗守形，上守神。神乎神，客在門。未睹其疾，惡知其原。刺之微，在速遲。粗守關，上守機。機之動，不離其空。
>
> *xiǎo zhēn zhī yào, yì chén ér nán rù. cū shǒu xíng, shàng shǒu shén. shén hū shén, kè zài mén. wèi dǔ qí jí, è zhī qí yuán. cì zhī wēi, zài sù chí. cū shǒu guān, shàng shǒu jī. jī zhī dòng, bù lí qí kōng.*
>
> The essence of the small needle is easy to state and hard to enter into. The crude practitioner guards the form; the superior guards the spirit. Spirit, and again spirit: the guest waits at the gate. Until you have seen the disease, how should you know its source? The fineness of needling lies in the quick and the slow. The crude guard the joint; the superior guard the trigger; and the trigger's movement never departs from the hollow of the point.

The small needle, it says, is easy to describe and hard to truly wield. The crude practitioner guards the form, keeping to the visible rules; the superior guards the spirit, attending to the living state of the qi. And the decisive moment is the mechanism, the instant the qi moves, which must be met neither too early nor too late. This is less a set of instructions than a warning that the art is one of timing and attention, not of technique alone.

LING SHU 3

所謂易陳者，易言也；難入者，難著於人也。麤守形者，守刺法也；上守神者，守人之血氣有餘不足，可補瀉也。神客者，正邪共會也；在門者，邪循正氣之所出入也。

suǒ wèi yì chén zhě, yì yán yě; nán rù zhě, nán zhù yú rén yě. cū shǒu xíng zhě, shǒu cì fǎ yě; shàng shǒu shén zhě, shǒu rén zhī xuè qì yǒu yú bù zú, kě bǔ xiè yě. shén kè zhě, zhèng xié gòng huì yě; zài mén zhě, xié xún zhèng qì zhī suǒ chū rù yě.

To say it is easy to state is to say it is easily put into words; to say it is hard to enter is to say it is hard to make take hold in a person. To say the crude guard the form means they keep only to the rules of needling; to say the superior guard the spirit means they watch whether a person's blood and qi are in excess or in want, so that they may fill or drain accordingly. The guest and the spirit together are the true qi and the evil meeting in one place; at the gate means the evil follows the very door by which the true qi goes out and comes in.

A companion chapter unfolds the saying line by line. To guard the form is to keep only to the rules of insertion; to guard the spirit is to watch whether the blood and qi stand in excess or in want, and to fill or drain accordingly. The evil and the true qi, it adds, meet at the very gate by which the qi enters and leaves the body, and the needler works precisely there, at the threshold, turning the balance one way or the other.

The saying it unfolds is famous for its bluntness: the essential of the small needle is easy to state and hard to master. Easy to state, because the rule is only to fill what is empty and drain what is full; hard to master, because knowing which is which in a living person, under the finger and not on the page, is the labour of a career. This is the same difference the chapter marks between guarding the form and guarding the spirit, and it, more than any point or technique, is what separates a skilled needler from a merely trained one.

> LING SHU 1
>
> 凡用鍼者，虛則實之，滿則泄之，宛陳則除之，邪勝則虛之。
>
> *fán yòng zhēn zhě, xū zé shí zhī, mǎn zé xiè zhī, wǎn chén zé chú zhī, xié shèng zé xū zhī.*
>
> In all use of the needle: where there is emptiness, fill it; where there is fullness, drain it; where the stale and stagnant has settled, clear it away; where the evil prevails, reduce it.

The aim is stated as plainly as a rule can be. Where there is emptiness, fill it; where there is fullness, drain it; where blood lies stagnant and pooled, remove it; where an evil prevails, deplete it. Every act of needling reduces to one of these four motions. The skill is not in knowing the rule but in reading a body accurately enough to know which of the four a given case requires.

> LING SHU 1
>
> 大要曰：徐而疾則實，疾而徐則虛。
>
> *dà yào yuē: xú ér jí zé shí, jí ér xú zé xū.*
>
> The great essential says: slow to enter and quick to withdraw fills the qi; quick to enter and slow to withdraw drains it.

How the motions are made is a matter of the needle's speed. Slow to enter and quick to withdraw fills; quick to enter and slow to withdraw drains. The same point and the same needle become a tonifying or a draining act according to the manner of the hand. This reversal, that technique and not location alone decides the effect, is among the subtlest things the classic has to teach, and among the easiest to get wrong.

LING SHU 1

刺之而氣不至，無問其數；刺之而氣至，乃去之，勿復鍼。刺之要，氣至而有效，效之信，若風之吹雲，明乎若見蒼天，刺之道畢矣。

cì zhī ér qì bù zhì, wú wèn qí shuò; cì zhī ér qì zhì, nǎi qù zhī, wù fù zhēn. cì zhī yào, qì zhì ér yǒu xiào, xiào zhī xìn, ruò fēng zhī chuī yún, míng hū ruò jiàn cāng tiān, cì zhī dào bì yǐ.

If you needle and the qi does not arrive, do not ask after the number of insertions; if you needle and the qi arrives, then withdraw, and needle no more. The key to needling is that the qi arrives, and then it works; and the proof of the working is sure, like wind blowing the clouds away, clear as the sight of the open sky. With this, the way of needling is whole.

The test of all of it is the arrival of the qi. If you needle and the qi does not come, do not count out a fixed number of manipulations and stop; wait for it, or seek it elsewhere. When the qi arrives the effect follows, and the needle is then withdrawn, for to keep working a point past that moment is to undo the good already done. The classic likens the clearing that comes to wind sweeping cloud from a sky: of a sudden the blue stands plain.

SU WEN 27

帝曰：候氣奈何？岐伯曰：夫邪去絡入於經也，舍於血脈之中，其寒溫未相得，如湧波之起也，時來時去，故不常在。故曰：方其來也，必按而止之，止而取之，無逢其衝而瀉之。真氣者，經氣也，經氣太虛，故曰其來不可逢，此之謂也。故曰：候邪不審，大氣已過，瀉之則真氣脫，脫則不復，邪氣復至，而病益蓄，故曰其往不可追，此之謂也。

dì yuē: hòu qì nài hé? qí bó yuē: fū xié qù luò rù yú jīng yě, shě yú xuè mài zhī zhōng, qí hán wēn wèi xiāng de, rú yǒng bō zhī qǐ yě, shí lái shí qù, gù bù cháng zài. gù yuē: fāng qí lái yě, bì àn ér zhǐ zhī, zhǐ ér qǔ zhī, wú féng qí chōng ér xiè zhī. zhēn qì zhě, jīng qì yě, jīng qì tài xū, gù yuē qí lái bù kě féng, cǐ zhī wèi yě. gù yuē: hòu xié bù shěn, dà qì yǐ guò, xiè zhī zé zhēn qì tuō, tuō zé bù fù, xié qì fù zhì, ér bìng yì xù, gù yuē qí wǎng bù kě zhuī, cǐ zhī wèi yě.

The Emperor asked: How does one watch for the qi? Qibo said: When an evil leaves the collaterals and enters a channel, it lodges within the blood-vessels; its cold and the body's warmth have not yet come to terms, and it rises like a surging wave, now coming, now going, never staying in one place. So it is said: at the moment of its coming, one must press and halt it, halt it and then take it, and not meet it at its onrush to drain it, for the true qi, which is the channel-qi, would then be left utterly empty. This is the meaning of the saying that its coming cannot be met head-on. And it is said: if the watching for the evil is not careful and the great evil-qi has already passed, then to drain there is to make the true qi escape; once it escapes it does not return, the evil comes again, and the disease only gathers the more. This is the meaning of the saying that its going cannot be chased.

Timing reaches to the disease itself. The Basic Questions describes watching for the moment an evil stirs within the vessels, coming and going like a swell on water, never quite fixed in one place. When it comes, the hand presses to halt it and then takes it; needled at the wrong instant, against the grain of its motion, the very same intervention does harm. To needle well, then, is to read three things at once, the state of the qi, the manner of the hand, and the moment, and to bring them together at a single point.

The Five Transport Points

If the method is the soul of needling, the points are its geography; and the classic orders the most important of them before it ever locates them on the body.

LING SHU 2

肺出於少商，少商者，手大指端內側也，為井木；溜於魚際，為滎；注於太淵，為輸；行於經渠，為經；入於尺澤，肘中之動脈也，為合。手太陰經也。

fèi chū yú shào shāng, shào shāng zhě, shǒu dà zhǐ duān nèi cè yě, wèi jǐng mù; liū yú yú jì, wèi xíng; zhù yú tài yuān, wèi shū; xíng yú jīng qú, wèi jīng; rù yú chǐ zé, zhǒu zhōng zhī dòng mài yě, wèi hé. shǒu tài yīn jīng yě.

The lung-channel issues at Shaoshang, on the inner side of the tip of the thumb, and this is the well; it glides at Yuji, the spring; pours at Taiyuan, the stream; passes at Jingqu, the river; and enters at Chize, the pulsating vessel in the crook of the elbow, the sea. Such is the hand greater-yin.

Near the end of every channel, at the hand or the foot, lie its five transport points, and the classic names them by a single rising image. The qi begins as a well at the very tip of a finger or toe, glides on as a spring, pours as a stream, runs as a river, and enters as a sea at the elbow or the knee. The picture is instruction, not decoration: the points farthest out are where the qi runs shallow and quick, those nearer the trunk where it runs deep and full. Each of the five has its own powers, the well for a sudden fullness below the heart and for reviving, the spring for fevers, the stream for a heavy body and aching joints, the river for cough and chills-and-fever, the sea for the rebellious qi and the disorders of its organ. To know a channel's five transports is to carry a small, versatile set of points, all near the limb and easy to reach.

Mapping the Points

Beyond the transport points the classic attempts a full map of the body's surface, and returns more than once to the same striking claim about how many points there are.

> SU WEN 58
>
> 黃帝問曰：余聞氣穴三百六十五，以應一歲，未知其所，願卒聞之。岐伯稽首再拜對曰：窘乎哉問也，其非聖帝，孰能窮其道焉，因請溢意盡言其處。
>
> *huáng dì wèn yuē: yú wén qì xué sān bǎi liù shí wǔ, yǐ yīng yī suì, wèi zhī qí suǒ, yuàn zú wén zhī. qí bó qǐ shǒu zài bài duì yuē: jiǒng hū zāi wèn yě, qí fēi shèng dì, shú néng qióng qí dào yān, yīn qǐng yì yì jǐn yán qí chù.*
>
> The Yellow Emperor asked: I have heard that the qi-points number three hundred and sixty-five, matching the year, but I do not know where they all lie; I wish to hear the whole of it. Qibo bowed his head twice and answered: A hard question. Were you not a sage sovereign, who could fathom its way? Let me then pour out all I know and tell their places in full.

They number three hundred and sixty-five, matched deliberately to the days of the year, so that the skin is imagined as a calendar of places where the qi may be reached. Whether the count is exact matters less than the principle behind it: the channels surface at fixed, nameable spots, and it is these, and not random skin, where the needle does its work.

SU WEN 59

足太陽脈氣所發者七十八穴：兩眉頭各一，入髮至項三寸半，傍五相去三寸，其浮氣在皮中者凡五行，行五，項中大筋兩傍各一，俠脊以下至尻尾二十一節十五間各一，循行於背腰之分，凡七十八穴。

zú tài yáng mài qì suǒ fā zhě qī shí bā xué: liǎng méi tóu gè yī, rù fà zhì xiàng sān cùn bàn, bàng wǔ xiāng qù sān cùn, qí fú qì zài pí zhōng zhě fán wǔ xíng, xíng wǔ, xiàng zhōng dà jīn liǎng bàng gè yī, xiá jí yǐ xià zhì kāo wěi èr shí yī jié shí wǔ jiān gè yī, xún xíng yú bèi yāo zhī fēn, fán qī shí bā xué.

The points where the qi of the foot great-yang vessel issues are seventy-eight: one at the head of each eyebrow; from the hairline to the nape, three and a half inches, with five to a side, three inches apart, the floating qi in the skin running in five rows of five; one on each side of the great sinew of the nape; one at each of the fifteen spaces of the twenty-one vertebrae from the flanks of the spine down to the tailbone; and so along the divisions of the back and loins, seventy-eight points in all.

A companion chapter does the bookkeeping, counting the points channel by channel, the foot greater-yang alone bearing seventy-eight where its qi emerges, and so on through the rest. Every point is thereby assigned to the channel whose qi issues there, which is what lets a sign at a point be read back to a channel, and a channel be treated at a chosen point along it.

SU WEN 60

帝曰：余聞骨空之名，願聞其處。岐伯曰：臂骨空在臂陽，去踝四寸兩骨空之間。股骨上空在股陽，出上膝四寸。骭骨空在輔骨之上端。股際骨空在毛中動下。尻骨空在髀骨之後相去四寸。髓空在腦後三分，在顱際銳骨之下。

dì yuē: yú wén gǔ kōng zhī míng, yuàn wén qí chù. qí bó yuē: bì gǔ kōng zài bì yáng, qù huái sì cùn liǎng gǔ kōng zhī jiān. gǔ gǔ shàng kōng zài gǔ yáng, chū shàng xī sì cùn. héng gǔ kōng zài fǔ gǔ zhī shàng duān. gǔ jì gǔ kōng zài máo zhōng dòng xià. kāo gǔ kōng zài bì gǔ zhī hòu xiāng qù sì cùn. suǐ kōng zài nǎo hòu sān fēn, zài lú jì ruì gǔ zhī xià.

The Emperor said: I have heard the names of the bone-holes; I wish to hear their places. Qibo said: The bone-hole of the arm lies on the yang side of the arm, four inches from the wrist, between two bone-holes. The upper bone-hole of the thigh lies on the yang side of the thigh, coming out four inches above the knee. The bone-hole of the shin lies at the upper end of the splint-bone. The bone-hole of the groin lies below the throbbing vessel in the pubic hair. The bone-holes of the sacrum lie behind the hip-bone, four inches apart. And the marrow-hole lies three parts behind the brain, below the pointed bone at the edge of the skull.

Many points sit in hollows of bone, and the classic catalogues these bone-holes by careful measurement from joint and landmark. The reason is practical: a point lodged in a hollow can be found by the feel of the bone even where the surface gives no sign, so the hand reads the bone for the hollow, and the hollow yields the point.

SU WEN 61

帝曰：諸水皆生於腎乎？岐伯曰：腎者，牝藏也，地氣上者屬於腎，而生水液也，故曰至陰。勇而勞甚則腎汗出，腎汗出逢於風，傳為胕腫，本之於腎，名曰風水。帝曰：水俞五十七處者，是何主也？岐伯曰：腎俞五十七穴，積陰之所聚也，水所從出入也。

dì yuē: zhū shuǐ jiē shēng yú shèn hū? qí bó yuē: shèn zhě, pìn cáng yě, dì qì shàng zhě shǔ yú shèn, ér shēng shuǐ yè yě, gù yuē zhì yīn. yǒng ér láo shèn zé shèn hàn chū, shèn hàn chū féng yú fēng, chuán wèi fǔ zhǒng, běn zhī yú shèn, míng yuē fēng shuǐ. dì yuē: shuǐ yú wǔ shí qī chù zhě, shì hé zhǔ yě? qí bó yuē: shèn yú wǔ shí qī xué, jī yīn zhī suǒ jù yě, shuǐ suǒ cóng chū rù yě.

The Emperor asked: Do all the waters arise from the kidney? Qibo said: The kidney is the female organ; the qi of the earth that rises belongs to the kidney and gives birth to the water-fluids, and so it is called the utmost yin. When one is bold and toils too hard, the kidney sweats, and the kidney-sweat meeting the wind passes on into a puffy swelling that has its root in the kidney, named wind-water. The Emperor asked: The fifty-seven water-points, what do they govern? Qibo said: The fifty-seven kidney-points are where the gathered yin collects, where the water comes out and goes in.

Certain points, finally, are gathered into working sets for whole classes of disease: fifty-seven points for the watery swellings the classic traces to the kidney, fifty-nine for the febrile heats. Here the map turns most practical of all, offering a named group of points to drain water or to clear heat, so that even a stubborn disease has a standing answer ready in the needle. Ordered as transports, counted against the year, lodged in the bone, and gathered into sets, the points are the ground on which the whole art stands.

Needling with the Seasons

The needle does not meet the body the same way all year. Because the qi shifts with the seasons, so must the depth and the site of the needle.

SU WEN 64

是故春氣在經脈，夏氣在孫絡，長夏氣在肌肉，秋氣在皮膚，冬氣在骨髓中。帝曰：余願聞其故。岐伯曰：春者，天氣始開，地氣始泄，凍解冰釋，水行經通，故人氣在脈。夏者，經滿氣溢，入孫絡受血，皮膚充實。長夏者，經絡皆盛，內溢肌中。秋者，天氣始收，腠理閉塞，皮膚引急。冬者蓋藏，血氣在中，內著骨髓，通於五藏。

shì gù chūn qì zài jīng mài, xià qì zài sūn luò, cháng xià qì zài jī ròu, qiū qì zài pí fū, dōng qì zài gǔ suǐ zhōng. dì yuē: yú yuàn wén qí gù. qí bó yuē: chūn zhě, tiān qì shǐ kāi, dì qì shǐ xiè, dòng jiě bīng shì, shuǐ xíng jīng tōng, gù rén qì zài mài. xià zhě, jīng mǎn qì yì, rù sūn luò shòu xuè, pí fū chōng shí. cháng xià zhě, jīng luò jiē shèng, nèi yì jī zhōng. qiū zhě, tiān qì shǐ shōu, còu lǐ bì sāi, pí fū yǐn jí. dōng zhě gài cáng, xuè qì zài zhōng, nèi zhù gǔ suǐ, tōng yú wǔ zàng.

And so in spring the qi is in the channel-vessels, in summer in the fine collaterals, in late summer in the flesh, in autumn in the skin, in winter deep in the bones and marrow. The Emperor said: I wish to hear the reason. Qibo said: In spring the qi of Heaven first opens and the qi of Earth first issues, the frost thaws and the ice melts, the waters run and the channels open, so the human qi is in the vessels. In summer the channels fill and the qi overflows, entering the fine collaterals to receive blood, and the skin is full and solid. In late summer the channels and collaterals are all abundant and overflow inward into the flesh. In autumn the qi of Heaven begins to gather, the pores shut, and the skin draws tight. In winter all is stored away, the blood and qi within, clinging deep to the bones and marrow and reaching to the five organs.

The classic places the qi at a different layer in each season: in spring in the channel-vessels, in summer in the fine collaterals, in late summer in the flesh, in autumn in the skin, in winter deep in the bone and marrow. The needle follows it there, set shallow in the warm months when the qi has risen toward the surface, and deeper in the cold ones when it has withdrawn inward. To needle in winter as one would in spring is to reach past the qi and trouble the depths.

> LING SHU 19
>
> 黃帝問於岐伯曰：夫四時之氣，各不同形，灸刺之道，何者為定？岐伯答曰：四時之氣，各有所在，灸刺之道，得氣穴為定。故春取經、血脈、分肉之間，夏取盛經孫絡，秋取經俞，冬取井滎。
>
> *huáng dì wèn yú qí bó yuē: fū sì shí zhī qì, gè bù tóng xíng, jiǔ cì zhī dào, hé zhě wèi dìng? qí bó dá yuē: sì shí zhī qì, gè yǒu suǒ zài, jiǔ cì zhī dào, dé qì xué wèi dìng. gù chūn qǔ jīng, xuè mài, fēn ròu zhī jiān, xià qǔ shèng jīng sūn luò, qiū qǔ jīng yú, dōng qǔ jǐng xíng.*
>
> The Yellow Emperor asked Qibo: The qi of the four seasons takes a different form in each, and the way of moxa and needle, by what is it fixed? Qibo said: The qi of the four seasons sits in a different place in each, and the way of moxa and needle is fixed by reaching the qi at its point. So in spring take the channels, the blood-vessels, and the spaces between the flesh; in summer the full channels and the fine network-vessels; in autumn the channel-transport points; and in winter the well and spring points.

A Spiritual Pivot chapter turns this into a plain rule for which points to choose: in spring the channels and the spaces of the flesh, in summer the full channels and the network-vessels, in autumn the transport points, in winter the well and spring points at the very ends of the limbs. The season chooses the class of point, so that the same complaint is met at different points in summer and in winter.

SU WEN 16

黃帝問曰：診要何如？岐伯對曰：正月二月，天氣始方，地氣始發，人氣在肝。三月四月，天氣正方，地氣定發，人氣在脾。五月六月，天氣盛，地氣高，人氣在頭。七月八月，陰氣始殺，人氣在肺。九月十月，陰氣始冰，地氣始閉，人氣在心。十一月十二月，冰復，地氣合，人氣在腎。

huáng dì wèn yuē: zhěn yào hé rú? qí bó duì yuē: zhēng yuè èr yuè, tiān qì shǐ fāng, dì qì shǐ fā, rén qì zài gān. sān yuè sì yuè, tiān qì zhèng fāng, dì qì dìng fā, rén qì zài pí. wǔ yuè liù yuè, tiān qì shèng, dì qì gāo, rén qì zài tóu. qī yuè bā yuè, yīn qì shǐ shā, rén qì zài fèi. jiǔ yuè shí yuè, yīn qì shǐ bīng, dì qì shǐ bì, rén qì zài xīn. shí yī yuè shí èr yuè, bīng fù, dì qì hé, rén qì zài shèn.

The Yellow Emperor asked: What are the essentials of diagnosis? Qibo answered: In the first and second months, the qi of Heaven begins to spread and the qi of Earth begins to issue, and the human qi is in the liver. In the third and fourth months, the qi of Heaven is fully spread and the qi of Earth steadily issues, and the human qi is in the spleen. In the fifth and sixth months, the qi of Heaven is at its height and the qi of Earth is high, and the human qi is in the head. In the seventh and eighth months, the yin qi begins to slay, and the human qi is in the lung. In the ninth and tenth months, the yin qi begins to freeze and the qi of Earth begins to close, and the human qi is in the heart. In the eleventh and twelfth months, the ice forms again and the qi of Earth joins shut, and the human qi is in the kidney.

The classic tracks the body's qi month by month as well, through liver and spleen and head and lung in their turn, so that the needler knows not only the layer to reach but the organ most exposed at a given time of year. To strike at an organ when the season has already drawn the qi toward it is to do harm; the calendar is a part of the method, not a frame around it.

The Cautions of the Needle

The classic is as careful to say what must not be done with the needle as what may, and gives several chapters over wholly to its cautions.

SU WEN 50

黃帝問曰：願聞刺要。岐伯對曰：病有浮沉，刺有淺深，各至其理，無過其道。過之則內傷，不及則生外壅，壅則邪從之。淺深不得，反為大賊，內動五藏，後生大病。

huáng dì wèn yuē: yuàn wén cì yào. qí bó duì yuē: bìng yǒu fú chén, cì yǒu qiǎn shēn, gè zhì qí lǐ, wú guò qí dào. guò zhī zé nèi shāng, bù jí zé shēng wài yōng, yōng zé xié cóng zhī. qiǎn shēn bù dé, fǎn wèi dà zéi, nèi dòng wǔ zàng, hòu shēng dà bìng.

The Yellow Emperor asked: I wish to hear the essentials of needling. Qibo answered: Diseases lie shallow or deep, and the needle goes shallow or deep; each must reach its proper layer and not pass beyond its way. Pass beyond, and there is injury within; fall short, and a blockage forms without, and where there is blockage the evil follows in. To miss the right depth, shallow or deep, is to do great harm, stirring the five organs within and breeding a great disease after.

The first caution is depth. A disease lies shallow or deep, and the needle must reach its level and go no further: too deep, it wounds within; too shallow, it leaves a blockage behind for the evil to follow. Wrong depth, the classic says without softening it, is a great thief that stirs the organs and breeds a worse disease. The rule is to read the level of the trouble first, and then set the depth to it exactly.

SU WEN 51

黃帝問曰：願聞刺淺深之分。岐伯對曰：刺骨者無傷筋，刺筋者無傷肉，刺肉者無傷脈，刺脈者無傷皮；刺皮者無傷肉，刺肉者無傷筋，刺筋者無傷骨。

huáng dì wèn yuē: yuàn wén cì qiǎn shēn zhī fēn. qí bó duì yuē: cì gǔ zhě wú shāng jīn, cì jīn zhě wú shāng ròu, cì ròu zhě wú shāng mài, cì mài zhě wú shāng pí; cì pí zhě wú shāng ròu, cì ròu zhě wú shāng jīn, cì jīn zhě wú shāng gǔ.

The Yellow Emperor asked: I wish to hear the dividing of shallow from deep in needling. Qibo answered: In needling the bone, do not injure the sinew; in needling the sinew, do not injure the flesh; in needling the flesh, do not injure the vessel; in needling the vessel, do not injure the skin. And the other way: in needling the skin, do not injure the flesh; in needling the flesh, do not injure the sinew; in needling the sinew, do not injure the bone.

A companion chapter makes the rule precise, layer by layer: needling to the bone, do not wound the sinew; to the sinew, do not wound the flesh; to the flesh, do not wound the vessel, and so on outward through the tissues. Each layer is a target to be reached cleanly and not passed through, and the hand must learn to know by feel the moment it has arrived.

SU WEN 53

黃帝問曰：願聞虛實之要。岐伯對曰：氣實形實，氣虛形虛，此其常也，反此者病。穀盛氣盛，穀虛氣虛，此其常也，反此者病。脈實血實，脈虛血虛，此其常也，反此者病。

huáng dì wèn yuē: yuàn wén xū shí zhī yào. qí bó duì yuē: qì shí xíng shí, qì xū xíng xū, cǐ qí cháng yě, fǎn cǐ zhě bìng. gǔ shèng qì shèng, gǔ xū qì xū, cǐ qí cháng yě, fǎn cǐ zhě bìng. mài shí xuè shí, mài xū xuè xū, cǐ qí cháng yě, fǎn cǐ zhě bìng.

The Yellow Emperor asked: I wish to hear the essential of emptiness and repletion. Qibo answered: When the qi is replete the body is replete, and when the qi is empty the body is empty: this is the norm, and the reverse is disease. When the grain is abundant the qi is abundant, and when the grain is scant the qi is scant: this is the norm, and the

> reverse is disease. When the pulse is replete the blood is replete, and when the pulse is empty the blood is empty: this is the norm, and the reverse is disease.

The needle must also match the body's fullness or emptiness. In health a full qi goes with a full form and an empty with an empty; where the two disagree, there is disease. The needler fills what is empty and drains what is full, and even the handling of the puncture differs, the hole held open to let an excess out, pressed closed to keep a deficiency in. The same point becomes a tonifying or a draining act by this reading of repletion and depletion.

> SU WEN 52
>
> 黃帝問曰：願聞禁數。岐伯對曰：藏有要害，不可不察。肝生於左，肺藏於右，心部於表，腎治於裏，脾為之使，胃為之市。鬲肓之上，中有父母，七節之傍，中有小心，從之有福，逆之有咎。
>
> *huáng dì wèn yuē: yuàn wén jìn shù. qí bó duì yuē: zàng yǒu yào hài, bù kě bù chá. gān shēng yú zuǒ, fèi cáng yú yòu, xīn bù yú biǎo, shèn zhì yú lǐ, pí wèi zhī shǐ, wèi wèi zhī shì. gé huāng zhī shàng, zhōng yǒu fù mǔ, qī jié zhī bàng, zhōng yǒu xiǎo xīn, cóng zhī yǒu fú, nì zhī yǒu jiù.*
>
> The Yellow Emperor asked: I wish to hear the count of prohibitions. Qibo answered: The organs have their vital and vulnerable places, which must be examined. The liver is born on the left, the lung is stored on the right, the heart governs the surface, the kidney rules the interior, the spleen serves as their envoy, and the stomach as their market. Above the diaphragm and the membrane there is the father and mother; beside the seventh vertebra there is the lesser heart. To follow these brings blessing; to go against them brings harm.

And some places must not be deeply pierced at all. The organs have their vital spots, and to drive a needle into the heart, the liver, or a great vessel is to kill, the classic naming even the day on which death would follow each wound. This is the hard limit of the whole art, a map of where the needle may not go, to be learned before any technique is practised.

SU WEN 55

刺家不診，聽病者言，在頭，頭疾痛，為藏鍼之，刺至骨病已，上無傷骨肉及皮，皮者道也。陰刺，入一傍四處，治寒熱。深專者，刺大藏，迫藏刺背，背俞也，刺之迫藏，藏會，腹中寒熱去而止。與刺之要，發鍼而淺出血。

cì jiā bù zhěn, tīng bìng zhě yán, zài tóu, tóu jí tòng, wèi cáng zhēn zhī, cì zhì gǔ bìng yǐ, shàng wú shāng gǔ ròu jí pí, pí zhě dào yě. yīn cì, rù yī bàng sì chù, zhì hán rè. shēn zhuān zhě, cì dà zàng, pò cáng cì bèi, bèi yú yě, cì zhī pò cáng, cáng huì, fù zhōng hán rè qù ér zhǐ. yǔ cì zhī yào, fā zhēn ér qiǎn chū xiě.

The skilled needler does not always diagnose, but listens to what the sick one says. When it is in the head, with a sharp headache, he needles deep, reaching the bone, and the disease ends; above, he injures neither bone, flesh, nor skin, the skin being only the road. The yin-needling, one needle in the centre and four around, treats cold and heat. For one that is deep and fixed, he needles the great organs, reaching toward an organ by needling the back at the back-transport points; needling there toward the organ, where the organ gathers, he stops when the cold and heat in the belly are gone. The essential in needling is to draw the needle and let a little blood out shallowly.

Yet within these limits the classic is practical and even bold. The skilled needler, it says, does not always work up a full diagnosis but listens to what the sufferer reports, and for a fixed pain in the head will needle deep to the bone and stop the moment the pain lifts. The cautions are a frame and not a paralysis; inside them, the hand acts directly on what the body says. Depth matched, the layers respected, fullness and emptiness read, and the forbidden places spared, the needle is left free to do its work.

Regulating the Channels

The rule to drain a surplus and to supplement a lack is simple to state; the classic gives a long chapter to making it precise.

SU WEN 62

黃帝問曰：余聞刺法言，有餘瀉之，不足補之，何謂有餘？何謂不足？岐伯對曰：有餘有五，不足亦有五，帝欲何問？帝曰：願盡聞之。岐伯曰：神有餘有不足，氣有餘有不足，血有餘有不足，形有餘有不足，志有餘有不足，凡此十者，其氣不等也。

huáng dì wèn yuē: yú wén cì fǎ yán, yǒu yú xiè zhī, bù zú bǔ zhī, hé wèi yǒu yú? hé wèi bù zú? qí bó duì yuē: yǒu yú yǒu wǔ, bù zú yì yǒu wǔ, dì yù hé wèn? dì yuē: yuàn jǐn wén zhī. qí bó yuē: shén yǒu yú yǒu bù zú, qì yǒu yú yǒu bù zú, xuè yǒu yú yǒu bù zú, xíng yǒu yú yǒu bù zú, zhì yǒu yú yǒu bù zú, fán cǐ shí zhě, qí qì bù děng yě.

The Yellow Emperor asked: I have heard the needling rule say, drain what has surplus and supplement what falls short; but what is called surplus, and what is called shortfall? Qibo answered: There are five surpluses and five shortfalls; which does the Emperor wish to ask of? The Emperor said: I wish to hear them all. Qibo said: The spirit may have surplus or shortfall, the qi surplus or shortfall, the blood surplus or shortfall, the form surplus or shortfall, the will surplus or shortfall; these ten, their qi are not alike.

There is not one surplus but five, and not one lack but five, in the spirit, the qi, the blood, the form, and the will; and each of the ten is met in its own way. A surplus of spirit is drained otherwise than a surplus of blood or of qi. So the needler must first name which of the five stands in excess or in want, and only then choose the stroke, since the wrong stroke on the wrong substance does as much harm as no treatment at all.

SU WEN 54

黃帝問曰：願聞九鍼之解，虛實之道。岐伯對曰：刺虛則實之者，鍼下熱也，氣實乃熱也。滿而泄之者，鍼下寒也，氣虛乃寒也。菀陳則除之者，出惡血也。邪勝則虛之者，出鍼勿按。

huáng dì wèn yuē: yuàn wén jiǔ zhēn zhī jiě, xū shí zhī dào. qí bó duì yuē: cì xū zé shí zhī zhě, zhēn xià rè yě, qì shí nǎi rè yě. mǎn ér xiè zhī zhě, zhēn xià hán yě, qì xū nǎi hán yě. wǎn chén zé chú zhī zhě, chū è xuè yě. xié shèng zé xū zhī zhě, chū zhēn wù àn.

The Yellow Emperor asked: I wish to hear the explanation of the nine needles and the way of emptiness and repletion. Qibo answered: To fill an emptiness in needling means that the qi grows warm beneath the needle, for the qi being replete it grows warm. To drain a fullness means that it grows cold beneath the needle, for the qi being emptied it grows cold. To clear away the stagnant and stale means to let out the bad blood. To empty where an evil prevails means to draw the needle and not press the hole shut.

But how is the needler to know the stroke has taken? The classic explains its own terms by sensation. To fill the empty is to bring a warmth beneath the needle, for the qi gathering there is felt as heat; to drain the full is to bring a coolness, the qi thinning felt as cold; to clear a stagnation is to let the dark blood out; to deplete an evil is to withdraw the needle and leave the hole unpressed. The proof of the technique is a felt change at the fingertip, warmth or coolness, not a counting of turns.

LING SHU 9

凡刺之道，畢於終始，明知終始，五藏為紀，陰陽定矣。持其脈口人迎，以知陰陽有餘不足，平與不平，天道畢矣。

fán cì zhī dào, bì yú zhōng shǐ, míng zhī zhōng shǐ, wǔ zàng wèi jì, yīn yáng dìng yǐ. chí qí mài kǒu rén yíng, yǐ zhī yīn yáng yǒu yú bù zú, píng yǔ bù píng, tiān dào bì yǐ.

The whole way of needling is completed in the beginning and the end; know the beginning and the end clearly, take the five organs as the thread, and yin and yang are

> settled. Hold the wrist-pulse and the man-ying pulse at the throat together, and you may know whether yin and yang stand in excess or in want, balanced or unbalanced; and in this the way of heaven is complete.

And the judgement of excess and lack rests on the pulses. The classic has the needler hold the wrist-pulse and the man-ying pulse at the throat together, comparing the two to read whether yin or yang is in surplus, and by how much; the whole art, it says, is completed in this reading of the beginning and the end. The two pulses, set against each other, tell which channel to fill and which to drain before ever the needle is placed.

The Special Punctures

Some disorders do not sit in the channels at all, and the classic keeps special punctures for them.

SU WEN 63

今邪客於皮毛，入舍於孫絡，留而不去，閉塞不通，不得入於經，流溢於大絡，而生奇病也。夫邪客大絡者，左注右，右注左，上下左右，與經相干，而布於四末，其氣無常處，不入於經俞，命曰繆刺。帝曰：願聞繆刺，以左取右，以右取左，奈何？岐伯曰：邪客於經，左盛則右病，右盛則左病，亦有移易者，左痛未已而右脈先病，如此者，必巨刺之，必中其經，非絡脈也。故絡病者，其痛與經脈繆處，故命曰繆刺。

jīn xié kè yú pí máo, rù shě yú sūn luò, liú ér bù qù, bì sāi bù tōng, bù dé rù yú jīng, liú yì yú dà luò, ér shēng qí bìng yě. fū xié kè dà luò zhě, zuǒ zhù yòu, yòu zhù zuǒ, shàng xià zuǒ yòu, yǔ jīng xiāng gān, ér bù yú sì mò, qí qì wú cháng chù, bù rù yú jīng yú, mìng yuē móu cì. dì yuē: yuàn wén móu cì, yǐ zuǒ qǔ yòu, yǐ yòu qǔ zuǒ, nài hé? qí bó yuē: xié kè yú jīng, zuǒ shèng zé yòu bìng, yòu shèng zé zuǒ bìng, yì yǒu yí yì zhě, zuǒ tòng wèi yǐ ér yòu mài xiān bìng, rú cǐ zhě, bì jù cì zhī, bì zhōng qí jīng, fēi luò mài yě. gù luò bìng zhě, qí tòng yǔ jīng mài móu chù, gù mìng yuē móu cì.

Now when an evil lodges in the skin and hair, enters the fine collaterals, and stays without leaving, it blocks the way and cannot enter the channel, so it overflows into the great collaterals and breeds a strange disease. An evil in the great collaterals pours from left to right and right to left, above and below, crossing the channels and spreading to the four extremities, its qi having no fixed place and not entering the channel-points; needling for this is called crossed needling. The Emperor said: I wish to hear how crossed needling takes the right to treat the left and the left to treat the right. Qibo said: When an evil lodges in a channel, a fullness on the left makes the right sick and a fullness on the right makes the left sick; and there are shifting cases, where the left pain has not ceased and yet the right vessel sickens first. For such, one must use the great needling, striking the channel itself and not the collateral. But in a disease of the

> collaterals, the pain lies crosswise from the channel-vessel, and so it is called crossed needling.

When an evil lodges not in a channel but in the great collateral, it crosses the body, the left pouring into the right and the right into the left, so that the pain shows on the side opposite its cause. For these the classic prescribes contralateral needling, treating the right by needling the left and the left by needling the right. Where a complaint will not answer to the needle on its own side, the mirror side is tried, following the crossing path of the collateral.

> LING SHU 39
>
> 黃帝曰：願聞奇邪之不在經者。岐伯曰：血絡是也。血絡盛者，刺之血出，其色必黑，黑則去之，血變而止。
>
> *huáng dì yuē: yuàn wén qí xié zhī bù zài jīng zhě. qí bó yuē: xuè luò shì yě. xuè luò shèng zhě, cì zhī xuè chū, qí sè bì hēi, hēi zé qù zhī, xuè biàn ér zhǐ.*
>
> The Yellow Emperor said: I wish to hear of the stray evils that do not lie in the channels. Qibo said: These are in the blood-collaterals. Where a blood-collateral is engorged, prick it and let the blood run out; its colour will be dark, and when the dark is gone and the blood turns to its true colour, stop.

And where the trouble is blood stagnant in the visible small vessels, the remedy is to prick them and let it run. The blood comes dark at first, and one stops only when it turns clear and true. The engorged collateral is opened directly and the spent blood released until the good appears, a plain and ancient technique still recognisable in practice today. By the mirror and by the lancet, the needle reaches what the ordinary puncture cannot.

First, the Spirit

For all its instruments and rules, the classic insists that needling begins not with the hand but with the mind, the needler's own.

SU WEN 25

帝曰：願聞其道。岐伯曰：凡刺之真，必先治神，五藏已定，九候已備，後乃存鍼。眾脈不見，眾凶弗聞，外內相得，無以形先，可玩往來，乃施於人。人有虛實，五虛勿近，五實勿遠，至其當發，間不容瞚。手動若務，鍼耀而勻，靜意視義，觀適之變，是謂冥冥，莫知其形，見其烏烏，見其稷稷，從見其飛，不知其誰，伏如橫弩，起如發機。

dì yuē: yuàn wén qí dào. qí bó yuē: fán cì zhī zhēn, bì xiān zhì shén, wǔ zàng yǐ dìng, jiǔ hòu yǐ bèi, hòu nǎi cún zhēn. zhòng mài bù jiàn, zhòng xiōng fú wén, wài nèi xiāng de, wú yǐ xíng xiān, kě wán wǎng lái, nǎi shī yú rén. rén yǒu xū shí, wǔ xū wù jìn, wǔ shí wù yuǎn, zhì qí dāng fā, jiān bù róng shùn. shǒu dòng ruò wù, zhēn yào ér yún, jìng yì shì yì, guān shì zhī biàn, shì wèi míng míng, mò zhī qí xíng, jiàn qí wū wū, jiàn qí jì jì, cóng jiàn qí fēi, bù zhī qí shuí, fú rú héng nǔ, qǐ rú fā jī.

The Emperor said: I wish to hear that Way. Qibo said: In the truth of all needling, one must first govern the spirit; only when the five organs are settled and the nine indicators read does one then take up the needle. The crowding pulses are not seen, the crowding alarms not heard, inside and outside answering each other, and one does not let the body's surface lead; one can play with the coming and going of the qi, and so apply the needle to a person. People have their emptiness and repletion: in the five emptinesses do not draw near, in the five repletions do not hold off, and at the moment for release the instant leaves no space even to blink. The hand moves as if intent on one thing, the needle gleaming and even; the mind held still, the physician watches the rightness of it, observing the fitness of the change. This is called the unseen: none can make out its shape. He sees the qi gather dark as a flock of crows, dense as ripening grain, and watches them take flight without knowing whose they are; he lies in wait like a drawn crossbow and releases like the springing of the trigger.

The truth of needling, it says, is to govern the spirit first: only when the organs are settled and the body fully read does the needler turn to the needle, working then with a stilled mind and a steady, gleaming stroke, catching the moment so exactly that an instant's delay would already be too long. Composure here is not a courtesy but a technique, for a wavering attention misreads the qi and mistimes the hand.

> SU WEN 26
>
> 黃帝問曰：用鍼之服，必有法則焉，今何法何則？岐伯對曰：法天則地，合以天光。帝曰：願卒聞之。岐伯曰：凡刺之法，必候日月星辰，四時八正之氣，氣定乃刺之。
>
> *huáng dì wèn yuē: yòng zhēn zhī fú, bì yǒu fǎ zé yān, jīn hé fǎ hé zé? qí bó duì yuē: fǎ tiān zé dì, hé yǐ tiān guāng. dì yuē: yuàn zú wén zhī. qí bó yuē: fán cì zhī fǎ, bì hòu rì yuè xīng chén, sì shí bā zhèng zhī qì, qì dìng nǎi cì zhī.*
>
> The Yellow Emperor asked: The practice of the needle must have its laws and standards; what now are its law and standard? Qibo answered: Take Heaven for the law and Earth for the model, and join them to the lights of Heaven. The Emperor said: I wish to hear the whole of it. Qibo said: In all the rules of needling, one must watch the sun and moon, the stars and constellations, and the qi of the four seasons and the eight cardinal times; only when that qi is settled does one needle.

And the timing reaches past the moment to the sky. The practice of the needle, the classic says, must pattern itself on heaven and earth and join with heaven's light, waiting on the sun and moon, the seasons and the eight nodes, and setting the needle only when the qi has settled. Elsewhere it is blunt about the moon: do not drain at the new moon when the blood runs thin, nor supplement at the full when it brims. The body's qi rises and ebbs with the month like a tide, and a needle that ignores the tide works against it.

The Fit Hand, and the Guest Within

Not every hand should hold a needle, and not every disturbance is what it seems; the classic is exact about both.

> LING SHU 73
>
> 明目者，可使視色；聰耳者，可使聽音；捷疾辭語者，可使傳論；徐而安靜、手巧而心審諦者，可使行鍼艾，理血氣而調諸逆順，察陰陽而兼諸方。
>
> *míng mù zhě, kě shǐ shì sè; cōng ěr zhě, kě shǐ tīng yīn; jié jí cí yǔ zhě, kě shǐ chuán lùn; xú ér ān jìng, shǒu qiǎo ér xīn shěn dì zhě, kě shǐ xíng zhēn ài, lǐ xuè qì ér diào zhū nì shùn, chá yīn yáng ér jiān zhū fāng.*
>
> One with clear eyes may be set to read the colours; one with sharp ears, to listen to the sounds; one quick and ready in speech, to hand down the teachings; and one unhurried and calm, deft of hand and exact of mind, may be set to ply the needle and the moxa, to order the blood and qi, to regulate what runs with and against, to watch the yin and yang and master all the methods together.

It matches the practitioner to the work. Clear eyes are set to read the colours, sharp ears to hear the sounds, a ready tongue to teach; but the needle and the moxa are given only to one unhurried and calm, deft of hand and exact of mind. The temperament is itself a qualification, and the classic would not put the needle in a restless or careless hand, whatever its knowledge.

LING SHU 7

凡刺之要，官鍼最妙。九鍼之宜，各有所為，長短大小，各有所施也，不得其用，病弗能移。

fán cì zhī yào, guān zhēn zuì miào. jiǔ zhēn zhī yí, gè yǒu suǒ wèi, cháng duǎn dà xiǎo, gè yǒu suǒ shī yě, bù dé qí yòng, bìng fú néng yí.

Of the essentials of needling, the matching of each needle to its office is the most subtle of all. Each of the nine needles has its own work, and long or short, large or small, each has its proper use; reach for the wrong one, and the disease will not be shifted.

It is exact, too, about matching the needle to the work. The fit hand reads first, by the means the diagnostic gates set out, and only then reaches for its instrument; for of all the essentials, the classic says, the fitting of the needle to its office is the subtlest. Each of the nine needles has its own task, long or short, large or small, and the wrong one will not shift the disease. From this follow the nine methods of needling, a shallow prick of the skin, the draining of a blood-collateral, a deep stroke between the muscles, and the rest, each answering a different kind of trouble; so the fit hand reaches for the right needle and the right method, never merely for a needle.

LING SHU 71

今厥氣客於五藏六府，則衛氣獨衛其外，行於陽，不得入於陰。行於陽則陽氣盛，陽氣盛則陽蹻陷，不得入於陰，陰虛，故目不瞑。

jīn jué qì kè yú wǔ zàng liù fǔ, zé wèi qì dú wèi qí wài, xíng yú yáng, bù dé rù yú yīn. xíng yú yáng zé yáng qì shèng, yáng qì shèng zé yáng juē xiàn, bù dé rù yú yīn, yīn xū, gù mù bù míng.

When a reversed qi lodges as a guest in the organs and palaces, the defensive qi alone guards the outside, running in the yang and unable to enter the yin. Running in the yang, the yang qi grows full; and the yang being full, the yin cannot be entered; the yin runs empty, and so the eyes do not close.

What is read is often a guest. When a stray qi lodges in the organs, it can hold the defensive qi out in the yang and bar it from the yin, so that the yin empties and the eyes will not close; sleeplessness, in this account, is an evil keeping the night-guard from coming home. The symptom is traced to where the qi has been forced, and the cure restores its proper passage.

> LING SHU 75
>
> 真氣者，所受於天，與穀氣並而充身者也。虛邪之中人也，洒淅動形；正邪之中人也微，先見於色，不知於身。
>
> *zhēn qì zhě, suǒ shòu yú tiān, yǔ gǔ qì bìng ér chōng shēn zhě yě. xū xié zhī zhōng rén yě, sǎ xī dòng xíng; zhèng xié zhī zhōng rén yě wēi, xiān jiàn yú sè, bù zhī yú shēn.*
>
> The true qi is what is received from heaven, joined with the qi of grain to fill the body. When a hollow evil strikes a person, it shakes the body with a shivering chill; but when a true-seeming evil strikes, it does so faintly, showing first in the colour before the body itself knows it.

And the needler must tell the body's true qi, received from heaven and fed by grain, from the evils that assail it: the gross evil that strikes with a shivering chill, and the subtle one that shows first only in the colour, before the body knows it is ill. The faint early evil is the one to catch, read in the complexion while the person still feels well, which is the whole advantage of a trained eye. With a fit hand, a careful reading, and the true told from the false, the needle is ready for any case this gate has named.

Fitting the Needle to the Person and the Hour

The same complaint is not met the same way in every body or at every moment, and the classic ends its teaching on the needle by fitting it to the case in hand.

LING SHU 38

廣肩腋、項肉薄、厚皮而黑色、脣臨臨然，其血黑以濁，其氣濇以遲，刺此者，深而留之，多益其數。瘦人者，皮薄色少，肉廉廉然，刺此者，淺而疾之。

guǎng jiān yè, xiàng ròu báo, hòu pí ér hēi sè, chún lín lín rán, qí xuè hēi yǐ zhuó, qí qì sè yǐ chí, cì cǐ zhě, shēn ér liú zhī, duō yì qí shù. shòu rén zhě, pí báo sè shǎo, ròu lián lián rán, cì cǐ zhě, qiǎn ér jí zhī.

For the stout person, broad in the shoulders, thick of skin and dark of colour, whose blood is dark and turbid and whose qi is sluggish and slow, needle deep and leave the needle in, and use the stroke more often. For the thin person, with thin skin and little colour and spare flesh, needle shallow and withdraw quickly.

It adjusts the stroke to the build. The stout, dark-skinned person whose blood runs thick and slow is needled deep, the needle left in and worked often; the thin, pale person is needled shallow and quick. Depth and retention are read from the body before the disease is even weighed, since a depth that suits a heavy frame would over-treat a slight one.

LING SHU 67

百姓之血氣，各不同形：或神動而氣先鍼行，或氣與鍼相逢，或鍼已出氣獨行，或數刺乃知，或發鍼而氣逆，或數刺病益劇。

bǎi xìng zhī xuè qì, gè bù tóng xíng: huò shén dòng ér qì xiān zhēn xíng, huò qì yǔ zhēn xiāng féng, huò zhēn yǐ chū qì dú xíng, huò shuò cì nǎi zhī, huò fā zhēn ér qì nì, huò shuò cì bìng yì jù.

The blood and qi of people are each of a different make. In one the spirit stirs and the qi runs ahead of the needle; in another the qi meets the needle as it enters; in another the qi moves only after the needle is drawn; in another only repeated needling is felt at

> all; in another the drawing of the needle sets the qi running the wrong way; and in another repeated needling makes the disease worse.

And people answer the needle differently. In one the qi runs ahead of the needle; in another it meets the needle entering; in another only repeated needling is felt; and in a few the needle drives the qi the wrong way or worsens the trouble. The needler reads the response and adjusts, gentle and sparing with the quick, more patient with the slow, and ready to stop the moment the qi turns adverse.

> LING SHU 34
>
> 清氣在陰，濁氣在陽，營氣順脈，衛氣逆行，清濁相干，亂於胸中，是謂大悗。故氣亂於心，則煩心密嘿，俛首靜伏；亂於肺，則俛仰喘喝，接手以呼；亂於腸胃，則為霍亂。
>
> *qīng qì zài yīn, zhuó qì zài yáng, yíng qì shùn mài, wèi qì nì xíng, qīng zhuó xiāng gān, luàn yú xiōng zhōng, shì wèi dà mán. gù qì luàn yú xīn, zé fán xīn mì hēi, fǔ shǒu jìng fú; luàn yú fèi, zé fǔ yǎng chuǎn hē, jiē shǒu yǐ hū; luàn yú cháng wèi, zé wèi huò luàn.*
>
> When the clear qi is in the yin and the turbid in the yang, the nutritive qi following the vessels while the defensive runs counter, the clear and the turbid interfere and fall into disorder in the chest, and this is called the great oppression. So when the qi is in disorder at the heart, there is a vexed heart and a heavy silence, the head bowed and still; at the lung, a gasping breath with the body bowing and rising and the hands pressed to it; at the stomach and intestines, a sudden turmoil of vomiting and flux.

Some disorders are neither an excess nor a lack but a confusion, the clear and the turbid qi crossed and tangled in the chest, showing as a vexed heart, a gasping breath, or a sudden turmoil of the gut. These are not drained or filled but gently set back in order, the needle restoring the right direction rather than adding or taking away.

LING SHU 55

兵法曰：無迎逢逢之氣，無擊堂堂之陣。刺法曰：無刺熇熇之熱，無刺漉漉之汗，無刺渾渾之脈，無刺病與脈相逆者。

bīng fǎ yuē: wú yíng féng féng zhī qì, wú jī táng táng zhī zhèn. cì fǎ yuē: wú cì hè hè zhī rè, wú cì lù lù zhī hàn, wú cì hún hún zhī mài, wú cì bìng yǔ mài xiāng nì zhě.

The art of war says: do not go to meet a host whose banners are massed, nor strike a formation drawn up in full array. The art of needling says: do not needle a blazing heat, do not needle a streaming sweat, do not needle a pulse running muddy and confused, and do not needle where the disease and the pulse run contrary to one another.

And the hour itself can forbid the needle. As the art of war does not strike a massed and ordered army, the art of needling does not needle a blazing fever, a streaming sweat, a pulse running muddy and confused, or a case where the disease and the pulse contradict each other. When the body is in violent flux the needle waits, for to intervene then is to be swept along with the disorder. Built to the person, and timed to the response and the hour, the same needle becomes a different instrument in every hand it meets.

The Weight of the Needle

The classic closes the matter of the needle where it should, on the gravity of the thing, and on the deepest reason a person stays well at all.

> LING SHU 60
>
> 黃帝曰：余以小鍼為細物也，夫子乃上合之於天，下合之於地，中合之於人，余以為過鍼之意矣。岐伯曰：何物大於天乎？夫大於鍼者，惟五兵者焉。五兵者，死之備也，非生之具。
>
> *huáng dì yuē: yú yǐ xiǎo zhēn wèi xì wù yě, fū zǐ nǎi shàng hé zhī yú tiān, xià hé zhī yú dì, zhōng hé zhī yú rén, yú yǐ wèi guò zhēn zhī yì yǐ. qí bó yuē: hé wù dà yú tiān hū? fū dà yú zhēn zhě, wéi wǔ bīng zhě yān. wǔ bīng zhě, sǐ zhī bèi yě, fēi shēng zhī jù.*
>
> The Yellow Emperor said: I had taken the small needle for a slight thing, yet you join it above to heaven, below to earth, and between to man; I think this makes too much of the needle. Qibo said: What is greater than heaven? Greater than the needle are only the five weapons; and the five weapons are the gear of death, not the instruments of life.

Small as it is, the needle is no slight instrument. Greater than it, the classic says, are only the weapons of war, and those are the gear of death while the needle serves life; to hold it is to hold a power over living and dying, and the classic means the weight of that to be felt. The seriousness is itself a discipline, the ground of the cautions, the prohibitions, and the long preparation the art asks for.

LING SHU 61

形肉已奪，是一奪也；大奪血之後，是二奪也；大汗出之後，是三奪也；大泄之後，是四奪也；新產及大血之後，是五奪也。此皆不可瀉。

xíng ròu yǐ duó, shì yī duó yě; dà duó xuè zhī hòu, shì èr duó yě; dà hán chū zhī hòu, shì sān duó yě; dà xiè zhī hòu, shì sì duó yě; xīn chǎn jí dà xuè zhī hòu, shì wǔ duó yě. cǐ jiē bù kě xiè.

When the flesh is already wasted, that is the first depletion; after a great loss of blood, the second; after a heavy sweat, the third; after a violent purging, the fourth; and after childbirth or a great bleeding, the fifth. In none of these five may the needle drain.

Hence its firm refusals. There are five states of depletion in which the needle must never drain: a wasted body, and the aftermath of great bleeding, of heavy sweat, of violent purging, and of childbirth. In these the body has already lost too much, and to drain further is to harm; the rule guards against the commonest fatal error, treating an emptiness as though it were a fullness.

LING SHU 51

肺腧在三焦之間，心腧在五焦之間，膈腧在七焦之間，肝腧在九焦之間，脾腧在十一焦之間，腎腧在十四焦之間。欲得而驗之，按其處，應在中而痛解，乃其腧也。

fèi shù zài sān jiāo zhī jiān, xīn shù zài wǔ jiāo zhī jiān, gé shù zài qī jiāo zhī jiān, gān shù zài jiǔ jiāo zhī jiān, pí shù zài shí yī jiāo zhī jiān, shèn shù zài shí sì jiāo zhī jiān. yù dé ér yàn zhī, àn qí chù, yīng zài zhōng ér tòng jiě, nǎi qí shù yě.

The lung-transport lies between the third vertebrae, the heart-transport between the fifth, the diaphragm-transport between the seventh, the liver-transport between the ninth, the spleen-transport between the eleventh, and the kidney-transport between the fourteenth. To find and confirm one, press the place; where the pressure answers within and the ache eases, there is the transport point.

It locates its steadiest points with care, the transport points of the five organs ranged down the back, each confirmed by pressing until the spot answers within and the ache eases. Gentle and reliable, these are often warmed rather than pierced, and are a mainstay where deep needling would be unsafe.

LING SHU 48

此先師之所禁，坐私傳之也，割臂歃血之盟也。子若欲得之，何不齋乎？雷公再拜而起曰：請聞命於是也，乃齋宿三日而請。

cǐ xiān shī zhī suǒ jìn, zuò sī chuán zhī yě, gē bì shà xuè zhī méng yě. zi ruò yù dé zhī, hé bù zhāi hū? léi gōng zài bài ér qǐ yuē: qǐng wén mìng yú shì yě, nǎi zhāi sù sān rì ér qǐng.

This is what the former masters forbade to be handed on lightly, sealed by the oath of cutting the arm and smearing the blood. If you would receive it, why not first purify yourself by fasting? Leigong bowed twice and rose, saying, Let me hear the charge; and he fasted and kept vigil three days before he asked again.

And it surrounds the whole art with an oath. The deepest teaching was not handed on lightly but sealed by cutting the arm and smearing the blood, and given only to one who had first fasted and kept vigil. The rite marks what the cautions imply, that this knowledge is grave enough to be received in earnest or not received at all.

SU WEN 72

黃帝曰：余聞五疫之至，皆相染易，無問大小，病狀相似，不施救療，如何可得不相移易者？岐伯曰：不相染者，正氣存內，邪不可干，避其毒氣。

huáng dì yuē: yú wén wǔ yì zhī zhì, jiē xiāng rǎn yì, wú wèn dà xiǎo, bìng zhuàng xiāng sì, bù shī jiù liáo, rú hé kě dé bù xiāng yí yì zhě? qí bó yuē: bù xiāng rǎn zhě, zhèng qì cún nèi, xié bù kě gàn, bì qí dú qì.

The Yellow Emperor said: I have heard that when the five pestilences arrive, all of them pass easily from one person to another, and whether the case be great or small the signs are alike; if no remedy is given, how may one keep from catching it? Qibo said: Those

> who are not infected, their true qi is preserved within, so the evil cannot assail them; and they keep away from its poisonous qi.

Beneath every technique lies one last teaching, set down where the classic turns to the pestilences that pass from person to person: those who do not fall ill are those whose true qi is kept whole within, so that the evil finds no opening. The needle, in the end, serves this, the keeping of an inner strength no evil can cross; which is why the first gate and this one meet here, and why the deepest medicine of all is the one that is never needed. Grave in the hand, firm in its refusals, sworn in its keeping, the needle is aimed at last not at the disease but at the strength that keeps disease away.

BEFORE THE NEEDLE IS SET

Whatever the complaint, a few questions come before the needle, and in roughly this order. Is the hour and the season one in which the qi may be safely reached, and is the body not in the violent flux, a high fever, a drenching sweat, a chaotic pulse, that the classic says to leave alone? Is the person depleted, by illness, bleeding, sweat, purging, or childbirth, so that the needle must not drain? Is the chosen point well clear of the forbidden spots over the organs and the great vessels? What is the level of the trouble, and so the depth to reach it cleanly? Only then does the hand act: fill what is empty, drain what is full, and wait for the answer, a warmth or a coolness, the arrival of the qi, before drawing the needle. The order protects the patient more surely than any single trick of technique.

ACUPUNCTURE AND THE NEEDLE

Essential Verses

These are among the gate's most quoted lines in the classic, gathered here for study.

SU WEN 52

藏有要害，不可不察。刺中心，一日死，其動為噫；刺中肝，五日死，其動為語；刺中腎，六日死，其動為嚏。刺跗上中大脈，血出不止死。

zàng yǒu yào hài, bù kě bù chá. cì zhōng xīn, yī rì sǐ, qí dòng wèi yī; cì zhōng gān, wǔ rì sǐ, qí dòng wèi yǔ; cì zhōng shèn, liù rì sǐ, qí dòng wèi tì. cì fū shàng zhōng dà mài, xuè chū bù zhǐ sǐ.

The organs have their vital and vulnerable places, which must be examined. Pierce the heart and death comes in one day, its sign a hiccup; pierce the liver and death comes in five days, its sign speech; pierce the kidney and death comes in six days, its sign sneezing. Pierce the great vessel on the instep so blood will not stop, and death follows.

This is the canon's charter of needling safety, the list of depths a needle must never reach. Strike the heart and death comes within a day, the liver in five, the kidney in six, each error announced by its own sign, a hiccup, a fit of speech, a sneeze, so that a wrong stroke betrays itself in the symptom that follows. Open the great vessel on the instep so the blood will not stop, and the patient is lost. What the line demands of the operator is knowledge of the vital structures lying beneath each point and a hand that judges depth, stopping the needle short of the organ or the artery. These prohibitions are not cautions but absolute limits, the boundary where skill ends and damage begins.

> SU WEN 59
>
> 脈氣所發者，氣穴也；浮氣在皮中者，衛氣也，不循經而行。手足之陽明各五，氣府者，氣之所注，脈氣所發之穴也。
>
> *mài qì suǒ fā zhě, qì xué yě; fú qì zài pí zhōng zhě, wèi qì yě, bù xún jīng ér xíng. shǒu zú zhī yáng míng gè wǔ, qì fǔ zhě, qì zhī suǒ zhù, mài qì suǒ fā zhī xué yě.*
>
> Where the channel-qi issues forth is a qi-point; the floating qi within the skin is the defensive qi, which runs without following the channels. The hand and foot yang-brightness each have their points. A qi-mansion is a point into which qi pours, where the channel-qi issues forth.

The chapter reads as a gazetteer of the points at which each channel's qi rises to the surface and can be reached, the qi-mansions, counted channel by channel. Its use is plain: it tells the practitioner exactly where a given channel offers a handle on its qi. Find the mansions where the chosen channel's qi emerges and work there to reach the deep current, while keeping in mind that the loose, floating qi just under the skin is defensive qi, running free of the channels and answered in a different way. For the needle-worker it is the difference between knowing a channel exists and knowing where to lay hands on it.

SU WEN 60

風從外入，令人振寒，汗出頭痛，身重惡寒，治在風府，調其陰陽，不足則補，有餘則瀉。衝脈者，起於氣街，並少陰之經，挾臍上行，至胸中而散。

fēng cóng wài rù, lìng rén zhèn hán, hàn chū tóu tòng, shēn zhòng è hán, zhì zài fēng fǔ, diào qí yīn yáng, bù zú zé bǔ, yǒu yú zé xiè. chōng mài zhě, qǐ yú qì jiē, bìng shào yīn zhī jīng, xié qí shàng háng, zhì xiōng zhōng ér sàn.

When wind enters from without it makes a person shiver and chill, sweat and ache in the head, the body heavy and averse to cold; the treatment lies at Wind-Mansion, regulating the yin and yang, supplementing what is deficient and draining what is in excess. The thoroughfare vessel arises at the qi-thoroughfare, runs alongside the lesser-yin channel, flanks the navel ascending, and disperses in the chest.

Two things sit side by side in this chapter, a named treatment and the deep anatomy that makes it possible. When wind enters from without it strikes high at the nape, bringing shiver, sweat, headache, and a body heavy and cold; the place to meet it is Wind-Mansion, where the yin-yang balance is restored, draining what is in excess and filling what is short. The chapter then charts the bone-holes and the course of the thoroughfare vessel, which rises from the qi-thoroughfare, flanks the navel, and disperses in the chest, so that disorders along the abdomen and chest can be reached by its mapped path. The practical point and the deep-vessel map belong together: one tells the physician what to do for wind, the other where the body's hidden roads run.

SU WEN 61

腎者，至陰也；至陰者，盛水也。肺者，太陰也。故其本在腎，其末在肺，皆積水也。腎者，胃之關也，關門不利，故聚水而從其類也。

shèn zhě, zhì yīn yě; zhì yīn zhě, shèng shuǐ yě. fèi zhě, tài yīn yě. gù qí běn zài shèn, qí mò zài fèi, jiē jī shuǐ yě. shèn zhě, wèi zhī guān yě, guān mén bù lì, gù jù shuǐ ér cóng qí lèi yě.

The kidney is the utmost yin, and the utmost yin abounds in water. The lung is the greater yin. Thus the root of water-disease lies in the kidney and its branch in the lung,

> both being accumulations of water. The kidney is the gate of the stomach; when that gate does not work freely, water gathers and follows its kind.

Water-swelling has a root and a branch, and the chapter places them precisely: the root below in the kidney, the branch above in the lung, with the kidney serving as the stomach's gate on the body's fluids. When that gate cannot open and close properly, the fluids it should pass are dammed and pool. Treatment therefore works at both ends, the root in the kidney and the branch in the lung, by needling the points the chapter assigns to water and to heat, opening the gate so the gathered water can move. Behind the swelling the line keeps a clear account of why and where fluid accumulates, which is what lets the needle address a cause rather than bail out a symptom.

> SU WEN 62
>
> 五藏之道，皆出於經隧，以行血氣。血氣不和，百病乃變化而生，是故守經隧焉。陽虛則外寒，陰虛則內熱，陽盛則外熱，陰盛則內寒。
>
> *wǔ zàng zhī dào, jiē chū yú jīng suì, yǐ xíng xuè qì. xuè qì bù hé, bǎi bìng nǎi biàn huà ér shēng, shì gù shǒu jīng suì yān. yáng xū zé wài hán, yīn xū zé nèi rè, yáng shèng zé wài rè, yīn shèng zé nèi hán.*
>
> The ways of the five organs all issue along the channel-tunnels, by which the blood and qi are moved. When blood and qi are not in harmony, the hundred diseases arise and transform; therefore one guards the channel-tunnels. Yang depletion gives outer cold, yin depletion inner heat; yang repletion outer heat, yin repletion inner cold.

All disease, the chapter says, arises from a disharmony of blood and qi moving in the channels, which is why the channels are what the physician must regulate. Four short formulas decode any presentation of heat or cold into its root, sorting outer from inner and excess from want: yang depletion gives outer cold, yin depletion inner heat, yang repletion outer heat, yin repletion inner cold. The work is then to hold to the channels as the place of intervention, read whether a patient's cold or heat is outer or inner, assign it to yang or yin and to repletion or depletion, and supplement or drain accordingly. It is the gate's clearest statement that regulating the channel-borne blood and qi is the whole of treatment.

SU WEN 63

邪之客於形也，必先舍於皮毛，留而不去，入舍於孫脈，留而不去，入舍於絡脈，留而不去，入舍於經脈。其入客於絡脈，留而不去，閉塞不通，不得入於經，流溢於大絡，而生奇病，繆刺之。

xié zhī kè yú xíng yě, bì xiān shě yú pí máo, liú ér bù qù, rù shě yú sūn mài, liú ér bù qù, rù shě yú luò mài, liú ér bù qù, rù shě yú jīng mài. qí rù kè yú luò mài, liú ér bù qù, bì sāi bù tōng, bù dé rù yú jīng, liú yì yú dà luò, ér shēng qí bìng, móu cì zhī.

When an evil settles in the body it first lodges in the skin and hair; staying, it enters the grandchild-vessels; staying, the network vessels; staying, the channels. When it lodges in the network vessels and stays, blocking the way so it cannot enter the channels, it overflows into the great networks and gives rise to anomalous disease; this is crossed-needling.

When an evil is trapped in the network vessels rather than the channels proper, the disease shows on one side while the channel itself stays sound, and for this the chapter prescribes crossed needling. Because the evil has overflowed into the great networks, which cross the body, the affected side is treated by needling the networks on the opposite side. The procedure is exact: confirm that pain is present while the channel pulse is undisturbed, find the involved networks, and needle the sound opposite side at the network level to release the blockage. It is a precise remedy for an otherwise puzzling class of one-sided complaints, where treating the obvious side would only chase the pain.

LING SHU 2

凡刺之道，必通十二經絡之所終始，絡脈之所別處，五輸之所留，六府之所與合。五藏之腧，五五二十五腧；六府之腧，六六三十六腧。

fán cì zhī dào, bì tōng shí èr jīng luò zhī suǒ zhōng shǐ, luò mài zhī suǒ bié chù, wǔ shū zhī suǒ liú, liù fǔ zhī suǒ yǔ hé. wǔ zàng zhī shù, wǔ wǔ èr shí wǔ shù; liù fǔ zhī shù, liù liù sān shí liù shù.

The way of needling requires knowing where the twelve channels begin and end, where the network vessels branch off, where the five transport-points lodge, and where the six bowels join. The transport-points of the five organs number five times five, twenty-five; those of the six bowels number six times six, thirty-six.

At the foundation of point-selection stands the small set of transport-points near the extremities, well, spring, stream, river, and sea, through which a channel's qi can be commanded. They are privileged because the channel-qi pools and surfaces at them, making them the most reliable handles on a channel. The physician learns the fixed roster of these points for the organs and the bowels, matches the point-type to the disorder, a well-point for fullness below the heart, a sea-point for counterflow, and needles there to govern the channel from its most accessible station. Everything later acupuncture builds rests on this scheme, in which a few commanding points stand for a whole channel.

LING SHU 39

血脈者，盛堅橫以赤，上下無常處，小者如鍼，大者如箸。刺而血出，黑而濁者止之，血出清而半為汁者去之。刺血絡而僕者，何也？血出而射者，何也？

xuè mài zhě, shèng jiān héng yǐ chì, shàng xià wú cháng chù, xiǎo zhě rú zhēn, dà zhě rú zhù. cì ér xuè chū, hēi ér zhuó zhě zhǐ zhī, xuè chū qīng ér bàn wèi zhī zhě qù zhī. cì xuè luò ér pú zhě, hé yě? xuè chū ér shè zhě, hé yě?

A blood-vessel that is full shows hard and crossways and red, with no fixed place above or below, the small ones like a needle, the large like a chopstick. When you needle and the blood comes out black and turbid, stop; when it comes out clear and half watery,

> drain it away. Why does one faint on needling a blood-network? Why does the blood spurt out?

Letting blood from a visible network vessel is a controlled procedure, and the chapter governs it by what the blood itself shows. An engorged vessel stands out hard and red, the small ones like a needle, the large like a chopstick; once opened, the blood is watched as it issues, and the operator stops when it turns from black and turbid to clear, since dark thick blood is stagnation to be released while clear watery blood signals depletion and a stroke to be ended. Fainting and spurting are anticipated so they can be managed. The skill lies not in the cut but in reading the changing blood and knowing the moment to halt.

> LING SHU 48
>
> 寸口主中，人迎主外，兩者相應，俱往俱來，若引繩大小齊等。春夏人迎微大，秋冬寸口微大，如是者名曰平人。人迎大一倍於寸口，病在足少陽。
>
> *cùn kǒu zhǔ zhōng, rén yíng zhǔ wài, liǎng zhě xiāng yīng, jù wǎng jù lái, ruò yǐn shéng dà xiǎo qí děng. chūn xià rén yíng wēi dà, qiū dōng cùn kǒu wēi dà, rú shì zhě míng yuē píng rén. rén yíng dà yī bèi yú cùn kǒu, bìng zài zú shào yáng.*
>
> The inch-mouth governs the interior, Man's-Welcome the exterior; the two answer each other, coming and going together, like a drawn cord equal at both ends. In spring and summer Man's-Welcome is slightly larger, in autumn and winter the inch-mouth slightly larger; one so balanced is called an even person. When Man's-Welcome is twice the inch-mouth, the disease is in the foot lesser-yang.

Pulse-taking here becomes a comparison: the carotid Man's-Welcome weighed against the wrist inch-mouth, balancing the exterior against the interior. Equality marks health, allowing for the slight seasonal shift, and a fixed degree of disproportion points to a particular channel and to whether the exterior or the interior should be drained. The physician feels both pulses together and reads the multiple by which one exceeds the other, a Man's-Welcome twice the inch-mouth sending the needle to the lesser-yang, and treats the channel and side that the ratio names. It turns the wrist from a single impression into a quantitative reading that directs the hand to a specific channel.

LING SHU 55

氣之逆順者，所以應天地陰陽四時五行也。脈之盛衰者，所以候血氣之虛實有餘不足。上工刺其未生者也，其次刺其未盛者也，其次刺其已衰者也。方其盛也，勿敢毀傷，刺其已衰，事必大昌。

qì zhī nì shùn zhě, suǒ yǐ yīng tiān dì yīn yáng sì shí wǔ xíng yě. mài zhī shèng shuāi zhě, suǒ yǐ hòu xuè qì zhī xū shí yǒu yú bù zú. shàng gōng cì qí wèi shēng zhě yě, qí cì cì qí wèi shèng zhě yě, qí cì cì qí yǐ shuāi zhě yě. fāng qí shèng yě, wù gǎn huǐ shāng, cì qí yǐ shuāi, shì bì dà chāng.

The counterflow and compliance of qi answer to heaven and earth, yin and yang, the four seasons and five phases. The flourishing and decline of the pulse are how one watches the deficiency or repletion of blood and qi. The superior physician needles before the disease arises, the next before it flourishes, the next when it has already declined. While it is at flood, dare not assail it; needle it once it has waned, and the work will surely prosper.

Needling has a right moment, bounded on one side by too early and on the other by too late, and the chapter makes the timing as decisive as the location. Qi rises and falls with the seasons and with the disease's own course, and the pulse reports where it stands; the physician reads it to place the illness on its curve. The needle is withheld while the qi is at full surge, the chapter's image of not striking a host drawn up in full array, and brought to bear before the disease has formed or once it has waned. The highest skill forestalls it altogether, needling what has not yet arisen, which is why the same chapter sets the physician who prevents above the one who waits for the disease to declare itself.

LING SHU 61

刺法曰：無刺熇熇之熱，無刺漉漉之汗，無刺渾渾之脈，無刺病與脈相逆者。上工平氣，中工亂脈，下工絕氣危生。故曰用鍼之要，無忘其神。

cì fǎ yuē: wú cì hè hè zhī rè, wú cì lù lù zhī hàn, wú cì hún hún zhī mài, wú cì bìng yǔ mài xiāng nì zhě. shàng gōng píng qì, zhōng gōng luàn mài, xià gōng jué qì wēi shēng. gù yuē yòng zhēn zhī yào, wú wàng qí shén.

The law of needling says: do not needle a blazing fever, a streaming sweat, a turbid chaotic pulse, or a case where disease and pulse run contrary. The superior physician levels the qi; the middling throws the pulse into disorder; the inferior cuts off the qi and endangers life. Therefore it is said: in wielding the needle, never forget the spirit.

There are moments when the needle must simply be withheld, and the chapter names four of them: a blazing fever, a pouring sweat, a turbid and chaotic pulse, and a disease at odds with its own pulse. At these crises the qi cannot bear intervention, and to force it is to harm; the chapter grades practitioners by exactly this, the superior levelling the qi, the middling throwing the pulse into disorder, the inferior cutting the qi off and endangering life. Before needling, then, the patient is checked against these four bars and the needle stayed if any is present, the patient's spirit held as the constant object of attention, and the hand moved only to settle the qi, never to scatter it. Knowing when not to needle is made the test of the master.

LING SHU 71

厥氣客於五藏六府，則衛氣獨衛其外，行於陽，不得入於陰。行於陽則陽氣盛，陽氣盛則陽蹻陷，不得入於陰，陰虛，故目不瞑。補其不足，瀉其有餘，調其虛實，以通其道而去其邪。

jué qì kè yú wǔ zàng liù fǔ, zé wèi qì dú wèi qí wài, xíng yú yáng, bù dé rù yú yīn. xíng yú yáng zé yáng qì shèng, yáng qì shèng zé yáng juē xiàn, bù dé rù yú yīn, yīn xū, gù mù bù míng. bǔ qí bù zú, xiè qí yǒu yú, diào qí xū shí, yǐ tōng qí dào ér qù qí xié.

When a reversal-qi lodges in the organs and bowels, the defensive qi guards the outside alone, moving in the yang and unable to enter the yin. Moving in the yang the yang-qi swells, the yang heel-vessel fills, it cannot cross into the yin, the yin is empty, and so the eyes do not close. Supplement what is deficient, drain what is in excess, regulate the emptiness and fullness, open the way and dispel the evil.

Sleeplessness gets a physiology here, and therefore a remedy. A reversal-qi lodged in the organs keeps the defensive qi out on the surface, so that at night it cannot cross from the yang into the yin; heaped in the yang it swells, fills the yang heel-vessel, and leaves the yin empty, and without the guard's nightly descent the eyes stay open. The treatment restores that crossing: drain the swollen yang, replenish the emptied yin, and open the road so the guard can complete its night circuit. Read this way, insomnia is not a mood to be sedated but a blocked passage to be cleared, which is why the chapter treats it as a disorder of the body's traffic rather than of the mind alone.

LING SHU 73

得其人乃傳，非其人勿言。明於陰陽，審於經絡，知其邪正，乃可言也。各得其能，方乃可行，其名乃彰。不得其人，其功不成，其師無名。

dé qí rén nǎi chuán, fēi qí rén wù yán. míng yú yīn yáng, shěn yú jīng luò, zhī qí xié zhèng, nǎi kě yán yě. gè dé qí néng, fāng nǎi kě xíng, qí míng nǎi zhāng. bù dé qí rén, qí gōng bù chéng, qí shī wú míng.

Transmit only to the right person; to the wrong one, say nothing. Only one clear about yin and yang, careful of the channels and networks, and able to tell the evil qi from the true may be spoken to. Let each be given the task he is fit for, and only then can the work go forward and his name be made bright. Given to the wrong person, the work fails and the teacher's name comes to nothing.

Two cautions sit together in this chapter, one about whom to teach and one about whom to set to a task. A method handed to someone without the grounding is wasted or dangerous, so the deeper technique is transmitted only to a student who already commands the fundamentals, yin and yang, the channels, the discernment of true qi from evil. The same judgement governs assignment: each worker is matched to the operation his skill can carry, so that the work goes forward and is not spoiled by being given to the wrong hands. The chapter sets the ethics and the pedagogy of the needling craft beside its techniques, as conditions of the work rather than asides to it.

LING SHU 75

刺有五節，有刺有五邪。五節者，一曰振埃，二曰發蒙，三曰去爪，四曰徹衣，五曰解惑。凡刺五邪之方，不過五章，癉熱消滅，腫聚散亡，寒痹益溫，小者益陽，大者必去。

cì yǒu wǔ jié, yǒu cì yǒu wǔ xié. wǔ jié zhě, yī yuē zhèn āi, èr yuē fā méng, sān yuē qù zhǎo, sì yuē chè yī, wǔ yuē jiě huò. fán cì wǔ xié zhī fāng, bù guò wǔ zhāng, dān rè xiāo miè, zhǒng jù sàn wáng, hán bì yì wēn, xiǎo zhě yì yáng, dà zhě bì qù.

There are five articulations of needling and five evils to be needled. The five articulations are: shaking off the dust, lifting the veil, cutting away the talon, stripping the garment, dissolving confusion. The methods for needling the five evils come to no more than five chapters: searing heat extinguished, swelling and gathering scattered, cold bi warmed, the small built up in yang, the great surely removed.

Advanced needling is organised here into five named manoeuvres, each a vivid figure for a distinct technique: shaking off the dust, lifting the veil, cutting away the talon, stripping the garment, dissolving confusion. The names are not ornament; each encodes the aim of its method, an obstruction cleared, the senses suddenly opened, and so on, and each answers a particular class of evil. The practitioner matches the disorder to its class, then performs the corresponding articulation, the technique suited to that evil's depth and seat, working through the small fixed repertoire the chapter lays out. It gives a set of named operations a physician can learn by heart and deploy by case, rather than a vague counsel to needle skilfully.

FROM THE AUTHOR

Patience is the temper this whole tradition asks for, and every gate teaches it in its own way. The pulse yields its meaning only to a quiet, unhurried hand; cultivation, slowest of all, is the work of a lifetime. The needle is simply where that patience shows most sharply, for here haste is not merely fruitless but dangerous. The classic spends as many words on governing the spirit, fitting the hand, and knowing when not to act as on where to place a point, and that emphasis is itself the lesson. Reading these chapters together, I came to see the long lists of cautions not as restrictions but as the gathered carefulness of people who took the power of a small piece of metal entirely seriously, and who wanted it, before anything else, to serve life rather than to display skill.

粗守形，上守神。

The crude practitioner guards the form; the superior guards the spirit.

WHERE THIS GATE LEADS

The needle works upon the rivers of *Gate Five, The Rivers of the Body*, and is guided by the readings of *Gate Four, Reading the Unspoken*. Its purpose is to restore the flow that illness, whose beginnings are traced in *Gate Seven, How Illness Begins*, has disturbed; and for the therapies that stand beside it, the herbs, the heat of moxa, and the regulating of the whole person, see *Gate Eight, The Physician's Hand*.

PART SEVEN

How Illness Begins

Disease and Its Causes

疾病

On disease. How sickness begins, where it comes from, and how it travels in the body. The evils of wind, cold, heat, and damp; the inner stirring of the emotions; and the bodily weakness without which, the classic insists, no evil can take hold.

GATE SEVEN · DISEASE AND ITS CAUSES

How Illness Begins

疾病

> *When the evil qi is abundant, there is repletion; when the essential qi is robbed, there is emptiness.*
>
> Su Wen 28

The gates so far have built the body and taught the reading of it; this one turns to what goes wrong with it. It is the largest gate in the book, for the Inner Classic returns to disease more often than to any other subject, and from many directions at once: the weather without, the feelings within, the food and labour of a life, and the strength or weakness of the body that meets them all.

Before any single disease, the classic sets down a principle that governs them all. Sickness is not simply an evil striking from without; it is an evil meeting a vacuity within. A body whose qi is whole turns aside the same wind that fells a body already weakened, so that the cause of an illness is always double, the evil and the opening it finds. This is why two people may meet the same cold and only one fall ill.

From this follow the chapters gathered here: how and where the evils enter, wind as the chief of them, the fevers of cold and the intermittent fevers, cough and pain, the impediments and the wiltings, the reversals, the distensions, and the disorders of the spirit and the senses. Each is read above all for one thing, how the disease forms and how it moves, since to know that is already to know where the treatment of the later gates must act.

How the Hundred Diseases Begin

The classic opens the subject of disease with its deepest and most characteristic claim, one that shapes everything said after it.

LING SHU 66

夫百病之始生也，皆生於風雨寒暑，清濕喜怒。風雨寒熱，不得虛，邪不能獨傷人。卒然逢疾風暴雨而不病者，蓋無虛，故邪不能獨傷人。此必因虛邪之風，與其身形，兩虛相得，乃客其形。

fū bǎi bìng zhī shǐ shēng yě, jiē shēng yú fēng yǔ hán shǔ, qīng shī xǐ nù. fēng yǔ hán rè, bù dé xū, xié bù néng dú shāng rén. zú rán féng jí fēng bào yǔ ér bù bìng zhě, gài wú xū, gù xié bù néng dú shāng rén. cǐ bì yīn xū xié zhī fēng, yǔ qí shēn xíng, liǎng xū xiāng de, nǎi kè qí xíng.

The hundred diseases, in their beginnings, all arise from wind and rain, cold and heat, dampness, and the swings of joy and anger. Yet wind and rain, cold and heat cannot harm a person who has no vacuity; the evil cannot do it alone. Those who meet a sudden fierce wind or violent rain and still do not fall ill are simply those with no vacuity, so the evil cannot harm them by itself. There must be a vacuity-evil wind meeting a vacuity in the body, the two vacuities coming together, before the evil lodges in the form.

The hundred diseases, it says, begin in the weather and the feelings, in wind and rain and cold and heat and damp, and in the swings of joy and anger. But none of these harms a whole body on its own. The person who meets a sudden storm and does not sicken is simply the one with no vacuity for the evil to enter; there must be a weakness in the body to meet the weakness in the weather, the two coming together, before an illness takes hold. The cause of disease, in this account, is never the evil alone but the meeting of an evil with an opening.

SU WEN 28

黃帝問曰：何謂虛實？岐伯對曰：邪氣盛則實，精氣奪則虛。帝曰：虛實何如？岐伯曰：氣虛者肺虛也，氣逆者足寒也，非其時則生，當其時則死。餘藏皆如此。

huáng dì wèn yuē: hé wèi xū shí? qí bó duì yuē: xié qì shèng zé shí, jīng qì duó zé xū. dì yuē: xū shí hé rú? qí bó yuē: qì xū zhě fèi xū yě, qì nì zhě zú hán yě, fēi qí shí zé shēng, dāng qí shí zé sǐ. yú zàng jiē rú cǐ.

The Yellow Emperor asked: What is meant by emptiness and repletion? Qibo answered: When the evil qi is abundant, there is repletion; when the essential qi is robbed, there is emptiness. The Emperor asked: How do they show? Qibo said: When the qi is empty, it is the lung that is empty; when the qi runs counter, the feet are cold. Out of its proper season the patient lives; in its own season he dies. It is so with all the other organs as well.

From this the classic draws the master distinction every later chapter leans on. When an evil is abundant, the condition is one of repletion; when the body's own essence is despoiled, it is one of vacuity. The whole of treatment will turn on telling these apart, for the full must be drained and the empty filled, and to mistake the one for the other is the gravest error in medicine. Almost every disease named in this gate is, at bottom, a state of too much or of too little.

LING SHU 4

黃帝曰：邪氣之中人，奈何？岐伯曰：邪氣之中人也高。身半已上者，邪中之也；身半已下者，濕中之也。故曰：邪之中人也無有常，中於陰則溜於府，中於陽則溜於經。

huáng dì yuē: xié qì zhī zhōng rén, nài hé? qí bó yuē: xié qì zhī zhōng rén yě gāo. shēn bàn yǐ shàng zhě, xié zhōng zhī yě; shēn bàn yǐ xià zhě, shī zhōng zhī yě. gù yuē: xié zhī zhōng rén yě wú yǒu cháng, zhōng yú yīn zé liū yú fǔ, zhōng yú yáng zé liū yú jīng.

The Yellow Emperor asked: How do evils strike a person? Qibo said: Evils strike a person high. From the waist up it is the airborne evils that strike; from the waist down it is the damp. So it is said that the striking of an evil keeps no fixed rule: striking the yin, it drains inward to the palaces; striking the yang, it travels along the channels.

The evils do not strike at random. The airborne ones, wind and cold and heat, tend to come in high and take the upper body, while damp rises into the lower; and where an evil enters decides its course, for striking the yin it drains inward to the organs, and striking the yang it runs along the channels. To know where and how an evil has come in is already to know which way it will travel, and where it may be met.

LING SHU 58

黃帝曰：今有其不離屏蔽，不出室穴之中，卒然病者，其故何也？岐伯曰：此皆嘗有所傷於濕氣，藏於血脈之中，分肉之間，久留而不去；若有所墮墜，惡血在內而不去，卒然喜怒不節，因加而發焉。

huáng dì yuē: jīn yǒu qí bù lí píng bì, bù chū shì xué zhī zhōng, zú rán bìng zhě, qí gù hé yě? qí bó yuē: cǐ jiē cháng yǒu suǒ shāng yú shī qì, cáng yú xuè mài zhī zhōng, fēn ròu zhī jiān, jiǔ liú ér bù qù; ruò yǒu suǒ duò zhuì, è xuè zài nèi ér bù qù, zú rán xǐ nù bù jié, yīn jiā ér fā yān.

The Yellow Emperor said: Here is someone who has not left the shelter of the house, who has stayed within four walls, and yet is suddenly taken ill; what is the reason? Qibo said: In every such case there was some earlier injury: a dampness lodged in the blood and vessels and the spaces of the flesh, long remaining and never dispersed; or a fall, leaving stagnant blood within that did not clear. Then an unguarded swing of joy or anger is added to it, and on that occasion the illness breaks out.

Nor is the cause always a fresh attack. The classic faces the puzzle of a person who has kept indoors, met no wind, and yet falls suddenly ill, and answers that the seed was laid long before: an old dampness lodged in the vessels, or stagnant blood from a forgotten fall, lying quietly in the body until some later upset sets it off. Much disease, in this view, is the flaring of a cause already present, which is why a careful history reaches back well before the day the symptoms began.

LING SHU 46

黃帝曰：一時遇風，同時得病，其病各異，願聞其故。少俞曰：夫一木之中，堅脆不同，堅者則剛，脆者易傷。人之有常病也，亦因其骨節皮膚腠理之不堅固者，邪之所舍也，故常為病也。

huáng dì yuē: yī shí yù fēng, tóng shí dé bìng, qí bìng gè yì, yuàn wén qí gù. shǎo yú yuē: fū yī mù zhī zhōng, jiān cuì bù tóng, jiān zhě zé gāng, cuì zhě yì shāng. rén zhī yǒu cháng bìng yě, yì yīn qí gǔ jié pí fū còu lǐ zhī bù jiān gù zhě, xié zhī suǒ shě yě, gù cháng wèi bìng yě.

The Yellow Emperor said: People meet the same wind at the same moment and fall ill together, yet their diseases differ; I wish to hear why. Shaoyu said: Within a single tree the wood is hard in one place and brittle in another, the hard part firm and the brittle easily harmed. So with a person: where the bones and joints, the skin, and the grain of the flesh are not firm, there the evil settles, and there the same illness comes again and again.

And the same evil does not make the same disease in everyone. The classic likens people to a stand of trees, where even a single tree is hard in one part and brittle in another, and different trees differ more; so where a person's bones and joints, skin, and the grain of the flesh are not firm, there the evil settles, and there the same illness tends to return. Susceptibility is written into the body's own terrain, and explains why one person's weakness is another's strength. With the evil, its point of entry, its hidden seed, and the body that meets it all accounted for, the classic is ready to take up the diseases one by one.

Wind, the Chief of the Hundred Evils

Of all the evils the classic gives wind the first place, and a chapter to itself.

SU WEN 42

黃帝問曰：風之傷人也，或為寒熱，或為熱中，或為寒中，或為癘風，或為偏枯，或為風也，其病各異，其名不同，或內至五藏六腑，不知其解，願聞其說。岐伯對曰：風氣藏於皮膚之間，內不得通，外不得泄。風者善行而數變，腠理開則洒然寒，閉則熱而悶，其寒也則衰食飲，其熱也則消肌肉，故使人怢慄而不能食，名曰寒熱。

huáng dì wèn yuē: fēng zhī shāng rén yě, huò wèi hán rè, huò wèi rè zhōng, huò wèi hán zhōng, huò wèi lì fēng, huò wèi piān kū, huò wèi fēng yě, qí bìng gè yì, qí míng bù tóng, huò nèi zhì wǔ zàng liù fǔ, bù zhī qí jiě, yuàn wén qí shuō. qí bó duì yuē: fēng qì cáng yú pí fū zhī jiān, nèi bù dé tōng, wài bù dé xiè. fēng zhě shàn xíng ér shuò biàn, còu lǐ kāi zé sǎ rán hán, bì zé rè ér mèn, qí hán yě zé shuāi shí yǐn, qí rè yě zé xiāo jī ròu, gù shǐ rén tū lì ér bù néng shí, míng yuē hán rè.

The Yellow Emperor asked: When wind injures a person, it becomes now cold and heat, now an inner-heat, now an inner-cold, now the pestilent wind, now a half-withering, now simply a wind; the diseases differ and the names differ, and some reach inward to the five organs and six palaces. I do not understand it, and wish to hear the explanation. Qibo answered: The wind-qi lodges between the skin and the flesh, where it can neither pass freely within nor vent without. Wind is good at moving and quick to change: when the pores open there is a shivering cold, when they close there is heat and oppression; in its cold it dulls the appetite, in its heat it wastes the flesh, so that a person shudders and cannot eat. This is named cold-and-heat.

Wind, it says, is good at moving and quick to change, and that is why it is the chief of the hundred diseases: it seldom stays one thing. Hidden in the skin, able neither to pass inward nor to vent outward, it becomes by turns a cold-and-heat, an inner heat or an inner cold, a pestilent wind, a half-withering of the body, each a different disorder under a different name, yet all of them wind wearing another face. To treat wind is therefore less to fix on a single disease than to recognise the one shifting evil behind many, and to follow it to wherever it has come to rest.

LING SHU 20

邪在肺，則病皮膚痛，寒熱，上氣喘，汗出，欬動肩背。邪在肝，則兩脅中痛。邪在脾胃，則病肌肉痛。邪在腎，則病骨痛、陰痹。邪在心，則病心痛，喜悲時眩仆。

xié zài fèi, zé bìng pí fū tòng, hán rè, shàng qì chuǎn, hàn chū, kài dòng jiān bèi. xié zài gān, zé liǎng xié zhōng tòng. xié zài pí wèi, zé bìng jī ròu tòng. xié zài shèn, zé bìng gǔ tòng, yīn bì. xié zài xīn, zé bìng xīn tòng, xǐ bēi shí xuàn pū.

When an evil is in the lung, there is aching skin, chills and fever, a rising panting breath, sweating, and a cough that shakes the shoulders and back. When it is in the liver, there is pain beneath the two flanks. When it is in the spleen and stomach, there is aching flesh. When it is in the kidney, there is aching bone and a hidden impediment. When it is in the heart, there is pain at the heart, with bouts of grief and sudden spells of dizziness and collapse.

The Spiritual Pivot sets this out organ by organ. An evil in the lung brings aching skin, chills and fever, a panting breath and a cough that shakes the shoulders; in the liver, pain beneath the two flanks; in the spleen and stomach, aching flesh; in the kidney, aching bone; in the heart, a pain at the heart with bouts of grief and sudden collapse. The same intruder declares itself differently according to which organ it has reached, so that the seat of the complaint names the organ to be treated, and one evil is tracked through the many signs it leaves.

Cold That Turns to Fever

The other great evil from without is cold, and the classic traces with unusual precision how a cold, once driven inward, becomes a fever.

SU WEN 31

黃帝問曰：今夫熱病者，皆傷寒之類也，或愈或死，其死皆以六七日之間，其愈皆以十日以上者，何也？不知其解，願聞其故。岐伯對曰：巨陽者，諸陽之屬也，其脈連於風府，故為諸陽主氣也。人之傷於寒也，則為病熱，熱雖甚不死；其兩感於寒而病者，必不免於死。

huáng dì wèn yuē: jīn fū rè bìng zhě, jiē shāng hán zhī lèi yě, huò yù huò sǐ, qí sǐ jiē yǐ liù qī rì zhī jiān, qí yù jiē yǐ shí rì yǐ shàng zhě, hé yě? bù zhī qí jiě, yuàn wén qí gù. qí bó duì yuē: jù yáng zhě, zhū yáng zhī shǔ yě, qí mài lián yú fēng fǔ, gù wèi zhū yáng zhǔ qì yě. rén zhī shāng yú hán yě, zé wèi bìng rè, rè suī shèn bù sǐ; qí liǎng gǎn yú hán ér bìng zhě, bì bù miǎn yú sǐ.

The Yellow Emperor asked: The fever diseases of today are all of the kind that come from cold-damage; some recover and some die, and those who die do so within six or seven days, while those who recover take ten days or more. Why is this? I do not understand it, and wish to hear the reason. Qibo answered: The great yang is the head of all the yang; its channel joins to the Wind Mansion, and so it governs the qi of all the yang. When a person is injured by cold, it becomes a fever-disease; and though the fever be severe, he does not die. But one who is doubly struck by cold and falls ill cannot escape death.

A fever of this kind, the classic says, is a sort of cold-damage, and it marches inward channel by channel on a daily schedule: the first day in the greater-yang, whose vessel joins the wind-mansion at the nape, the second in the yang-brightness, the third in the lesser-yang, and then into the three yin in turn. The day of the illness thus tells which channel holds the evil, so the physician needles the channel the disease has reached and reads recovery or decline by whether it halts there or sinks deeper. This daily march of cold through the six channels is the seed from which a whole later tradition of fever medicine would grow.

SU WEN 32

肝熱病者，小便先黃，腹痛多臥身熱。熱爭，則狂言及驚，脅滿痛，手足躁，不得安臥。庚辛甚，甲乙大汗，氣逆則庚辛死。刺足厥陰、少陽。其逆則頭痛員員，脈引衝頭也。

gān rè bìng zhě, xiǎo biàn xiān huáng, fù tòng duō wò shēn rè. rè zhēng, zé kuáng yán jí jīng, xié mǎn tòng, shǒu zú zào, bù dé ān wò. gēng xīn shèn, jiǎ yǐ dà hán, qì nì zé gēng xīn sǐ. cì zú jué yīn, shào yáng. qí nì zé tóu tòng yuán yuán, mài yǐn chōng tóu yě.

In a liver heat-disease, the urine first turns yellow, the belly aches, the patient lies about much, and the body is hot. When the heat contends, there is raving and fright, the flanks are full and painful, the hands and feet are restless, and he cannot lie at ease. It is worst on the days geng and xin, and breaks in a great sweat on jia and yi; when the qi runs counter, death comes on geng and xin. Needle the foot reverting-yin and lesser-yang. When it runs counter, the headache throbs round and round, for the pulse draws upward and surges to the head.

When the heat settles in a particular organ it announces itself before the fever is full. A heat-disease of the liver begins with yellowed urine, a sore belly, much lying about, and a hot body, and only then, as the heat contends, comes the raving and fright; each organ has its own early signs in this way. Catching them, the classic needles the organ's own channels, here the foot reverting-yin and lesser-yang, treating the heat as it gathers rather than waiting for its height.

SU WEN 33

黃帝問曰：有病溫者，汗出輒復熱，而脈躁疾，不為汗衰，狂言不能食，病名為何？岐伯對曰：病名陰陽交，交者死也。帝曰：願聞其說。岐伯曰：人所以汗出者，皆生於穀，穀生於精。今邪氣交爭於骨肉而得汗者，是邪卻而精勝也。精勝則當能食而不復熱。復熱者邪氣也，汗者精氣也，今汗出而輒復熱者，是邪勝也，不能食者，精無俾也，病而留者，其壽可立而傾也。

huáng dì wèn yuē: yǒu bìng wēn zhě, hàn chū zhé fù rè, ér mài zào jí, bù wèi hàn shuāi, kuáng yán bù néng shí, bìng míng wèi hé? qí bó duì yuē: bìng míng yīn yáng jiāo, jiāo zhě sǐ yě. dì yuē: yuàn wén qí shuō. qí bó yuē: rén suǒ yǐ hàn chū zhě, jiē shēng yú gǔ, gǔ shēng yú jīng. jīn xié qì jiāo zhēng yú gǔ ròu ér dé hàn zhě, shì xié què ér jīng shèng yě. jīng shèng zé dāng néng shí ér bù fù rè. fù rè zhě xié qì yě, hàn zhě jīng qì yě, jīn hàn chū ér zhé fù rè zhě, shì xié shèng yě, bù néng shí zhě, jīng wú bǐ yě, bìng ér liú zhě, qí shòu kě lì ér qīng yě.

The Yellow Emperor asked: There is a warm disease in which the sweat breaks and at once the fever returns, the pulse is restless and rapid and does not wane with the sweat, the patient raves and cannot eat. What is this disease called? Qibo answered: It is called the crossing of yin and yang, and one who crosses thus dies. The Emperor said: I wish to hear the explanation. Qibo said: The reason a person sweats is that the sweat is born of the grain, and the grain is born of the essence. Now when the evil qi and the body contend in the bones and flesh and a sweat is won, it means the evil has retreated and the essence has prevailed. When the essence prevails, the patient should be able to eat and the fever should not return. That the fever returns is the evil qi; that there is sweat is the essence qi; so when the sweat breaks and at once the fever returns, it means the evil has prevailed, and that he cannot eat means the essence has nothing to draw on. With the disease thus lodged, his life may topple in a moment.

Not every fever can be turned, and the classic names the worst of them exactly. In one, the sweat breaks and the fever at once returns, the pulse stays rapid and does not wane with the sweat, and the patient raves and cannot eat. This it calls the crossing of yin and yang, and says without hedging that the crossing brings death, for sweat is made from the body's own essence, and here the essence pours out while the evil stays behind. The lesson is one of prognosis: to know the pattern that will not yield, and not to mistake a doomed fever for a treatable one.

LING SHU 23

熱病已得汗出，而脈尚躁盛，此陰脈之極也，死；其得汗而脈靜者，生。熱病者，脈尚盛躁而不得汗者，此陽脈之極也，死。

rè bìng yǐ dé hàn chū, ér mài shàng zào shèng, cǐ yīn mài zhī jí yě, sǐ; qí dé hàn ér mài jìng zhě, shēng. rè bìng zhě, mài shàng shèng zào ér bù dé hàn zhě, cǐ yáng mài zhī jí yě, sǐ.

When a febrile disease has already brought sweat, yet the pulse is still agitated and full, this is the extreme of the yin vessels, and death follows; but if the sweat comes and the pulse grows quiet, the patient lives. When in a febrile disease the pulse is still full and agitated and yet no sweat comes, this is the extreme of the yang vessels, and death follows.

The Spiritual Pivot draws the same line between the fevers that can be helped and those that cannot. If the sweat comes and the pulse then grows quiet, the patient lives; but if the pulse stays agitated and full after the sweat, or if no sweat comes at all while the pulse races, the vessels have reached their extreme and death follows. The needle is used to vent a heat while the body can still answer it, and withheld where these signs show the essence already spent. Cold driven inward becomes fever; read by its daily march, by its organ signs, and above all by whether the body can still respond, it is met early with the needle or, when the signs are fatal, recognised and let be.

The Intermittent Fevers

Some fevers do not stay but come and go on a clock of their own, and the classic gives the malarias two chapters to explain that strange timing and to needle it.

SU WEN 35

黃帝問曰：夫痎瘧皆生於風，其蓄作有時者何也？岐伯對曰：瘧之始發也，先起於毫毛，伸欠乃作，寒慄鼓頷，腰脊俱痛，寒去則內外皆熱，頭痛如破，渴欲冷飲。

huáng dì wèn yuē: fū jiē nüè jiē shēng yú fēng, qí xù zuò yǒu shí zhě hé yě? qí bó duì yuē: nüè zhī shǐ fā yě, xiān qǐ yú háo máo, shēn qiàn nǎi zuò, hán lì gǔ hàn, yāo jí jù tòng, hán qù zé nèi wài jiē rè, tóu tòng rú pò, kě yù lěng yǐn.

The Yellow Emperor asked: The malarial fevers all arise from wind, yet they gather and break out at set times. Why is this? Qibo answered: When a malaria first breaks out, it begins in the body hair: the patient stretches and yawns, then shivers and his jaw chatters, the loins and spine all ache; and when the cold goes, inside and outside both burn, the head aches as if splitting, and he is thirsty for cold drink.

A malaria, the classic says, arises from wind, yet breaks out only at set times. Each attack begins in the fine body-hairs with yawning and stretching, then a shivering cold that sets the jaw chattering and aches the spine; and when the cold passes the whole body turns to heat, the head splitting, the patient craving cold water. The disease is a single thing swinging between two opposite states, and the swing, not either state alone, is what marks it.

SU WEN 35

夫瘧之未發也，陰未並陽，陽未並陰，因而調之，真氣得安，邪氣乃亡，故工不能治其已發，為其氣逆也。其間日而作者，由邪氣內薄於五藏，橫連募原也，其道遠，其氣深，其行遲，不能與衛氣俱行，不得皆出，故間日乃作也。

fū nüè zhī wèi fā yě, yīn wèi bìng yáng, yáng wèi bìng yīn, yīn ér diào zhī, zhēn qì dé ān, xié qì nǎi wáng, gù gōng bù néng zhì qí yǐ fā, wèi qí qì nì yě. qí jiān rì ér zuò zhě, yóu xié qì nèi báo yú wǔ zàng, héng lián mù yuán yě, qí dào yuǎn, qí qì shēn, qí xíng chí, bù néng yǔ wèi qì jù xíng, bù dé jiē chū, gù jiān rì nǎi zuò yě.

Before a malaria breaks out, the yin has not yet gathered into the yang nor the yang into the yin; regulate it then, and the true qi is set at ease and the evil qi perishes. So the physician cannot treat it once it has broken out, because the qi is then in counterflow. As for the malaria that breaks out every other day: the evil qi has pressed inward against the five organs and spread crosswise to the membrane-source; its road is far, its qi deep, its movement slow, so that it cannot travel together with the defensive qi nor all come out at once, and so it breaks out only every other day.

Why it returns on a schedule the classic explains by the meeting of the defensive qi with the lodged evil: only when the two come together does an attack break, and where the evil sits deep, drawn back into the organs, it meets the defensive qi but every second day, so the fever skips one. The practical lesson follows at once. Treat in the lull, before the attack, while yin and yang have not yet gathered to clash; for once the fever is breaking, the qi runs counter and the moment is lost.

SU WEN 36

足太陽之瘧，令人腰痛頭重，寒從背起，先寒後熱，熇熇暍暍然，熱止汗出，難已，刺郄中出血。足少陽之瘧，令人身體解㑊，寒不甚，熱不甚，惡見人，見人心惕惕然，熱多汗出甚，刺足少陽。足陽明之瘧，令人先寒，洒淅洒淅，寒甚久乃熱，熱去汗出，喜見日月光火氣乃快然，刺足陽明跗上。

zú tài yáng zhī nüè, lìng rén yāo tòng tóu zhòng, hán cóng bèi qǐ, xiān hán hòu rè, hè hè yē yē rán, rè zhǐ hàn chū, nán yǐ, cì qiè zhōng chū xiě. zú shào yáng zhī nüè, lìng rén shēn tǐ jiě yì, hán bù shèn, rè bù shèn, è jiàn rén, jiàn rén xīn tì tì rán, rè duō hàn chū shèn, cì zú shào yáng. zú yáng míng zhī nüè, lìng rén xiān hán, sǎ xī sǎ xī, hán shèn jiǔ nǎi rè, rè qù hàn chū, xǐ jiàn rì yuè guāng huǒ qì nǎi kuài rán, cì zú yáng míng fū shàng.

A malaria of the foot great yang makes the loins ache and the head heavy, the cold rising from the back, cold first and heat after, blazing and sweltering; when the heat stops, the sweat breaks, and it is hard to end. Needle the hollow of the knee and let out blood. A malaria of the foot lesser yang makes the body slack and weary, the cold not severe and the heat not severe; the patient loathes the sight of people, and seeing them his heart starts in fright; the heat is much and the sweating heavy. Needle the foot lesser yang. A malaria of the foot bright yang makes the patient cold first, shivering and shrinking; the cold is severe and lasts long before the heat comes, and when the heat goes the sweat breaks; he delights in the light of sun and moon and the warmth of fire, which ease him. Needle the foot bright yang on the instep.

The needling is matched to the channel the malaria has taken. The foot greater-yang form aches the loins and weighs the head; for it the classic opens a vessel behind the knee and lets blood. Each form has its own channel and point, so the pattern, by where it strikes and how its cold and heat balance, chooses where to needle, struck in the lull rather than the blaze.

Cough

A complaint as ordinary as a cough the classic treats with characteristic breadth, refusing to lay it all at one door.

SU WEN 38

黃帝問曰：肺之令人欬何也？岐伯對曰：五藏六腑皆令人欬，非獨肺也。帝曰：願聞其狀。岐伯曰：皮毛者，肺之合也，皮毛先受邪氣，邪氣以從其合也。其寒飲食入胃，從肺脈上至於肺則肺寒，肺寒則外內合邪，因而客之，則為肺欬。

huáng dì wèn yuē: fèi zhī lìng rén kài hé yě? qí bó duì yuē: wǔ zàng liù fǔ jiē lìng rén kài, fēi dú fèi yě. dì yuē: yuàn wén qí zhuàng. qí bó yuē: pí máo zhě, fèi zhī hé yě, pí máo xiān shòu xié qì, xié qì yǐ cóng qí hé yě. qí hán yǐn shí rù wèi, cóng fèi mài shàng zhì yú fèi zé fèi hán, fèi hán zé wài nèi hé xié, yīn ér kè zhī, zé wèi fèi kài.

The Yellow Emperor asked: How is it that the lung makes a person cough? Qibo answered: All five organs and six palaces can make a person cough, not the lung alone. The Emperor said: I wish to hear how. Qibo said: The skin and body hair are the lung's match; the skin and hair receive the evil qi first, and the evil follows that match inward. And when cold food and drink enter the stomach, they rise along the lung channel to the lung, so the lung turns cold; the cold lung joins an evil within to one without, and being thus lodged in, it becomes a lung-cough.

The lung is not the only cause of a cough, it insists; all five organs and the six palaces can bring one on. Cold taken in through the skin does reach the lung, but each organ, struck in its own season, passes its disorder to the lung in turn, so that a cough may be a liver-cough or a kidney-cough by the signs that come with it, and if it lasts it moves on again from the organ to its paired palace. A cough is therefore read for its source and treated at the organ behind it rather than at the throat, which is why the same symptom asks for different points in different patients, and why even a cough is a sign pointing inward.

The Roots of Pain

Pain the classic treats not as one thing but as a sign with causes, and two of them it singles out: cold, and the movements of the feelings.

> SU WEN 39
>
> 黃帝問曰：願聞人之五藏卒痛，何氣使然？岐伯對曰：經脈流行不止，環周不休，寒氣入經而稽遲，泣而不行，客於脈外則血少，客於脈中則氣不通，故卒然而痛。
>
> *huáng dì wèn yuē: yuàn wén rén zhī wǔ zàng zú tòng, hé qì shǐ rán? qí bó duì yuē: jīng mài liú xíng bù zhǐ, huán zhōu bù xiū, hán qì rù jīng ér jī chí, qì ér bù xíng, kè yú mài wài zé xuè shǎo, kè yú mài zhōng zé qì bù tōng, gù zú rán ér tòng.*
>
> The Yellow Emperor asked: I wish to hear of the sudden pains in a person's five organs; what qi makes them? Qibo answered: The channel-vessels flow on without stopping, circling the body without rest; when cold qi enters a channel it makes the flow halt and lag, congealing so that it does not move. Lodging outside the vessel, it leaves the blood scant; lodging within the vessel, it stops the qi from passing; and so pain comes on suddenly.

The channel-vessels flow on without stopping, the classic says, until cold enters and makes them lag: the blood congeals and will not move, and where it is blocked, outside the vessel or within, the qi cannot pass, and a sudden pain arises. Pain, in this account, is most often a stoppage, and cold its commonest cause, which is why warmth so often eases it and cold deepens it.

The same chapter holds one of the classic's most quoted sentences: the hundred diseases arise from qi. It then lists how the feelings move it: anger drives the qi up, joy loosens it, grief consumes it, fear sends it down, fright scatters it, cold contracts it, overwork wears it out, and brooding knots it. It is a plain map of how a mood or a strain becomes a disorder of the body, and it is why this medicine asks after a person's life and feelings as closely as it asks after their symptoms.

SU WEN 39

帝曰：善。余知百病生於氣也，怒則氣上，喜則氣緩，悲則氣消，恐則氣下，寒則氣收，炅則氣泄，驚則氣亂，勞則氣耗，思則氣結，九氣不同，何病之生？

dì yuē: shàn. yú zhī bǎi bìng shēng yú qì yě, nù zé qì shàng, xǐ zé qì huǎn, bēi zé qì xiāo, kǒng zé qì xià, hán zé qì shōu, jiǒng zé qì xiè, jīng zé qì luàn, láo zé qì hào, sī zé qì jié, jiǔ qì bù tóng, hé bìng zhī shēng?

The Emperor said: Good. I know that the hundred diseases arise from the qi. Anger sends the qi upward; joy slackens it; grief consumes it; fear sends it down; cold draws it in; heat lets it leak out; fright throws it into disorder; toil wears it away; and pondering knots it. These nine are not alike; what diseases arise from them?

But the same chapter widens to one of the classic's most quoted lines, that the hundred diseases arise from the qi, and lists how the feelings move it: anger drives the qi up, joy slackens it, grief consumes it, fear sends it down, fright throws it into disorder, and brooding ties it in a knot. Pain and much else besides are thus traced to a qi pushed the wrong way by feeling, so that the physician asks after the state of mind as well as the body, and treats a knotted or a risen qi as a real cause and not a mood.

SU WEN 41

足太陽脈令人腰痛，引項脊尻背如重狀，刺其郄中太陽正經出血，春無見血。

zú tài yáng mài lìng rén yāo tòng, yǐn xiàng jí kāo bèi rú zhòng zhuàng, cì qí qiè zhōng tài yáng zhèng jīng chū xiě, chūn wú jiàn xuè.

The foot great-yang vessel makes the loins ache, drawing at the nape, spine, buttocks, and back as though they were weighed down. Needle the proper great-yang channel at the hollow of the knee and let out blood; but in spring let no blood.

Where the pain is fixed, the classic needles by the channel that bears it. A low-back pain of the foot greater-yang drags at the nape, spine, and buttocks as though they were weighted, and is met by opening that channel behind the knee; other backs ache along other channels and are needled along them. The line of the pain names the channel, and the channel gives the point.

> LING SHU 53
>
> 黃帝曰：人之耐痛與不耐痛，何以知之？少俞曰：人之骨強、筋弱、肉緩、皮膚厚者耐痛，其於鍼石之痛，火焫亦然。堅肉薄皮者，不耐鍼石之痛，於火焫亦然。
>
> *huáng dì yuē: rén zhī nài tòng yǔ bù nài tòng, hé yǐ zhī zhī? shǎo yú yuē: rén zhī gǔ qiáng, jīn ruò, ròu huǎn, pí fū hòu zhě nài tòng, qí yú zhēn shí zhī tòng, huǒ ruò yì rán. jiān ròu báo pí zhě, bù nài zhēn shí zhī tòng, yú huǒ ruò yì rán.*
>
> The Yellow Emperor said: How is one to know who will bear pain and who will not? Shaoyu said: Those whose bone is strong, whose sinew is yielding, whose flesh is slack and whose skin is thick will bear pain, and bear likewise the pain of the needle, the lancet, and the burning moxa. Those with firm flesh and thin skin do not bear the pain of the needle or the lancet, nor that of the moxa either.

And pain, the classic notes finally, is not felt the same by all. A strong bone, a yielding sinew, slack flesh, and thick skin bear pain well, the needle and the moxa with it; firm flesh under thin skin bears them poorly. The practitioner judges a person's tolerance before reaching for needle or moxa, fitting the force of the treatment to the body that must endure it. Cold and feeling at its root, named by its channel, and weighed against the patient's own endurance, pain becomes for the classic not a thing to silence but a sign to read.

The Impediments

A whole family of disorders the classic groups under one name, the impediment, where something settles in the body and blocks the free movement of qi and blood.

> SU WEN 43
>
> 黃帝問曰：痺之安生？岐伯對曰：風寒濕三氣雜至，合而為痺也。其風氣勝者為行痺，寒氣勝者為痛痺，濕氣勝者為著痺也。
>
> *huáng dì wèn yuē: bì zhī ān shēng? qí bó duì yuē: fēng hán shī sān qì zá zhì, hé ér wèi bì yě. qí fēng qì shèng zhě wèi xíng bì, hán qì shèng zhě wèi tòng bì, shī qì shèng zhě wèi zhù bì yě.*
>
> The Yellow Emperor asked: How does blockage arise? Qibo answered: When the three qi of wind, cold, and damp arrive mingled together, they join to make a blockage. Where the wind-qi prevails, it is a moving blockage; where the cold-qi prevails, a painful blockage; where the damp-qi prevails, a fixed blockage.

The impediment arises, it says, when the three evils of wind, cold, and damp arrive together and join, and its character follows whichever of the three prevails: wind dominant makes a wandering impediment that shifts from joint to joint; cold dominant a painful impediment, fixed and aching; damp dominant a heavy, lodged impediment that will not move. To treat one is therefore first to weigh which evil leads, since the wandering, the painful, and the heavy ask for different handling though they share a single cause.

> LING SHU 27
>
> 周痹者，在於血脈之中，隨脈以上，隨脈以下，不能左右，各當其所。
>
> *zhōu bì zhě, zài yú xuè mài zhī zhōng, suí mài yǐ shàng, suí mài yǐ xià, bù néng zuǒ yòu, gè dāng qí suǒ.*
>
> The all-over impediment lies within the blood-vessels; it follows a vessel upward and follows it downward, but cannot cross from side to side, keeping each time to its own place.

One form travels. The all-over impediment, the Spiritual Pivot says, lies within the blood-vessels and moves along them, up a vessel and down it, but cannot cross from side to side, keeping to the line of the channel it has entered. Because it follows the vessel, it is met along that vessel's course, its travelling read as the evil carried by the blood rather than spreading at random. Wind, cold, and damp combined, named by which leads and by whether it stays or travels, the impediment is a blockage to be traced and freed.

The Wiltings

Against the impediments the classic sets the wiltings, where the limbs do not ache but fail, losing their strength until they can no longer be used.

SU WEN 44

黃帝問曰：五藏使人痿何也？岐伯對曰：肺主身之皮毛，心主身之血脈，肝主身之筋膜，脾主身之肌肉，腎主身之骨髓。故肺熱葉焦，則皮毛虛弱急薄，著則生痿躄也。

huáng dì wèn yuē: wǔ zàng shǐ rén wěi hé yě? qí bó duì yuē: fèi zhǔ shēn zhī pí máo, xīn zhǔ shēn zhī xuè mài, gān zhǔ shēn zhī jīn mó, pí zhǔ shēn zhī jī ròu, shèn zhǔ shēn zhī gǔ suǐ. gù fèi rè yè jiāo, zé pí máo xū ruò jí báo, zhù zé shēng wěi bì yě.

The Yellow Emperor asked: How do the five organs make a person waste and wilt? Qibo answered: The lung governs the skin and body hair, the heart the blood vessels, the liver the sinews and their sheaths, the spleen the flesh, and the kidney the bones and marrow. So when the lung is hot and its lobes scorched, the skin and hair grow weak, taut, and thin, and once this sets in, there arises a wilting-lameness.

Each organ governs a tissue, the lung the skin and hair, the heart the vessels, the liver the sinews, the spleen the flesh, the kidney the bones; and a wilting begins, characteristically, when heat in the lung scorches its leaves, so that the skin and hair thin and weaken and the legs give way beneath the body. The wilting is read back to a heat drying the tissue an organ feeds, most often the lung, so the cause sought is a scorching dryness and not a blockage.

SU WEN 44

帝曰：論言治痿者獨取陽明何也？岐伯曰：陽明者，五藏六腑之海，主潤宗筋，宗筋主束骨而利機關也。衝脈者，經脈之海也，主滲灌谿谷，與陽明合於宗筋。陽明虛則宗筋縱，帶脈不引，故足痿不用也。帝曰：治之奈何？岐伯曰：各補其滎而通其俞，調其虛實，和其逆順，筋脈骨肉，各以其時受月，則病已矣。

dì yuē: lùn yán zhì wěi zhě dú qǔ yáng míng hé yě? qí bó yuē: yáng míng zhě, wǔ zàng liù fǔ zhī hǎi, zhǔ rùn zōng jīn, zōng jīn zhǔ shù gǔ ér lì jī guān yě. chōng mài zhě, jīng mài zhī hǎi yě, zhǔ shèn guàn xī gǔ, yǔ yáng míng hé yú zōng jīn. yáng míng xū zé zōng jīn zòng, dài mài bù yǐn, gù zú wěi bù yòng yě. dì yuē: zhì zhī nài hé? qí bó yuē: gè bǔ qí xíng ér tōng qí yú, diào qí xū shí, hé qí nì shùn, jīn mài gǔ ròu, gè yǐ qí shí shòu yuè, zé bìng yǐ yǐ.

The Emperor asked: The discourse says that in treating wilting one takes the bright yang alone; why? Qibo said: The bright yang is the sea of the five organs and six palaces, and it governs the moistening of the ancestral sinew, which binds the bones and frees the joints. The thrusting vessel is the sea of the channels, governing the irrigation of the larger and smaller hollows, and it joins the bright yang at the ancestral sinew. When the bright yang is empty, the ancestral sinew slackens and the belt-vessel cannot draw it taut, so the foot wilts and will not serve. The Emperor asked: How is it treated? Qibo said: Supplement each organ at its spring point and free its transport point, regulate its emptiness and repletion, harmonise what runs counter and what runs with, and let the sinews, vessels, bones, and flesh each receive treatment in the month of its season; then the disease ends.

And the classic gives the wiltings a single famous rule of treatment, to take the yang-brightness alone. The yang-brightness is the sea of the organs and palaces and the source that moistens the great sinews which bind the joints and work the limbs; let it run empty and the sinews slacken and the legs fail. To restore a wilting, then, the physician nourishes the yang-brightness, rebuilding the stomach and its sea so that the tissues are fed and fill again, a rule still central to the treatment of weakness in the limbs.

The Reversals

A third family the classic calls reversal, where the qi runs counter to its proper course, with sudden and sometimes grave effects.

> SU WEN 45
>
> 黃帝問曰：厥之寒熱者何也？岐伯對曰：陽氣衰於下，則為寒厥；陰氣衰於下，則為熱厥。
>
> *huáng dì wèn yuē: jué zhī hán rè zhě hé yě? qí bó duì yuē: yáng qì shuāi yú xià, zé wèi hán jué; yīn qì shuāi yú xià, zé wèi rè jué.*
>
> The Yellow Emperor asked: As for the cold and the heat of reversal, what are they? Qibo answered: When the yang qi wanes below, there is cold-reversal; when the yin qi wanes below, there is heat-reversal.

In its plainest form the reversal is a failure of warmth or of cooling at the body's foundation: when the yang wanes below, a cold-reversal follows, the limbs turning cold from the feet up; when the yin wanes below, a heat-reversal, a burning rising instead. The chill or the heat of the extremities is read as the qi reversed at the root, and treated by restoring the waning yang or yin rather than the limb itself.

SU WEN 37

黃帝問曰：五藏六腑，寒熱相移者何？岐伯曰：腎移寒於肝，癰腫少氣。脾移寒於肝，癰腫筋攣。肝移寒於心，狂，膈中。心移寒於肺，肺消，肺消者飲一溲二，死不治。肺移寒於腎，為湧水，湧水者，按腹不堅，水氣客於大腸，疾行則鳴濯濯，如囊裹漿，水之病也。

huáng dì wèn yuē: wǔ zàng liù fǔ, hán rè xiāng yí zhě hé? qí bó yuē: shèn yí hán yú gān, yōng zhǒng shǎo qì. pí yí hán yú gān, yōng zhǒng jīn luán. gān yí hán yú xīn, kuáng, gé zhōng. xīn yí hán yú fèi, fèi xiāo, fèi xiāo zhě yǐn yī sōu èr, sǐ bù zhì. fèi yí hán yú shèn, wèi yǒng shuǐ, yǒng shuǐ zhě, àn fù bù jiān, shuǐ qì kè yú dà cháng, jí xíng zé míng zhuó zhuó, rú náng guǒ jiāng, shuǐ zhī bìng yě.

The Yellow Emperor asked: When the five organs and six palaces pass cold and heat to one another, what comes of it? Qibo said: When the kidney passes cold to the liver, there are abscesses, swelling, and scant qi. When the spleen passes cold to the liver, there are abscesses, swelling, and cramping sinews. When the liver passes cold to the heart, there is mania and a blockage in the diaphragm. When the heart passes cold to the lung, there is lung-wasting; in lung-wasting the patient drinks one measure and passes two, and it is fatal and cannot be treated. When the lung passes cold to the kidney, there is surging-water; in surging-water, pressing the belly finds it not firm, the water qi having lodged as a guest in the large intestine, so that walking briskly makes a sloshing sound, like a bag holding fluid; it is a disease of water.

The classic then traces how a disorder passes from organ to organ, each handing its cold or its heat to the next: the kidney passing cold to the liver, the liver to the heart, and so along a chain, some of the transfers mild and some, like the wasting of the lung in which a person drinks once and passes water twice, fatal. A disease is followed along the organs it moves through, so that a sign in one is read as cold or heat received from another, and the chain, not the single organ, is what must be treated.

LING SHU 24

厥頭痛，面若腫起而煩心，取之足陽明、太陰。真頭痛，頭痛甚，腦盡痛，手足寒至節，死不治。

jué tóu tòng, miàn ruò zhǒng qǐ ér fán xīn, qǔ zhī zú yáng míng, tài yīn. zhēn tóu tòng, tóu tòng shèn, nǎo jǐn tòng, shǒu zú hán zhì jié, sǐ bù zhì.

In a reversal headache the face seems swollen and the heart is vexed; take it at the foot yang-brightness and greater-yin. In a true headache the pain is severe, the whole brain aches, and the hands and feet are cold up to the joints; this is fatal and beyond treatment.

And the reversals reach the head. A reversal-headache swells the face and vexes the heart, and is met at the foot yang-brightness and greater-yin; but the classic carefully sets apart from it a true headache, where the pain is severe, the whole brain aches, and the hands and feet turn cold to the joints, and says plainly that this one is fatal and beyond the needle. The distinction is prognostic above all, parting a reversal that can be turned from a collapse of the qi at the head that cannot. Counter-running at the root, along the organs, or risen to the head, the reversal is read by its direction and met by turning the qi back, wherever it can still be turned.

Distension and Water

A swollen belly may be filled with qi or with water, and the classic is at pains to tell the two apart, since they look alike yet ask for opposite treatment.

LING SHU 35

黃帝曰：脹者焉生？何因而有？岐伯曰：厥氣在下，營衛留止，寒氣逆上，真邪相攻，兩氣相搏，乃合為脹也。

huáng dì yuē: zhàng zhě yān shēng? hé yīn ér yǒu? qí bó yuē: jué qì zài xià, yíng wèi liú zhǐ, hán qì nì shàng, zhēn xié xiāng gōng, liǎng qì xiāng bó, nǎi hé wèi zhàng yě.

The Yellow Emperor said: Where do distensions come from, and by what cause do they arise? Qibo said: A reversed qi sits below, the nutritive and defensive are held up and stalled, a cold qi rises counter against them, and the true and the evil fall to fighting; the two forces grapple, and from their meeting a distension is formed.

A distension, it says, forms when a reversed qi sits low and the nutritive and defensive are stalled, a cold rising counter against them until the true and the evil grapple and their struggle swells the body. The qi-distension is thus read as a blockage of the circulating qi, relieved by freeing the stalled flow and settling the counter-rising cold, not by drawing off any fluid, for there is none to draw.

LING SHU 57

水始起也，目窠上微腫，如新臥起之狀，頸脈動，時欬，足脛腫，腹乃大，其水已成矣。以手按其腹，隨手而起，如裹水之狀，此其候也。

shuǐ shǐ qǐ yě, mù kē shàng wēi zhǒng, rú xīn wò qǐ zhī zhuàng, jǐng mài dòng, shí kài, zú jìng zhǒng, fù nǎi dà, qí shuǐ yǐ chéng yǐ. yǐ shǒu àn qí fù, suí shǒu ér qǐ, rú guǒ shuǐ zhī zhuàng, cǐ qí hòu yě.

When water-swelling first begins, there is a slight puffiness above the eye-sockets, as in one just risen from sleep; the neck vessel throbs, there is an occasional cough, the shins

> swell, and at last the belly grows large, the water now fully formed. Press the belly with the hand and it rises back at once, as though it wrapped water; this is its sign.

Water is another matter, and the classic gives a bedside test for it. A water-swelling begins with a faint puffiness above the eyes, a throbbing neck-vessel and an occasional cough, then swollen shins and at last a great belly; and pressed with the hand, such a belly springs back at once, as though it wrapped water, where a qi-distension instead stays pitted as the finger lifts. The single act of pressing the belly and watching whether it rebounds or holds the dent separates water from qi, and so decides whether to drain a fluid or to move a stalled qi.

> SU WEN 40
>
> 黃帝問曰：有病心腹滿，旦食則不能暮食，此為何病？岐伯對曰：名為鼓脹。帝曰：治之奈何？岐伯曰：治之以雞矢醴，一劑知，二劑已。帝曰：其時有復發者何也？岐伯曰：此飲食不節，故時有病也。雖然其病且已時，故當病氣聚於腹也。
>
> *huáng dì wèn yuē: yǒu bìng xīn fù mǎn, dàn shí zé bù néng mù shí, cǐ wèi hé bìng? qí bó duì yuē: míng wèi gǔ zhàng. dì yuē: zhì zhī nài hé? qí bó yuē: zhì zhī yǐ jī shǐ lǐ, yī jì zhī, èr jì yǐ. dì yuē: qí shí yǒu fù fā zhě hé yě? qí bó yuē: cǐ yǐn shí bù jié, gù shí yǒu bìng yě. suī rán qí bìng qiě yǐ shí, gù dāng bìng qì jù yú fù yě.*
>
> The Yellow Emperor asked: There is a disease in which the heart and belly are full, so that one who eats in the morning cannot eat at evening. What disease is this? Qibo answered: It is named drum-distension. The Emperor asked: How is it treated? Qibo said: Treat it with the chicken-dropping ferment: one dose and it answers, two and it is over. The Emperor asked: Why does it sometimes return? Qibo said: This comes of food and drink without measure, and so the disease returns from time to time. Even when the disease is about to end, the disease-qi still gathers in the belly.

The Basic Questions adds a named case and, unusually, a prescription. A heart and belly so full that a morning meal cannot be followed by an evening one it calls drum-distension, and treats with a ferment, one dose to take effect and a second to finish; yet it warns that the disease returns where eating stays unmeasured. Even a specific remedy is bound to its cause, so the cure is paired with a change of habit, the ferment relieving the present distension and restraint forestalling the next.

The Spirit Astray

The classic counts disorders of the mind and the senses among diseases like any other, with causes in the body and signs to be read, not set apart as afflictions of another kind.

> LING SHU 22
>
> 癲疾始生，先不樂，頭重痛，視舉目赤，甚作極已而煩心。狂始發，少臥不飢，自高賢也，自辨智也，自尊貴也，善罵詈，日夜不休。
>
> *diān jí shǐ shēng, xiān bù lè, tóu zhòng tòng, shì jǔ mù chì, shèn zuò jí yǐ ér fán xīn. kuáng shǐ fā, shǎo wò bù jī, zì gāo xián yě, zì biàn zhì yě, zì zūn guì yě, shàn mà lì, rì yè bù xiū.*
>
> When the withdrawal-disease first arises, there is first a joylessness, a heavy aching head, the gaze lifted and the eyes reddened, and at its height a vexation of the heart. When mania first breaks out, the person sleeps little and feels no hunger; he holds himself a sage, calls himself wise, exalts himself as noble, and rails and curses without stopping, day and night.

It distinguishes two great disturbances of the spirit. The withdrawal-disease begins in joylessness, a heavy aching head and reddened, lifted eyes, rising to a vexed heart; mania breaks out the other way, in sleeplessness without hunger, the person grown grandiose, calling himself wise and noble and railing and cursing day and night. Each is read by its onset and its bearing, the one sunk and clouded, the other raised and overflowing, and each traced to the qi, withdrawal to a sinking and mania to an excess, so that the treatment moves to lift or to drain accordingly.

LING SHU 80

五藏六府之精氣，皆上注於目而為之精。邪中於項，因逢其身之虛，深入則隨眼系入於腦，入於腦則腦轉，腦轉則引目系急，目系急則目眩以轉矣。

wǔ zàng liù fǔ zhī jīng qì, jiē shàng zhù yú mù ér wèi zhī jīng. xié zhōng yú xiàng, yīn féng qí shēn zhī xū, shēn rù zé suí yǎn xì rù yú nǎo, rù yú nǎo zé nǎo zhuǎn, nǎo zhuǎn zé yǐn mù xì jí, mù xì jí zé mù xuàn yǐ zhuǎn yǐ.

The essence-qi of the five organs and six palaces all pours upward into the eyes and becomes their seeing-essence. When an evil strikes the nape and meets a vacuity in the body, it sinks deep along the eye-stalk into the brain; once in the brain it sets the brain turning, the turning drags the eye-stalk tight, and the tightened stalk makes the eyes swim and the head spin.

And it grounds even dizziness in the body's plumbing. The essence of all the organs pours upward into the eyes to become their power of sight; so when an evil strikes the nape, meets a weakness, and follows the eye-stalk into the brain, it sets the brain turning, drags the eye-stalk tight, and the world swims and spins. A clouded head and a reeling sight are read as the essence at the eyes disturbed at its root in the brain and organs, and treated there, rather than dismissed as a vagueness of the mind. Sunk or overflowing in the spirit, or set spinning at the eyes, these too are diseases of qi and essence, met in the body that produces them.

The Lesser Disorders

The classic does not hold the smallest complaints beneath explanation, and gives a chapter to the body's involuntary tics, each traced to a movement of qi.

LING SHU 28

黃帝曰：人之欠者，何氣使然？岐伯曰：陰陽相引，故數欠。人之太息者，何氣使然？岐伯曰：憂思則心系急，心系急則氣道約，約則不利，故太息以伸出之。

huáng dì yuē: rén zhī qiàn zhě, hé qì shǐ rán? qí bó yuē: yīn yáng xiāng yǐn, gù shuò qiàn. rén zhī tài xī zhě, hé qì shǐ rán? qí bó yuē: yōu sī zé xīn xì jí, xīn xì jí zé qì dào yuē, yuē zé bù lì, gù tài xī yǐ shēn chū zhī.

The Yellow Emperor said: When a person yawns, what qi brings it on? Qibo said: The yin draws downward and the yang upward, and as the two pull against each other one yawns again and again. The Emperor said: And the long sigh, what qi brings that? Qibo said: Worry and brooding tighten the cords of the heart, the tightened cords narrow the passage of the qi, the narrowed passage will not run free, and so one draws a long sigh to stretch it open.

A yawn, it says, comes when the yin draws the qi down and the yang draws it up and the two pull against each other; a long sigh, when worry tightens the cords of the heart and narrows the passage of the qi, so that one sighs to stretch the passage open again. Even a reflex is read as a small contest of forces, and a frequent yawn or sigh becomes a sign of where the qi is pulled or pent, not a thing to pass over.

SU WEN 34

帝曰：人有逆氣不得臥而息有音者，有不得臥而息無音者，有起居如故而息有音者，有得臥行而喘者，有不得臥不能行而喘者，有不得臥臥而喘者，皆何藏使然？願聞其故。岐伯曰：不得臥而息有音者，是陽明之逆也。足三陽者下行，今逆而上行，故息有音也。陽明者胃脈也，胃者六腑之海，其氣亦下行，陽明逆，不得從其道，故不得臥也。下經曰：胃不和則臥不安，此之謂也。

dì yuē: rén yǒu nì qì bù dé wò ér xī yǒu yīn zhě, yǒu bù dé wò ér xī wú yīn zhě, yǒu qǐ jū rú gù ér xī yǒu yīn zhě, yǒu dé wò xíng ér chuǎn zhě, yǒu bù dé wò bù néng xíng ér chuǎn zhě, yǒu bù dé wò wò ér chuǎn zhě, jiē hé zàng shǐ rán? yuàn wén qí gù. qí bó yuē: bù dé wò ér xī yǒu yīn zhě, shì yáng míng zhī nì yě. zú sān yáng zhě xià xíng, jīn nì ér shàng háng, gù xī yǒu yīn yě. yáng míng zhě wèi mài yě, wèi zhě liù fǔ zhī hǎi, qí qì yì xià xíng, yáng míng nì, bù dé cóng qí dào, gù bù dé wò yě. xià jīng yuē: wèi bù hé zé wò bù ān, cǐ zhī wèi yě.

The Emperor asked: Some have counterflowing qi and cannot lie down, and their breath makes a sound; some cannot lie down and their breath makes no sound; some go about as usual yet their breath makes a sound; some can lie down but pant when they walk; some can neither lie down nor walk and they pant; and some cannot lie down, and pant when they do lie. Which organ makes each of these? I wish to hear the reason. Qibo said: To be unable to lie down with the breath making a sound is a counterflow of the bright yang. The three yang of the foot run downward; here they run counter and rise, so the breath makes a sound. The bright yang is the stomach channel, and the stomach is the sea of the six palaces, whose qi also runs downward; when the bright yang runs counter and cannot follow its road, the patient cannot lie down. The lower canon says: when the stomach is not in harmony, the lying is not at peace. This is its meaning.

The same attention falls on sleep. When the qi runs counter and a person cannot lie down without the breath rasping, the classic traces it to the yang-brightness, the stomach's channel, whose qi should descend but here pushes upward; an unsettled stomach, in short, unsettles rest. Sleeplessness with a noisy breath is therefore treated at its source in the stomach and its descending qi, the rest restored by settling the organ beneath it.

Voice and the Gullet

Two passages take up the throat, the one for the voice it carries and the other for the food.

> LING SHU 69
>
> 會厭者，音聲之戶也。寒氣客於會厭，則開闔不利，厭不能發，故卒然無音。
>
> *huì yàn zhě, yīn shēng zhī hù yě. hán qì kè yú huì yàn, zé kāi hé bù lì, yàn bù néng fā, gù zú rán wú yīn.*
>
> The epiglottis is the door of the voice. When a cold qi lodges at the epiglottis, its opening and closing no longer work smoothly and it cannot sound, and so the voice is suddenly lost.

The voice has its door at the epiglottis, and when a cold lodges there its opening and closing falter, it cannot sound, and the voice is suddenly lost; grief and anger, the chapter's title reminds us, are what often drive the cold or the pent qi that shuts it. A lost voice is thus traced to the gate that makes it, and freed there, rather than treated as a failure of the lungs alone.

> LING SHU 68
>
> 氣為上膈者，食飲入而還出；其下膈者，食晬時乃出。喜怒不適，寒溫不時，邪氣稽留，積聚乃成，下管約而不通也。
>
> *qì wèi shàng gé zhě, shí yǐn rù ér hái chū; qí xià gé zhě, shí zuì shí nǎi chū. xǐ nù bù shì, hán wēn bù shí, xié qì jī liú, jī jù nǎi chéng, xià guǎn yuē ér bù tōng yě.*
>
> In a blockage above the diaphragm, food and drink are taken in and at once come back up; in a blockage below, the food returns only after a full day. Joy and anger ill-governed, and cold and warmth met out of season, let an evil qi linger until a gathering forms, and the lower passage is bound and will not let things through.

The gullet can close as well. Where food is swallowed and at once returned, the blockage sits high; where it comes back only after a full day, it sits low; and behind either, the classic says, lies a gathering formed by ill-governed feeling and untimely cold, binding the passage until nothing can pass. The level at which food is rejected locates the blockage, and the treatment is aimed at the gathering that has bound the passage, not at the swallowing itself. Voice and food share one narrow road, and the classic reads a failure of either by where along the road the qi has shut.

The Brave and the Timid

The classic ends this run of disorders by turning from the disease to the person, and asks why courage itself should differ from one body to the next.

> LING SHU 50
>
> 勇士者，目深以固，其心端直，其肝大以堅，其膽滿以傍，怒則氣盛而胸張，肝舉而膽橫。怯士者，其肝系緩，其膽不滿而縱，脅下空，雖方大怒，氣不能滿其胸，故不能久怒。
>
> *yǒng shì zhě, mù shēn yǐ gù, qí xīn duān zhí, qí gān dà yǐ jiān, qí dǎn mǎn yǐ bàng, nù zé qì shèng ér xiōng zhāng, gān jǔ ér dǎn héng. qiè shì zhě, qí gān xì huǎn, qí dǎn bù mǎn ér zòng, xié xià kōng, suī fāng dà nù, qì bù néng mǎn qí xiōng, gù bù néng jiǔ nù.*
>
> The brave man has deep, steady eyes, an upright heart, a liver large and firm, and a gallbladder full and set square; when he is angered the qi swells and the chest expands, the liver lifts and the gallbladder squares itself. The timid man has slack liver-cords and a gallbladder neither full nor firm, with a hollow beneath the ribs; even in a great rage the qi cannot fill his chest, and so his anger cannot last.

The brave man, it says, has deep steady eyes, an upright heart, a large firm liver, and a full square gallbladder, so that anger swells his chest and lifts the liver; the timid man has slack liver-cords, a gallbladder neither full nor firm, and a hollow beneath the ribs, so that even in a rage the qi cannot fill his chest and his anger soon fails. Temperament is read from the make of the organs, above all the liver and the gallbladder, so that courage and timidity are bodily facts, and how a person will meet fear, pain, and illness is part of the physician's reckoning. How one bears disease is written in the same organs that produce it, and the classic counts that bearing among the things to be known before treatment begins.

Cold-Heat Nodes and Sores

A set of disorders sits between the seasonal fevers and the open wound, where a cold and heat lodges in the flesh and will not pass.

LING SHU 70

黃帝曰：寒熱瘰癧在於頸腋者，皆何氣使生？岐伯曰：此皆鼠瘻寒熱之毒氣也，留於脈而不去者也。其本在臟，其末上出於頸腋之間。

huáng dì yuē: hán rè luǒ lì zài yú jǐng yè zhě, jiē hé qì shǐ shēng? qí bó yuē: cǐ jiē shǔ lòu hán rè zhī dú qì yě, liú yú mài ér bù qù zhě yě. qí běn zài zàng, qí mò shàng chū yú jǐng yè zhī jiān.

The Yellow Emperor said: The cold-and-heat scrofula that beads the neck and the armpits, what qi brings it into being? Qibo said: In every case it is the poison-qi of the rat-fistula's cold and heat, lodged in the vessels and refusing to leave; its root is in an organ, and its end is pushed up into the space of the neck and the armpit.

The scrofula that beads the neck and armpits the classic names a rat-fistula, a poison-qi of cold and heat lodged in the vessels and refusing to leave, its root set in an organ and only its end pushed up where it shows. The nodes are therefore read not as a local growth but as the surfacing of a deep, lodged evil, so that treatment reaches for the root in the organ as well as for the swelling at the surface.

LING SHU 21

皮寒熱者，不可附席，毛髮焦，鼻槁臘；肌寒熱者，肌痛，毛髮焦而唇槁臘；骨寒熱者，病無所安，汗注不休。

pí hán rè zhě, bù kě fù xí, máo fà jiāo, bí gǎo là; jī hán rè zhě, jī tòng, máo fà jiāo ér chún gǎo là; gǔ hán rè zhě, bìng wú suǒ ān, hàn zhù bù xiū.

In a cold-and-heat of the skin, the patient cannot bear to lie against the mat, the hair is scorched and the nostrils dry and withered; in a cold-and-heat of the flesh, the flesh aches, the hair scorched and the lips dry and withered; in a cold-and-heat of the bone, there is no rest anywhere, and the sweat pours without ceasing.

A wasting cold-and-heat can sit at three depths, and the classic reads the depth from the signs: in the skin, the patient cannot bear the touch of the mat and the hair is scorched and the nose dry; in the flesh, the flesh itself aches; in the bone, there is no rest anywhere and the sweat pours without stop. The deeper the cold-heat, the graver and more restless the picture, and the depth named guides how far the treatment must reach.

LING SHU 81

營衛稽留於經脈之中，則血泣而不行，不行則衛氣從之而不通，壅遏而不得行，故熱。大熱不止，熱勝則肉腐，肉腐則為膿。

yíng wèi jī liú yú jīng mài zhī zhōng, zé xuè qì ér bù xíng, bù xíng zé wèi qì cóng zhī ér bù tōng, yōng è ér bù dé xíng, gù rè. dà rè bù zhǐ, rè shèng zé ròu fǔ, ròu fǔ zé wèi nóng.

When the nutritive and defensive are held up within the channels, the blood congeals and will not move; and unmoving, the defensive qi too is stopped behind it, dammed and unable to flow, and so it turns to heat. Where the great heat does not abate, the heat prevailing rots the flesh, and the rotted flesh becomes pus.

Where such a stagnation turns to a sore, the classic gives its mechanism plainly: the nutritive and defensive held up in the channels, the blood congealed and dammed until it heats, and the heat, unabating, rotting the flesh into pus. An abscess is thus the end of a blockage gone to heat, and the teaching looks behind the visible sore to the stalled blood and qi that bred it, and would move the stasis before the flesh is lost. Lodged in the vessels, sunk to skin, flesh, or bone, or ripened into a sore, the cold-heat is one process at different stages, read by its depth and met before it rots.

The Course of a Disease

The classic closes its long survey of disease by stepping back from any single illness to the shape disease takes in time.

> LING SHU 42
>
> 病先發於心，一日而之肺，三日而之肝，五日而之脾，三日不已，死。冬夜半，夏日中。
>
> *bìng xiān fā yú xīn, yī rì ér zhī fèi, sān rì ér zhī gān, wǔ rì ér zhī pí, sān rì bù yǐ, sǐ. dōng yè bàn, xià rì zhōng.*
>
> A disease that first breaks out in the heart passes in one day to the lung, in three days to the liver, in five to the spleen; and if in three days more it is not resolved, death follows, at midnight in winter and at midday in summer.

A disease, it observes, travels. One breaking out in the heart passes in a day to the lung, in three days to the liver, in five to the spleen, and if it is not checked in three more, the patient dies; each organ has such a chain, with its own intervals and its own fatal term. The schedule lets the physician forecast a disease's path and judge how long remains to turn it, treating ahead of the next organ rather than behind the last.

LING SHU 44

朝則人氣始生，病氣衰，故旦慧；日中人氣長，長則勝邪，故安；夕則人氣始衰，邪氣始生，故加；夜半人氣入藏，邪氣獨居於身，故甚也。

cháo zé rén qì shǐ shēng, bìng qì shuāi, gù dàn huì; rì zhōng rén qì zhǎng, zhǎng zé shèng xié, gù ān; xī zé rén qì shǐ shuāi, xié qì shǐ shēng, gù jiā; yè bàn rén qì rù zàng, xié qì dú jū yú shēn, gù shèn yě.

At dawn the human qi begins to rise and the disease-qi wanes, so the patient is brightest in the morning; at midday the human qi is at its height and masters the evil, so there is ease; at dusk the human qi begins to wane and the evil to stir, so the illness gains; and at midnight the human qi withdraws into the organs, leaving the evil alone in the body, so it is at its worst.

And a disease breathes with the day. At dawn, as the body's qi rises and the disease-qi wanes, the patient is brightest; at midday the qi is full and masters the evil, and there is ease; at dusk the body's qi begins to fail and the evil to stir, and the illness gains; at midnight the qi withdraws into the organs, leaving the evil alone, and it is at its worst. The day is itself a small year, and reading where in that cycle a patient sits explains the morning's ease and the night's crisis, and tells the physician when to expect the worst and when to act. Moving organ by organ and rising and falling with the hours, disease has a course in time as well as a seat in the body, and to know that course is to meet it before it arrives.

The Strange and the Miscellaneous

The classic keeps several chapters for diseases that do not fit the main families, the strange, the named oddities, and the everyday miscellany, and explains even these by the principles already laid down.

SU WEN 47

帝曰：有病口甘者，病名為何？何以得之？岐伯曰：此五氣之溢也，名曰脾癉。夫五味入口，藏於胃，脾為之行其精氣，津液在脾，故令人口甘也，此肥美之所發也，此人必數食甘美而多肥也，肥者令人內熱，甘者令人中滿，故其氣上溢，轉為消渴，治之以蘭，除陳氣也。帝曰：有病口苦，名曰膽癉。夫肝者中之將也，取決於膽，咽為之使，此人者，數謀慮不決，故膽虛氣上溢，而口為之苦，治之以膽募俞。

dì yuē: yǒu bìng kǒu gān zhě, bìng míng wèi hé? hé yǐ dé zhī? qí bó yuē: cǐ wǔ qì zhī yì yě, míng yuē pí dān. fū wǔ wèi rù kǒu, cáng yú wèi, pí wèi zhī xíng qí jīng qì, jīn yè zài pí, gù lìng rén kǒu gān yě, cǐ féi měi zhī suǒ fā yě, cǐ rén bì shuò shí gān měi ér duō féi yě, féi zhě lìng rén nèi rè, gān zhě lìng rén zhōng mǎn, gù qí qì shàng yì, zhuǎn wèi xiāo kě, zhì zhī yǐ lán, chú chén qì yě. dì yuē: yǒu bìng kǒu kǔ, míng yuē dǎn dān. fū gān zhě zhōng zhī jiāng yě, qǔ jué yú dǎn, yàn wèi zhī shǐ, cǐ rén zhě, shuò móu lǜ bù jué, gù dǎn xū qì shàng yì, ér kǒu wèi zhī kǔ, zhì zhī yǐ dǎn mù yú.

The Emperor asked: There is a disease of a sweet taste in the mouth; what is it named, and how is it got? Qibo said: This is an overflow of the five qi, named spleen-heat. The five flavours enter the mouth and are stored in the stomach, and the spleen moves their essence-qi; when the fluids stay in the spleen, the mouth tastes sweet. It is brought on by rich and dainty food: such a person has surely eaten much that is sweet and fat, for the fat breeds inner heat and the sweet fills the centre, so the qi overflows upward and turns into wasting-thirst. Treat it with eupatorium, to clear away the stale qi. The Emperor asked about a bitter taste in the mouth, named gallbladder-heat. The liver is the general within, and its decision rests with the gallbladder, the throat serving as its envoy; such a person ponders and plans much without deciding, so the gallbladder grows empty and its qi overflows upward, and the mouth turns bitter. Treat it at the alarm and transport points of the gallbladder.

A sweet taste in the mouth it calls a spleen-overflow, and traces without moralising to a diet of rich and fatty food: the richness breeds an inner heat and the sweetness a fullness, until the qi spills upward and the disease turns to a wasting thirst. A modern-sounding chain, from over-rich eating to a wasting, sugar-craving illness, is set out plainly, and the treatment begins at the table.

SU WEN 46

帝曰：有病怒狂者，此病安生？岐伯曰：生於陽也。帝曰：陽何以使人狂？岐伯曰：陽氣者，因暴折而難決，故善怒也，病名曰陽厥。帝曰：何以知之？岐伯曰：陽明者常動，巨陽少陽不動，不動而動大疾，此其候也。帝曰：治之奈何？岐伯曰：奪其食即已。夫食入於陰，長氣於陽，故奪其食即已。使之服以生鐵落為飲，夫生鐵落者，下氣疾也。

dì yuē: yǒu bìng nù kuáng zhě, cǐ bìng ān shēng? qí bó yuē: shēng yú yáng yě. dì yuē: yáng hé yǐ shǐ rén kuáng? qí bó yuē: yáng qì zhě, yīn bào zhé ér nán jué, gù shàn nù yě, bìng míng yuē yáng jué. dì yuē: hé yǐ zhī zhī? qí bó yuē: yáng míng zhě cháng dòng, jù yáng shào yáng bù dòng, bù dòng ér dòng dà jí, cǐ qí hòu yě. dì yuē: zhì zhī nài hé? qí bó yuē: duó qí shí jí yǐ. fū shí rù yú yīn, zhǎng qì yú yáng, gù duó qí shí jí yǐ. shǐ zhī fú yǐ shēng tiě luò wèi yǐn, fū shēng tiě luò zhě, xià qì jí yě.

The Emperor asked: There are those with a raging madness; where is this disease born? Qibo said: It is born of the yang. The Emperor asked: How does the yang make a person mad? Qibo said: The yang qi, broken off suddenly and hard to resolve, makes him quick to rage; the disease is named yang-reversal. The Emperor asked: How is it known? Qibo said: The bright yang beats always, while the great yang and lesser yang do not; when those that should not beat beat with a great rapidity, that is its sign. The Emperor asked: How is it treated? Qibo said: Take away his food, and it ends, for food entering the yin nourishes the qi of the yang, so to take away the food ends it. And give him a draught of iron-filings water, for iron-filings drive the qi down swiftly.

A raging madness it derives from the yang: a yang qi suddenly checked and unable to discharge turns to anger, and this it names a yang-reversal. Even a violent disturbance of behaviour is read as a blocked and reversed qi, to be drained and freed rather than merely restrained.

> SU WEN 30
>
> 帝曰：或喘而死者，或喘而生者，何也？岐伯曰：厥逆連藏則死，連經則生。帝曰：善。病甚則棄衣而走，登高而歌，或至不食數日，踰垣上屋，所上之處，皆非其素所能也，病反能者何也？岐伯曰：四支者，諸陽之本也，陽盛則四支實，實則能登高也。
>
> *dì yuē: huò chuǎn ér sǐ zhě, huò chuǎn ér shēng zhě, hé yě? qí bó yuē: jué nì lián zàng zé sǐ, lián jīng zé shēng. dì yuē: shàn. bìng shèn zé qì yī ér zǒu, dēng gāo ér gē, huò zhì bù shí shù rì, yú yuán shàng wū, suǒ shàng zhī chù, jiē fēi qí sù suǒ néng yě, bìng fǎn néng zhě hé yě? qí bó yuē: sì zhī zhě, zhū yáng zhī běn yě, yáng shèng zé sì zhī shí, shí zé néng dēng gāo yě.*
>
> The Emperor asked: Of those who pant, some die and some live; why? Qibo said: When the reversal reaches the organs, the patient dies; when it reaches only the channels, he lives. The Emperor said: Good. When the disease is severe, the patient casts off his clothes and runs, climbs to high places and sings, or goes several days without eating, leaps over walls and onto roofs, all places he could never reach in his usual state; why can the disease give him such powers? Qibo said: The four limbs are the root of all the yang; when the yang is abundant the four limbs are replete, and being replete, he can climb to high places.

And the startling strength of some fevered patients, who cast off their clothes and run, climb walls and roofs and sing from the heights, far past their ordinary power, the classic explains by the same yang: the limbs are the root of the yang, and a yang in excess fills them with a vigour the calm body never had. A sign that might look like possession is traced to a measurable excess of yang in the limbs, and treated as such.

SU WEN 49

太陰所謂病脹者，太陰子也，十一月萬物氣皆藏於中，故曰病脹。所謂上走心為噫者，陰盛而上走於陽明，陽明絡屬心，故曰上走心為噫也。所謂得後與氣則快然如衰者，十二月陰氣下衰，而陽氣且出，故曰得後與氣則快然如衰也。

tài yīn suǒ wèi bìng zhàng zhě, tài yīn zi yě, shí yī yuè wàn wù qì jiē cáng yú zhōng, gù yuē bìng zhàng. suǒ wèi shàng zǒu xīn wèi yī zhě, yīn shèng ér shàng zǒu yú yáng míng, yáng míng luò shǔ xīn, gù yuē shàng zǒu xīn wèi yī yě. suǒ wèi dé hòu yǔ qì zé kuài rán rú shuāi zhě, shí èr yuè yīn qì xià shuāi, ér yáng qì qiě chū, gù yuē dé hòu yǔ qì zé kuài rán rú shuāi yě.

In the greater yin, what is called a disease of distension: the greater yin is the branch zi, the eleventh month, when the qi of all things is stored within, and so it is called a disease of distension. The rising to the heart that becomes belching: the yin is abundant and rises to the bright yang, whose collateral belongs to the heart, so it rises to the heart and becomes belching. That passing stool and wind brings a pleasant sense of relief: in the twelfth month the yin qi wanes below and the yang qi is about to come out, so passing stool and wind brings the pleasant sense as of the disease waning.

A whole chapter is given to explaining why each channel's disorder yields just the signs it does, tying them to the month and the state of the qi: a greater-yin distension to the eleventh month, when all things store inward, and a belching that runs up to the heart to the same inward turn. The classic will not leave a symptom unexplained, but grounds each in the season and the movement of qi behind it, so the sign is understood and not merely noted.

LING SHU 26

嗌乾，口中熱如膠，取足少陰。喉痺不能言，取足陽明；能言，取手陽明。瘧不渴，間日而作，取足陽明；渴而日作，取手陽明。

ài qián, kǒu zhōng rè rú jiāo, qǔ zú shào yīn. hóu bì bù néng yán, qǔ zú yáng míng; néng yán, qǔ shǒu yáng míng. nüè bù kě, jiān rì ér zuò, qǔ zú yáng míng; kě ér rì zuò, qǔ shǒu yáng míng.

For a dry throat with a heat in the mouth like glue, take the foot lesser-yin. For a throat-block that takes away speech, take the foot yang-brightness; if speech remains, the hand yang-brightness. For a malaria without thirst that comes every other day, take the foot yang-brightness; for one with thirst that comes daily, the hand yang-brightness.

And for the ordinary miscellany it simply pairs complaint with point: a dry throat hot as glue taken at the foot lesser-yin, a throat-block that steals speech at the foot yang-brightness, a malaria with or without thirst at one channel or another. The everyday disorders are met with direct, tested point-prescriptions, the practical residue of the whole tradition. Strange or common, each disease is brought under the one reading, a cause, a site, a movement of qi, and a point or a change of life that answers it.

READING ANY DISEASE

The gate names a great many diseases, but it reads them all by a few questions, and those questions are worth carrying as a set. What is the evil, if any, and where did it enter? Is the trouble a repletion, an abundant evil, or a vacuity, a robbed essence, since the one is drained and the other filled? At what depth does it sit, skin, flesh, channel, organ, or bone? In which direction is the qi disordered, risen, sunk, stalled, or reversed? Where is the disease in its course, early or late, easing at dawn or gaining at night? And what manner of body has met it, firm or frail, brave or timid, easily pained or not? A disease answered by its name alone is barely answered; a disease set against these questions is already half treated, for each one points to where the later gates must act.

DISEASE AND ITS CAUSES

Essential Verses

These are among the gate's most quoted lines in the classic, gathered here for study.

SU WEN 30

足陽明之脈病，惡人與火，聞木音則惕然而驚。陽明者胃脈也，胃者土也，故聞木音而驚者，土惡木也。陽盛則使人妄言罵詈，不避親疏而不欲食。

zú yáng míng zhī mài bìng, è rén yǔ huǒ, wén mù yīn zé tì rán ér jīng. yáng míng zhě wèi mài yě, wèi zhě tǔ yě, gù wén mù yīn ér jīng zhě, tǔ è mù yě. yáng shèng zé shǐ rén wàng yán mà lì, bù bì qīn shū ér bù yù shí.

In disease of the foot yang-brightness channel the person dreads people and fire, and starts in alarm at the sound of wood. The yang-brightness is the stomach-channel, and the stomach is earth; so to start at the sound of wood is earth's aversion to wood. When the yang is at its height it makes a person rave and curse, sparing neither kin nor stranger, and wanting no food.

The strange behaviours of yang-brightness disease, a dread of people and of fire, a start at the sound of wood, raving and refusal of food, look senseless until the five phases decode them. The stomach is earth, and earth is conquered by wood, so the patient flinches at wood's sound while loud bells leave him calm. Read this way, each particular aversion or excess becomes a pointer: the raving and the refusal of food mark yang at its flood-tide in the yang-brightness, and the treatment drains that excess. The chapter is a small demonstration of how a baffling cluster of symptoms resolves into a clean channel diagnosis once the phase-relations behind it are seen.

> SU WEN 33
>
> 邪之所湊，其氣必虛。陰虛者陽必湊之，故少氣時熱而汗出也。人所以汗出者，皆生於穀，穀生於精。今邪氣交爭於骨肉而得汗者，是邪卻而精勝也。
>
> *xié zhī suǒ còu, qí qì bì xū. yīn xū zhě yáng bì còu zhī, gù shǎo qì shí rè ér hàn chū yě. rén suǒ yǐ hàn chū zhě, jiē shēng yú gǔ, gǔ shēng yú jīng. jīn xié qì jiāo zhēng yú gǔ ròu ér dé hàn zhě, shì xié què ér jīng shèng yě.*
>
> Where an evil gathers, the qi there is surely deficient. Where the yin is empty the yang will crowd in, and so there is shortness of qi, intermittent heat, and sweating. The reason a person can sweat at all is that sweat is born of grain, and grain is born of essence. When the evil contends with the bone and flesh and sweat is won, it is the evil giving way and the essence prevailing.

Here the canon states its deepest principle of disease in a single breath: an evil settles only where the body's qi is already empty, so illness is finally a matter of vacancy. That principle reframes even a fever's sweat. Sweat draws on grain and essence, so a sweat broken during the struggle is good news, the sign that the essence has reserves and is driving the evil back; the body with nothing to sweat with is the one in danger. The physician therefore looks beneath any evil for the deficiency that admitted it and supports that, reads a sweat as favourable when it marks the essence prevailing, and works to reinforce the upright qi as much as to expel the intruder. Strengthening the host, not assaulting the guest, becomes the heart of treating disease.

SU WEN 46

人病胃脘癰者，診當何如？診此者當候胃脈，其脈當沉細，沉細者氣逆，逆者人迎甚盛，甚盛則熱。人迎者胃脈也，逆而盛則熱聚於胃口而不行，故胃脘為癰也。

rén bìng wèi wǎn yōng zhě, zhěn dāng hé rú? zhěn cǐ zhě dāng hòu wèi mài, qí mài dāng chén xì, chén xì zhě qì nì, nì zhě rén yíng shèn shèng, shèn shèng zé rè. rén yíng zhě wèi mài yě, nì ér shèng zé rè jù yú wèi kǒu ér bù xíng, gù wèi wǎn wèi yōng yě.

When a person has an abscess of the stomach cavity, how should it be diagnosed? One should examine the stomach pulse; it should be sunken and thin, and sunken and thin means the qi is counterflowing; counterflowing, Man's-Welcome is very full, and very full means heat. Man's-Welcome is the stomach pulse; counterflowing and full, the heat gathers at the stomach's mouth and does not move on, and so the stomach cavity forms an abscess.

The chapter works a diagnosis from the disagreement between two pulses, deducing an internal stomach abscess that no eye could see. A deep, thin stomach pulse signals counterflow; a flooding Man's-Welcome signals heat; and the two together mean heat dammed at the stomach's mouth, where it gathers and festers. The method is to take the stomach pulse and Man's-Welcome together, read the deep-thin against the over-full as counterflow plus heat, and infer the lesion forming where the heat cannot move on. It is a model of reasoning from combined pulse signs to a hidden structural disease, the kind of inference that lets the hand reach what the eye cannot.

SU WEN 47

人有重身，九月而瘖，此為何也？胞之絡脈絕也。胞絡者繫於腎，少陰之脈貫腎繫舌本，故不能言。無治也，當十月復。無損不足，益有餘，以成其疹，然後調之。

rén yǒu chóng shēn, jiǔ yuè ér yīn, cǐ wèi hé yě? bāo zhī luò mài jué yě. bāo luò zhě xì yú shèn, shào yīn zhī mài guàn shèn xì shé běn, gù bù néng yán. wú zhì yě, dāng shí yuè fù. wú sǔn bù zú, yì yǒu yú, yǐ chéng qí zhěn, rán hòu diào zhī.

A woman is with child, and in the ninth month loses her voice; what is this? The network vessel of the womb is cut off. The womb-network connects to the kidney, and the lesser-yin channel threads the kidney and ties to the root of the tongue, so she cannot speak. There is nothing to treat; in the tenth month it will return. Do not drain what is deficient nor add to what is in excess, lest you make her ailment; afterward, regulate her.

Some cases call for no treatment at all, and the hardest skill is recognising them. A woman late in pregnancy loses her voice because the womb-network, tied through the kidney channel to the root of the tongue, is briefly cut off; the condition is structural and temporary and will right itself at term. To drain or supplement an already stretched system here would only do harm, the very error of injuring the deficient or stuffing the full. So the physician names the self-limiting case by its mechanism, withholds the needle, and simply waits, regulating gently only afterward. The chapter teaches restraint as a clinical act, the discipline of doing nothing when nothing is the wise treatment.

SU WEN 49

太陽所謂腫腰脽痛者，正月太陽寅，寅太陽也，正月陽氣出在上而陰氣盛，陽未得自次也，故腫腰脽痛也。所謂強上引背者，陽氣大上而爭，故強上也。

tài yáng suǒ wèi zhǒng yāo shuí tòng zhě, zhēng yuè tài yáng yín, yín tài yáng yě, zhēng yuè yáng qì chū zài shàng ér yīn qì shèng, yáng wèi dé zì cì yě, gù zhǒng yāo shuí tòng yě. suǒ wèi qiáng shàng yǐn bèi zhě, yáng qì dà shàng ér zhēng, gù qiáng shàng yě.

As for the greater-yang so-called swelling and pain of the loin and buttock: the first month is the greater-yang, the tiger-month; in the first month the yang-qi comes forth above while the yin-qi is still abundant, and the yang has not yet taken its place, so there is swelling and pain of the loin and buttock. As for stiffness above drawing the back, the yang-qi rises greatly and contends, and so there is stiffness above.

This chapter is less a list of cures than a demonstration of how to reason, deriving each channel-complaint from the contest of yin and yang at a particular month of the year. The channels wax with the seasonal qi, so a symptom's very form follows from where the yang stands in its yearly rise: in the first month, the greater-yang's month, the yang comes forth while the yin is still strong, and the swelling and pain of the loin are the predictable result of yang emerging against it. The physician matches the channel to its season and reads the symptom as the expected outcome of that contest, letting the calendar name both the cause and the likely course. It trains a way of seeing rather than offering a lookup of remedies.

LING SHU 4

諸急者多寒，緩者多熱，大者多氣少血，小者血氣皆少，滑者陽氣盛微有熱，澀者多血少氣微有寒。是故刺急者，深內而久留之；刺緩者，淺內而疾發鍼。

zhū jí zhě duō hán, huǎn zhě duō rè, dà zhě duō qì shǎo xuè, xiǎo zhě xuè qì jiē shǎo, huá zhě yáng qì shèng wēi yǒu rè, sè zhě duō xuè shǎo qì wēi yǒu hán. shì gù cì jí zhě, shēn nèi ér jiǔ liú zhī; cì huǎn zhě, qiǎn nèi ér jí fā zhēn.

A tense pulse means much cold; a slack one, much heat; a large one, much qi and little blood; a small one, both blood and qi scant; a slippery one, yang-qi flourishing with

> slight heat; a rough one, much blood and little qi with slight cold. Therefore in needling a tense pulse, insert deep and retain long; in needling a slack pulse, insert shallow and withdraw quickly.

What makes this passage so useful is that it carries the reading straight through to the hand: the same pulse that names a disorder also prescribes how the needle should be set. A tense pulse means much cold, a slack one much heat, and so on through size, slipperiness, and roughness; each translates into a balance of cold and heat, blood and qi. From there the needle is matched to the finding, set deep and retained long for the cold-bound tense pulse, shallow and swift for the hot slack one. The chapter closes the usual gap between diagnosis and treatment in a single rule, so that feeling the pulse and choosing the technique become one motion.

> LING SHU 23
>
> 熱病三日，氣口靜、人迎躁者，取之諸陽，五十九刺，以瀉其熱而出其汗，實其陰以補其不足者。熱病七日八日，脈口動喘而短者，急刺之，汗且自出，淺刺手大指間。
>
> *rè bìng sān rì, qì kǒu jìng, rén yíng zào zhě, qǔ zhī zhū yáng, wǔ shí jiǔ cì, yǐ xiè qí rè ér chū qí hàn, shí qí yīn yǐ bǔ qí bù zú zhě. rè bìng qī rì bā rì, mài kǒu dòng chuǎn ér duǎn zhě, jí cì zhī, hàn qiě zì chū, qiǎn cì shǒu dà zhǐ jiān.*
>
> In heat disease of three days, when the qi-mouth is quiet but Man's-Welcome agitated, treat at the yang channels, the fifty-nine needlings, to drain the heat and bring out the sweat, filling the yin to supplement what is deficient. In heat disease of seven or eight days, when the pulse-mouth throbs panting and short, needle at once, the sweat about to break of itself; needle shallowly between the thumb and its neighbour.

Febrile disease is treated here in stages, the day of illness and the two pulses together choosing where and how to needle. Early on, a quiet wrist against an agitated Man's- Welcome shows heat still held in the yang exterior, and the fifty-nine heat-draining points are used to force a sweat while the yin is replenished; later, a panting, short pulse marks a crisis that demands immediate, shallow needling at the hand. So the physician counts the days, compares qi-mouth and Man's-Welcome, and times the needle to where the fever has reached, draining the yang and filling the yin to break a sweat at one turn and releasing the sweat the body is already moving toward at the next. The fever is met as a moving target, not a fixed one.

> LING SHU 27
>
> 周痹者，在於血脈之中，隨脈以上，隨脈以下，不能左右，各當其所。痛從上下者，先刺其下以過之，後刺其上以脫之；痛從下上者，先刺其上以過之，後刺其下以脫之。
>
> *zhōu bì zhě, zài yú xuè mài zhī zhōng, suí mài yǐ shàng, suí mài yǐ xià, bù néng zuǒ yòu, gè dāng qí suǒ. tòng cóng shàng xià zhě, xiān cì qí xià yǐ guò zhī, hòu cì qí shàng yǐ tuō zhī; tòng cóng xià shàng zhě, xiān cì qí shàng yǐ guò zhī, hòu cì qí xià yǐ tuō zhī.*
>
> The wandering bi lies within the blood-vessels, following the vessel upward, following it downward, unable to cross side to side, each in its own track. When the pain runs from above downward, first needle below it to head it off, then needle above to release it; when the pain runs from below upward, first needle above it to head it off, then needle below to release it.

A pain that travels along a vessel rather than settling is hard to pin, and the chapter catches it by needling in step with its motion. Because the pain moves in one direction, the first needle is set ahead of it to block its advance and the second behind it to discharge what remains; the order reverses for a pain that climbs rather than descends. The practitioner first determines the direction the pain is travelling, then places the downstream needle to intercept it and the upstream needle to release it. A frustrating, moving complaint becomes a tractable target once the needle is timed to where the pain is going, not to where it happens to be at the moment.

LING SHU 28

夫百病之始生也，皆生於風雨寒暑，陰陽喜怒，飲食居處。故邪之所在，皆為不足。上氣不足，腦為之不滿，耳為之苦鳴，頭為之苦傾，目為之眩。中氣不足，溲便為之變，腸為之苦鳴。

fū bǎi bìng zhī shǐ shēng yě, jiē shēng yú fēng yǔ hán shǔ, yīn yáng xǐ nù, yǐn shí jū chù. gù xié zhī suǒ zài, jiē wèi bù zú. shàng qì bù zú, nǎo wèi zhī bù mǎn, ěr wèi zhī kǔ míng, tóu wèi zhī kǔ qīng, mù wèi zhī xuàn. zhōng qì bù zú, sōu biàn wèi zhī biàn, cháng wèi zhī kǔ míng.

The hundred diseases all begin from wind and rain, cold and heat, the yin and yang of joy and anger, from food and drink and dwelling. Thus wherever an evil lodges, there is deficiency. When the qi above is insufficient, the brain is not filled, the ears ring, the head hangs heavy, the eyes grow dizzy. When the middle qi is insufficient, the stool and urine alter and the intestines rumble.

Many small, everyday troubles, ringing ears, a heavy head, dizziness, altered stools, are read here not as diseases in themselves but as a local insufficiency of qi showing at the surface. An evil settles only where qi is wanting, so these complaints are signs of qi falling short in a particular region, the head and senses when the upper qi is empty, the gut when the middle qi is. The physician localises the shortfall by the symptom and supplements the depleted region, rather than attacking a complaint that is merely emptiness made visible. The lesson is that slight and chronic troubles are often best met by quietly filling a deficiency, not by draining or forcing.

LING SHU 35

夫心脹者，煩心短氣，臥不安；肺脹者，虛滿而喘咳；肝脹者，脅下滿而痛引小腹；脾脹者，善噦，四肢煩悗，體重不能勝衣，臥不安。三里而瀉，近者一下，遠者三下。

fū xīn zhàng zhě, fán xīn duǎn qì, wò bù ān; fèi zhàng zhě, xū mǎn ér chuǎn ké; gān zhàng zhě, xié xià mǎn ér tòng yǐn xiǎo fù; pí zhàng zhě, shàn yuě, sì zhī fán mán, tǐ zhòng bù néng shèng yī, wò bù ān. sān lǐ ér xiè, jìn zhě yī xià, yuǎn zhě sān xià.

In heart-distension there is vexation, shortness of breath, and unrest in lying down; in lung-distension, an empty fullness with panting and cough; in liver-distension, fullness below the ribs with pain drawing into the lower belly; in spleen-distension, frequent retching, the four limbs vexed and the body too heavy to bear its clothes. Drain at the three-mile point, once for a recent case, thrice for an old one.

The distensions are sorted here by organ, each with its own cluster of signs, and then met at a single point. Heart-distension brings vexation and breathlessness, lung-distension an empty fullness with panting, liver-distension flank pain drawing into the lower belly, spleen-distension retching and a body too heavy to bear its clothes; the symptom-set names which organ is swollen. The physician identifies the organ from its signs, then drains at the three-mile point, dosing the number of needlings to the age of the disease, once for a recent case and thrice for an old one. A careful differential and a concrete, dosed protocol are set side by side, so that naming the trouble and treating it become parts of one procedure.

LING SHU 53

人之骨強筋弱肉緩皮膚厚者耐痛，其於鍼石之痛，火焫亦然。堅肉薄皮者，不耐鍼石之痛，於火焫亦然。同時而傷，其身多熱者易已，多寒者難已。

rén zhī gǔ qiáng jīn ruò ròu huǎn pí fū hòu zhě nài tòng, qí yú zhēn shí zhī tòng, huǒ ruò yì rán. jiān ròu báo pí zhě, bù nài zhēn shí zhī tòng, yú huǒ ruò yì rán. tóng shí ér shāng, qí shēn duō rè zhě yì yǐ, duō hán zhě nán yǐ.

One whose bones are strong, sinews supple, flesh loose, and skin thick can bear pain, and so too the pain of needle and stone, and of moxa burning. One of firm flesh and

> thin skin cannot bear the pain of needle and stone, nor of moxa. Of those injured at the same time, the body that runs hot mends easily, the one that runs cold mends with difficulty.

The same techniques land differently on different bodies, and this chapter asks the physician to read the patient's build before choosing the strength of a treatment. One with strong bones, supple sinews, loose flesh, and thick skin can bear hard needling and moxa; one of firm flesh and thin skin cannot, and the same wound mends quickly in a warm constitution and slowly in a cold one. So the practitioner weighs bone, sinew, flesh, skin, and complexion before reaching for needle, stone, or moxa, sparing the thin-skinned and firm-fleshed, and adjusts the prognosis by whether the body tends hot or cold. It fits the intensity of treatment to the person, not to the disease alone, which is part of why two patients with the same complaint may need very different hands.

> LING SHU 57
>
> 水與膚脹、鼓脹、腸覃、石瘕、石水，何以別之？腸覃者，寒氣客於腸外，與衛氣相搏，瘜肉乃生。石瘕者，生於胞中，寒氣客於子門，惡血當瀉不瀉，衃以留止，日以益大，狀如懷子。
>
> *shuǐ yǔ fū zhàng, gǔ zhàng, cháng tán, shí jiǎ, shí shuǐ, hé yǐ bié zhī? cháng tán zhě, hán qì kè yú cháng wài, yǔ wèi qì xiāng bó, xī ròu nǎi shēng. shí jiǎ zhě, shēng yú bāo zhōng, hán qì kè yú zi mén, è xuè dāng xiè bù xiè, pēi yǐ liú zhǐ, rì yǐ yì dà, zhuàng rú huái zi.*
>
> Water-swelling, skin-distension, drum-distension, the intestinal growth, the stony concretion, and stone-water, how are they told apart? The intestinal growth arises when cold settles outside the intestines and contends with the defensive qi, and a fleshy mass grows. The stony concretion arises in the womb when cold settles at its mouth, the bad blood that should be discharged is not, the clots remain, and day by day it grows until it looks like a pregnancy.

Several swellings of the belly look alike and demand wholly different responses, so the chapter teaches the physician to tell them apart before acting. Water-swelling and drum-distension are fluid; the intestinal growth is a fleshy mass bred when cold lodges outside the intestine; the stony concretion forms in the womb when cold holds blood that should have been discharged, hardening day by day until it resembles a pregnancy. Each is read from its history and the nature of the swelling, and only then treated, water to be moved, a stagnant-blood mass to be broken, a true pregnancy never to be touched. The whole value of the chapter is the discrimination it gives, the difference between draining what should be drained and assaulting what should be left alone.

> LING SHU 69
>
> 人卒然無音者，寒氣客於厭，則厭不能發，發不能下，至其開闔不致，故無音。會厭者，音聲之戶也；口脣者，音聲之扇也；舌者，音聲之機也。
>
> *rén zú rán wú yīn zhě, hán qì kè yú yàn, zé yàn bù néng fā, fā bù néng xià, zhì qí kāi hé bù zhì, gù wú yīn. huì yàn zhě, yīn shēng zhī hù yě; kǒu chún zhě, yīn shēng zhī shàn yě; shé zhě, yīn shēng zhī jī yě.*
>
> When a person suddenly loses the voice, cold has settled at the epiglottis, so that it cannot rise, and rising cannot descend, and its opening and closing fail to meet, and so there is no voice. The epiglottis is the door of the voice; the lips are its leaves; the tongue is its trigger.

Sudden voicelessness is located here not in the lung in the abstract but in the working parts of the throat, seized by cold. The chapter names the apparatus, the epiglottis as the door of the voice, the lips as its leaves, the tongue as its trigger, so the fault can be placed exactly at the failed opening and closing of that door. Treatment follows from the diagnosis: identify cold lodged at the epiglottis as the cause, and restore the free motion of the gate, warming and freeing the throat until its opening and closing meet again. A frightening, sudden symptom becomes a definite mechanical fault with a definite target, which is what makes it treatable rather than mysterious.

LING SHU 80

目者，五藏六府之精也，營衛魂魄之所常營也，神氣之所生也。故神勞則魂魄散，志意亂。是故瞳子黑眼法於陰，白眼赤脈法於陽也，故陰陽合傳而精明也。

mù zhě, wǔ zàng liù fǔ zhī jīng yě, yíng wèi hún pò zhī suǒ cháng yíng yě, shén qì zhī suǒ shēng yě. gù shén láo zé hún pò sàn, zhì yì luàn. shì gù tóng zi hēi yǎn fǎ yú yīn, bái yǎn chì mài fǎ yú yáng yě, gù yīn yáng hé chuán ér jīng míng yě.

The eyes are the essence of the five organs and six bowels, where the nutritive and defensive qi, the ethereal and bodily souls, are constantly at work, and where the spirit-qi is born. Thus when the spirit is overtaxed the souls scatter and the will is thrown into confusion. The pupil and dark of the eye follow the yin, the white and its red vessels follow the yang, and so yin and yang join and transmit, and the eye sees clear and bright.

The eye gathers the essence of every organ and is where the spirit shows itself, so the chapter reads clouded vision and confusion as disorders of the spirit, not merely of the eye. Pupil and dark belong to the yin, the white and its red vessels to the yang, and clear sight depends on their meeting; when the spirit is overtaxed the souls scatter and the will is thrown into disorder. The physician therefore takes disturbed or unfocused eyes as a sign of a taxed and scattering spirit, traces dizziness and bewilderment to the exhaustion of the essence feeding the eyes, and treats by settling the spirit and restoring that essence rather than the eye alone. Failing vision and confusion are rooted in the spirit behind the gaze.

LING SHU 81

寒氣客於經脈之中，則血泣，血泣則不通，不通則衛氣歸之，不得復反，故癰腫。寒氣化為熱，熱勝則肉腐，肉腐則為膿，故命曰癰。

hán qì kè yú jīng mài zhī zhōng, zé xuè qì, xuè qì zé bù tōng, bù tōng zé wèi qì guī zhī, bù dé fù fǎn, gù yōng zhǒng. hán qì huà wèi rè, rè shèng zé ròu fǔ, ròu fǔ zé wèi nóng, gù mìng yuē yōng.

When a cold evil settles within the channels, the blood congeals; congealing, it does not flow; not flowing, the defensive qi gathers to it and cannot return, and so an abscess swells. The cold turns to heat, and when the heat prevails the flesh rots and becomes pus, and so it is named an abscess.

An abscess is given a whole genesis here, traced from its cold beginning to its final pus. Cold settling in the channels congeals the blood; congealed, it ceases to flow; the defensive qi gathers to the obstruction and cannot return; the cold then turns to heat, and when the heat prevails the flesh rots into pus. Because the process moves through stages, each stage offers a different point of intervention: caught early, while it is still congealed blood and stalled qi, the lesion can be warmed and moved to disperse it before heat takes hold; once heat prevails and pus forms, management shifts to releasing it. Reading suppuration as a traceable progression, rather than a sudden event, is what lets the physician meet it at the right moment.

FROM THE AUTHOR

What stays with me in these chapters is how rarely the classic blames the evil alone. Again and again it pairs the wind or the cold with a weakness that let it in, the rich meal with the heat it bred, the grief with the qi it knotted. Disease, in this telling, is something the body and the world make together. That is a humbling thought, for no way of living leaves us proof against everything. It is also a hopeful one. Part of the cause is always how we live and how we are cared for, and that part we can still reach. In arranging these treatises I have tried to keep both halves in view, for to my mind they are the practical heart of the whole medicine.

邪之所湊，其氣必虛。

Where an evil gathers, the qi there is surely deficient.

WHERE THIS GATE LEADS

Every disease named here is read so that it may be treated: by the needle of *Gate Six, The Point of the Needle*, guided by the diagnosis of *Gate Four, Reading the Unspoken*, and by the wider art of *Gate Eight, The Physician's Hand*, where the herbs, the heat of moxa, and the regulating of the whole person take up what the needle cannot reach alone. Behind all treatment stands *Gate One, The Hundred Years*, for the surest answer to disease is to leave it no vacuity to enter.

PART EIGHT

The Physician's Hand

The Art of Treatment

論治

On treatment. How the physician chooses and combines the methods, needle and stone, moxa and herb, diet and massage, fitting each to the land, the person, and the hour, and treating always the root beneath the branch.

GATE EIGHT · THE ART OF TREATMENT

The Physician's Hand

論治

> *One who knows root and branch acts ten thousand times and is right ten thousand times.*
>
> Su Wen 65

The diseases of the last gate are named in order to be answered, and this gate is about the answering: the art of treatment itself, how a physician chooses among the methods, combines them, and fits them to the case. The Inner Classic is famous for the needle, yet it never pretends the needle is the whole of medicine. Stone and moxa, herb and broth, diet, massage, and the right ordering of a life all have their place, and the mark of a good physician is knowing which the case before them asks for.

Two ideas run through everything here. The first is that treatment is plural and fitted: there is no single remedy for a disease, but a remedy for this disease in this person in this place, and the sage is the one who combines the methods, each to what it suits. The second is that treatment has an order, a root and a branch, a cause beneath a symptom, and to take them in the wrong sequence is to fail however good the remedy.

From these follow the chapters gathered here: the methods that suit different lands, the treating of the root before the branch, food and the five flavours as medicine, broths and ferments and the limits of what any treatment can do, and, not least, the faults and failings of physicians themselves, for the classic is as concerned with how the healer goes wrong as with how the body does.

Different Methods for Different Lands

The classic begins its account of treatment with a question that could stand as its motto: why does the same disease, treated in quite different ways, get better in all of them?

> SU WEN 12
>
> 黃帝問曰：醫之治病也，一病而治各不同，皆愈何也？岐伯對曰：地勢使然也。
>
> *huáng dì wèn yuē: yī zhī zhì bìng yě, yī bìng ér zhì gè bù tóng, jiē yù hé yě? qí bó duì yuē: dì shì shǐ rán yě.*
>
> The Yellow Emperor asked: When physicians treat illness, one and the same disease is treated in different ways, and all are cured. Why is this? Qibo answered: It is the lie of the land that makes it so.

Physicians in different regions, it observes, treat one and the same disease by quite different means, and yet all of them cure; the reason, it says, lies in the lay of the land. Each region breeds its own disorders and its own remedy, and what works is what fits the place. The lesson is not that any method works anywhere, but that the right method is local, grown from the diet, the climate, and the life of the people it serves.

The classic then maps the five. From the east, a land of fish and salt by the sea, came the lancing stone, for the sores that its rich diet bred; from the west, a country of metal and stone where the wind is hard, came the medicines and herbs, for the diseases that arise within; from the cold north, where the people camp in the open and live on milk, came the burning moxa, for the fullness that cold breeds; from the warm, damp south came the fine needle, for the cramps and impediments of that wet heat; and from the central plain, level and damp, where people eat a mixed diet and do not toil, came the guiding exercises and the massage that loosen a wilting, reversing limb. Each therapy is a local answer to a local cause, which is why the complete physician inherits all five and insists on none.

SU WEN 12

中央者，其地平以濕，天地所以生萬物也眾。其民食雜而不勞，故其病多痿厥寒熱，其治宜導引按蹻。故導引按蹻者，亦從中央出也。故聖人雜合以治，各得其所宜，故治所以異而病皆愈者，得病之情，知治之大體也。

zhōng yāng zhě, qí dì píng yǐ shī, tiān dì suǒ yǐ shēng wàn wù yě zhòng. qí mín shí zá ér bù láo, gù qí bìng duō wěi jué hán rè, qí zhì yí dǎo yǐn àn juē. gù dǎo yǐn àn juē zhě, yì cóng zhōng yāng chū yě. gù shèng rén zá hé yǐ zhì, gè dé qí suǒ yí, gù zhì suǒ yǐ yì ér bìng jiē yù zhě, dé bìng zhī qíng, zhī zhì zhī dà tǐ yě.

The central region is level and damp, where Heaven and Earth bring forth the ten thousand things in abundance. Its people eat a mixed diet and do not toil hard, so their diseases are mostly wilting, reversal, and alternating cold and heat, best treated by guiding-and-stretching exercises and massage. And so the arts of guiding the qi and pressing the limbs came from the centre. Therefore the sage blends all these methods together in treatment, each fitted to where it suits, so that though the treatments differ, all the diseases are cured: he has grasped the true state of the illness and knows the great body of the art of healing.

And the classic draws the conclusion plainly: the sage combines the methods in treatment, each fitted to what it suits, so that the treatments differ and yet the disease is healed in every case. The art is not to master one therapy but to hold them all and to match, choosing for each case the method, or the blend of methods, that its cause and its setting call for. Treatment, then, begins not with a favourite remedy but with a question, what does this case, in this body and this place, actually ask for; and the rest of the gate is the classic's attempt to answer it.

Root and Branch

The classic's second great rule of treatment is one of order: that a disease has a root and a branch, and the two must be taken in their right sequence.

SU WEN 65

故知逆與從，正行無問，知標本者，萬舉萬當，不知標本，是謂妄行。夫陰陽逆從標本之為道也，小而大，言一而知百病之害，少而多，淺而博，可以言一而知百也。以淺而知深，察近而知遠，言標與本，易而勿及。

gù zhī nì yǔ cóng, zhèng xíng wú wèn, zhī biāo běn zhě, wàn jǔ wàn dāng, bù zhī biāo běn, shì wèi wàng xíng. fū yīn yáng nì cóng biāo běn zhī wèi dào yě, xiǎo ér dà, yán yī ér zhī bǎi bìng zhī hài, shǎo ér duō, qiǎn ér bó, kě yǐ yán yī ér zhī bǎi yě. yǐ qiǎn ér zhī shēn, chá jìn ér zhī yuǎn, yán biāo yǔ běn, yì ér wù jí.

So one who knows the against and the with proceeds straight and need not ask; one who knows root and branch acts ten thousand times and is right ten thousand times, while one who does not is said to act blindly. The way of yin and yang, the against and the with, the root and the branch, is small yet great: say one thing and know the harm of a hundred diseases; it is little yet much, shallow yet broad, so that to speak of one is to know a hundred. By the shallow to know the deep, by examining the near to know the far, to speak of branch and root is easy and yet seldom mastered.

One who knows root from branch, the classic says, acts rightly ten thousand times, while one who does not is said to act blindly; the whole of treatment turns on telling the cause beneath a symptom from the symptom itself. Before acting, the physician asks which is root and which is branch here, the original disorder or the trouble it has thrown up, and treats in the order the case allows.

LING SHU 25

先病而後逆者，治其本；先逆而後病者，治其本。先寒而後生病者，治其本；先病而後生寒者，治其本。惟先病而後生中滿者，治其標。

xiān bìng ér hòu nì zhě, zhì qí běn; xiān nì ér hòu bìng zhě, zhì qí běn. xiān hán ér hòu shēng bìng zhě, zhì qí běn; xiān bìng ér hòu shēng hán zhě, zhì qí běn. wéi xiān bìng ér hòu shēng zhōng mǎn zhě, zhì qí biāo.

When the disease comes first and the counterflow after, treat the root; when the counterflow comes first and the disease after, still treat the root. When cold comes first and the disease after, treat the root; when the disease comes first and cold after, treat the root. Only when the disease comes first and a fullness of the middle arises after it does one treat the branch.

The rule is usually to treat the root: whether the disease came before the counterflow or after it, before a cold or after, it is the root that is taken first, and the branch follows once the root is settled. The classic allows one telling exception: when the disease comes first and a fullness of the middle arises after, the branch, the fullness, is treated first, because a blocked and swollen middle is urgent and will not wait. Root before branch as a rule, branch before root only when the branch would kill first, the judgement resting on which threatens the patient soonest. A right remedy in the wrong order is a wrong treatment.

Food as Medicine: The Five Flavors

Among the methods, the classic gives food a place beside the needle and the herb, and works out the actions of the five flavours with care.

> SU WEN 22
>
> 辛散，酸收，甘緩，苦堅，鹹軟。毒藥攻邪，五穀為養，五果為助，五畜為益，五菜為充，氣味合而服之，以補精益氣。此五者，有辛酸甘苦鹹，各有所利，或散或收，或緩或急，或堅或軟，四時五藏，病隨五味所宜也。
>
> *xīn sàn, suān shōu, gān huǎn, kǔ jiān, xián ruǎn. dú yào gōng xié, wǔ gǔ wèi yǎng, wǔ guǒ wèi zhù, wǔ chù wèi yì, wǔ cài wèi chōng, qì wèi hé ér fú zhī, yǐ bǔ jīng yì qì. cǐ wǔ zhě, yǒu xīn suān gān kǔ xián, gè yǒu suǒ lì, huò sàn huò shōu, huò huǎn huò jí, huò jiān huò ruǎn, sì shí wǔ zàng, bìng suí wǔ wèi suǒ yí yě.*
>
> The pungent disperses, the sour gathers in, the sweet relaxes, the bitter firms, the salty softens. Potent drugs attack the evil; the five grains nourish, the five fruits assist, the five domestic animals enrich, the five vegetables fill out; taken with their qi and flavours joined together, they supplement the essence and boost the qi. These five flavours, pungent, sour, sweet, bitter, and salty, each have their benefit, dispersing or gathering, relaxing or tautening, firming or softening; through the four seasons and the five organs, the disease is treated according to the flavour that suits it.

Each flavour has a direction: the pungent disperses, the sour gathers in, the sweet relaxes, the bitter firms, the salty softens; and food is ranked by its office, the potent drugs to attack an evil, the grains to nourish, the fruits to assist, the meats to benefit, the vegetables to fill. A diet is thus composed as a treatment is, choosing flavours for what they do, dispersing or gathering or softening as the disorder requires, with drugs held in reserve for the evil and ordinary food doing the daily work of nourishment.

> LING SHU 56
>
> 五味各走其所喜：酸先走肝，苦先走心，甘先走脾，辛先走肺，鹹先走腎。
>
> *wǔ wèi gè zǒu qí suǒ xǐ: suān xiān zǒu gān, kǔ xiān zǒu xīn, gān xiān zǒu pí, xīn xiān zǒu fèi, xián xiān zǒu shèn.*
>
> Each of the five flavours runs to the organ it favours: sour runs first to the liver, bitter to the heart, sweet to the spleen, acrid to the lung, and salt to the kidney.

Each flavour, the classic adds, runs first to a particular organ: sour to the liver, bitter to the heart, sweet to the spleen, pungent to the lung, salt to the kidney. Knowing where a flavour goes lets the physician feed or spare an organ through the diet, sending sour to a liver that needs gathering, or keeping salt from a strained kidney.

> LING SHU 63
>
> 酸走筋，多食之令人癃；鹹走血，多食之令人渴；辛走氣，多食之令人洞心；苦走骨，多食之令人變嘔；甘走肉，多食之令人悗心。
>
> *suān zǒu jīn, duō shí zhī lìng rén lóng; xián zǒu xuè, duō shí zhī lìng rén kě; xīn zǒu qì, duō shí zhī lìng rén dòng xīn; kǔ zǒu gǔ, duō shí zhī lìng rén biàn ǒu; gān zǒu ròu, duō shí zhī lìng rén mán xīn.*
>
> Sour runs to the sinews, and eaten to excess it brings on a dribbling stoppage of water; salt runs to the blood, and in excess brings thirst; acrid runs to the qi, and in excess a hollow burning at the heart; bitter runs to the bone, and in excess turns the stomach to retching; sweet runs to the flesh, and in excess an oppression at the heart.

But every flavour in excess harms the very tissue it serves: too much sour brings a dribbling stoppage, too much salt a thirst, too much pungent a hollow burning at the heart, too much bitter a turning of the stomach, too much sweet an oppression. The dose is everything, for the same flavour that nourishes in measure injures in excess, so dietary therapy is as much a matter of restraint as of choice. Chosen for its direction, aimed at its organ, and kept within measure, food becomes in the classic's hands a true and careful medicine, the one the patient takes three times a day.

Broths, Ferments, and the Limits of the Art

One chapter the classic gives to the made remedies, the broths and the ferments, and to a sober truth about all treatment: that there are limits no remedy crosses.

> SU WEN 14
>
> 帝曰：形弊血盡而功不立者何？岐伯曰：神不使也。帝曰：何謂神不使？岐伯曰：鍼石，道也。精神不進，志意不治，故病不可愈。今精壞神去，榮衛不可復收。何者？嗜欲無窮，而憂患不止，精氣弛壞，榮泣衛除，故神去之而病不愈也。
>
> *dì yuē: xíng bì xuè jǐn ér gōng bù lì zhě hé? qí bó yuē: shén bù shǐ yě. dì yuē: hé wèi shén bù shǐ? qí bó yuē: zhēn shí, dào yě. jīng shén bù jìn, zhì yì bù zhì, gù bìng bù kě yù. jīn jīng huài shén qù, róng wèi bù kě fù shōu. hé zhě? shì yù wú qióng, ér yōu huàn bù zhǐ, jīng qì chí huài, róng qì wèi chú, gù shén qù zhī ér bìng bù yù yě.*
>
> The Emperor asked: When the body is worn and the blood is spent and yet no cure takes hold, why is that? Qibo said: It is that the spirit no longer answers. The Emperor asked: What is meant by the spirit not answering? Qibo said: The needle and the stone are only a Way, a means. When the essence and spirit do not come forward and the will and intent are not set in order, the disease cannot be cured. Now if the essence is ruined and the spirit gone, the nutritive and defensive qi cannot be gathered back. Why? Because desire was without end and worry without rest, the essence-qi slackened and broke down, the nutritive qi dried and the defensive qi was stripped away; so the spirit has departed, and the disease will not be cured.

In the highest antiquity, the chapter says, such broths were prepared but rarely needed, for a well-ordered life kept disease away; later they were needed, and later still even strong medicine failed. Why does a worn and bled body sometimes refuse all cure? Because, the classic answers, the spirit no longer answers. The needle and the herb are only a Way, and where endless craving and ceaseless worry have wrecked the essence and driven the spirit out, the nutritive and defensive cannot be gathered back, and no treatment takes hold. A remedy works through the patient's own vitality, so when that vitality is spent the remedy has nothing to work upon, and the physician must know that point and not flog a body past it.

> SU WEN 14
>
> 帝曰：其有不從毫毛而生，五臟陽以竭也，津液充郭，其魄獨居，孤精於內，氣耗於外，形不可與衣相保，此四極急而動中，是氣拒於內，而形施於外，治之奈何？岐伯曰：平治於權衡，去宛陳莝，微動四極，溫衣，繆刺其處，以復其形。開鬼門，潔淨府，精以時服，五陽已布，疏滌五臟，故精自生，形自盛，骨肉相保，巨氣乃平。
>
> *dì yuē: qí yǒu bù cóng háo máo ér shēng, wǔ zàng yáng yǐ jié yě, jīn yè chōng guō, qí pò dú jū, gū jīng yú nèi, qì hào yú wài, xíng bù kě yǔ yī xiāng bǎo, cǐ sì jí jí ér dòng zhōng, shì qì jù yú nèi, ér xíng shī yú wài, zhì zhī nài hé? qí bó yuē: píng zhì yú quán héng, qù wǎn chén cuò, wēi dòng sì jí, wēn yī, móu cì qí chù, yǐ fù qí xíng. kāi guǐ mén, jié jìng fǔ, jīng yǐ shí fú, wǔ yáng yǐ bù, shū dí wǔ zàng, gù jīng zì shēng, xíng zì shèng, gǔ ròu xiāng bǎo, jù qì nǎi píng.*
>
> The Emperor asked: There are cases that do not arise from the body hair, where the yang of the five organs is exhausted, the fluids swell against the body's walls, the bodily soul dwells alone, the essence is orphaned within while the qi is spent without, and the body can no longer be kept within its clothes; the four limbs are taut and the trouble stirs the centre. This is qi shut up within while the form is swollen without. How is it treated? Qibo said: Treat by bringing it back to balance and measure: clear away what is stagnant and stale, gently move the four limbs, keep the clothing warm, and needle the affected places by the crossing method to restore the form. Open the ghost gate and cleanse the clean palace, so that the essence is taken up in season; when the five yang are spread again and the five organs washed clean, the essence is born of itself, the form fills of itself, bone and flesh keep each other whole, and the great qi comes back to its level.

Where treatment can still reach, the classic is concrete. For a swelling where the organs' yang is spent and fluid floods the body, it prescribes a whole regimen: balance the body, clear away the stale and the stagnant, move the limbs gently, warm the clothing, and open the two doors by which water leaves, the pores and the bladder. Even a grave edema is met not by one act but by a coordinated set, draining the water by sweat and urine while warming and moving the body to restore its yang, a model of treatment as a campaign rather than a single stroke. A made remedy is powerful but not omnipotent; it works where the spirit still answers and the body can still respond, and the wise physician reads that limit as carefully as the disease.

The Physician's Faults

The classic ends its account of treatment, remarkably, by turning the examination upon the physician, and cataloguing the ways a healer fails.

> SU WEN 77
>
> 凡欲診病者，必問飲食居處，暴樂暴苦，始樂後苦，皆傷精氣。嘗貴後賤，雖不中邪，病從內生，名曰脫營。
>
> *fán yù zhěn bìng zhě, bì wèn yǐn shí jū chù, bào lè bào kǔ, shǐ lè hòu kǔ, jiē shāng jīng qì. cháng guì hòu jiàn, suī bù zhōng xié, bìng cóng nèi shēng, míng yuē tuō yíng.*
>
> Whoever would examine a disease must ask after the patient's food and dwelling, and after any sudden joy or sudden grief, for a joy that turns to grief injures the essence-qi. One who was honoured and is now brought low, though no evil has struck him, breeds a disease from within, named the loss of the nutritive.

The first faults are faults of inquiry. Whoever would examine a disease, it says, must ask after the patient's life, the food and the dwelling, the sudden joys and griefs, for a fall from honour to low estate breeds a wasting from within though no evil ever struck. A physician who treats the body and never asks after the life will miss the cause entirely, and the classic counts that incuriosity among the gravest errors.

> SU WEN 78
>
> 診不知陰陽逆從之理，此治之一失矣。受師不卒，妄作雜術，謬言為道，此治之二失也。診病不問其始，憂患飲食之失節，而卒持寸口，何病能中，妄言作名，此治之四失也。
>
> *zhěn bù zhī yīn yáng nì cóng zhī lǐ, cǐ zhì zhī yī shī yǐ. shòu shī bù zú, wàng zuò zá shù, miù yán wèi dào, cǐ zhì zhī èr shī yě. zhěn bìng bù wèn qí shǐ, yōu huàn yǐn shí zhī shī jié, ér zú chí cùn kǒu, hé bìng néng zhōng, wàng yán zuò míng, cǐ zhì zhī sì shī yě.*
>
> To examine without knowing the principle of yin and yang, of going with the current and against it, is the first failing of treatment. To leave a teacher's instruction half-learned, dabble in scattered arts, and call the muddle the Way, is the second. And to examine a disease without asking how it began, the griefs and the lapses of diet behind it, but to seize at once upon the wrist-pulse, by which what disease could be rightly struck, and then to invent a name regardless, is the fourth failing of treatment.

Others are faults of discipline. To examine without grasping the principle of yin and yang is the first failing; to leave a teacher half-heard and dabble in scattered tricks, calling the muddle the Way, the second; and to seize at once on the wrist-pulse without asking how the disease began, then pin a name on it regardless, the fourth. The classic faults not only ignorance but haste and pretension, the practitioner who reaches for the pulse before the history and for a diagnosis before the facts.

> LING SHU 29
>
> 入國問俗，入家問諱，上堂問禮，臨病人問所便。
>
> *rù guó wèn sú, rù jiā wèn huì, shàng táng wèn lǐ, lín bìng rén wèn suǒ biàn.*
>
> Entering a country, ask its customs; entering a house, ask what is forbidden there; ascending into the hall, ask its manners; and coming to the side of a patient, ask what eases him.

And against these failings it sets a single rule of bearing. Entering a country, ask its customs; entering a house, ask what is forbidden there; and coming to the side of a patient, ask what eases him. The physician adapts to the person, learning what they can bear and what comforts them before prescribing, so that treatment is fitted to a life and a temper and not imposed upon them. Knowing the principle, learning it fully, asking after the whole life, and adapting to the person, the physician escapes the faults the classic names, and earns the trust on which the cure, in the end, depends.

BEFORE CHOOSING A TREATMENT

Once a disease is read, the gate's counsel can be gathered into a few questions before any remedy is chosen. Which method, or blend of methods, does this case in this body and this place call for, needle or stone, moxa or herb, diet, movement, or the ordering of a life? Is the root or the branch the thing to treat first, and would taking them in the wrong order do harm? If food is part of the answer, which flavours, toward which organ, and in what measure? Does the patient's own vitality still answer, or has the spirit withdrawn past the reach of any cure? And have I asked enough, of the life as well as the body, to know what I am treating? The remedy matters, but the questions around it matter more, for they decide whether the remedy meets the disease at all.

THE ART OF TREATMENT

Essential Verses

These are among the gate's most quoted lines in the classic, gathered here for study.

> SU WEN 14
>
> 病為本，工為標，標本不得，邪氣不服。形弊血盡而功不立者何？神不使也。鍼石，道也。精神不進，志意不治，故病不可愈。
>
> *bìng wèi běn, gōng wèi biāo, biāo běn bù dé, xié qì bù fú. xíng bì xuè jǐn ér gōng bù lì zhě hé? shén bù shǐ yě. zhēn shí, dào yě. jīng shén bù jìn, zhì yì bù zhì, gù bìng bù kě yù.*
>
> The patient is the root, the physician the branch; when root and branch do not meet, the evil qi is not subdued. Why is it that, with the body worn and the blood spent, no cure is established? Because the spirit will not serve. Needle and stone are but the method. When essence and spirit do not advance, when the will is not set in order, the disease cannot be healed.

The physician is only the branch; the patient is the root, and no technique takes hold unless the patient's own spirit answers to it. This is why a cure can fail even when the treatment is right: where essence and spirit are gone and the will is broken, there is nothing left in the patient for the method to work upon. So the physician's first task is to secure the patient's spirit and will, through reassurance, regimen, and engagement, before expecting needle and stone, the mere instruments, to do their part. The line is a reminder that healing is a partnership in which the patient's own spirit does the decisive work, and that the most skilful hand is helpless against a spirit that will not return.

> SU WEN 22
>
> 合人形以法四時五行而治。肝苦急，急食甘以緩之；心苦緩，急食酸以收之；脾苦濕，急食苦以燥之；肺苦氣上逆，急食苦以洩之；腎苦燥，急食辛以潤之。
>
> *hé rén xíng yǐ fǎ sì shí wǔ xíng ér zhì. gān kǔ jí, jí shí gān yǐ huǎn zhī; xīn kǔ huǎn, jí shí suān yǐ shōu zhī; pí kǔ shī, jí shí kǔ yǐ zào zhī; fèi kǔ qì shàng nì, jí shí kǔ yǐ xiè zhī; shèn kǔ zào, jí shí xīn yǐ rùn zhī.*
>
> Treat by matching the human form to the law of the four seasons and five phases. The liver suffers from tension; quickly eat sweet to relax it. The heart suffers from slackness; quickly eat sour to gather it. The spleen suffers from damp; quickly eat bitter to dry it. The lung suffers from qi rising in counterflow; quickly eat bitter to drain it. The kidney suffers from dryness; quickly eat acrid to moisten it.

Each organ has a characteristic affliction, and the chapter answers each with a particular taste: sweet to relax a tense liver, sour to gather a slack heart, bitter to dry a damp spleen or drain a lung's rising qi, acrid to moisten a dry kidney. The five tastes act on the organs in fixed ways, so a flavour can correct an organ's besetting fault, which makes food and the tastes of medicines into instruments of treatment rather than mere nourishment. The physician identifies the organ at fault and its mode of suffering, prescribes the flavour that opposes it, and times the regimen to the season and phase. It is the canon's systematic ground for treating with diet and with the flavours of the materia medica.

SU WEN 65

病有標本，刺有逆從。先病而後逆者治其本，先逆而後病者治其本；先寒而後生病者治其本，先病而後生寒者治其本。謹察間甚，以意調之，間者並行，甚者獨行。

bìng yǒu biāo běn, cì yǒu nì cóng. xiān bìng ér hòu nì zhě zhì qí běn, xiān nì ér hòu bìng zhě zhì qí běn; xiān hán ér hòu shēng bìng zhě zhì qí běn, xiān bìng ér hòu shēng hán zhě zhì qí běn. jǐn chá jiān shèn, yǐ yì diào zhī, jiān zhě bìng xíng, shèn zhě dú xíng.

Disease has its root and its branch, and needling has its going-against and going-along. When disease comes first and counterflow after, treat the root; when counterflow comes first and disease after, treat the root; when cold comes first and disease after, treat the root; when disease comes first and cold after, treat the root. Carefully judge the mild from the severe, and regulate by understanding: for the mild, treat root and branch together; for the severe, treat one alone.

Disease has a root and a branch, and the order in which they are treated decides the outcome, since treating the branch while the root still stands only invites the trouble back. The chapter's rule of thumb is to trace which complaint arose first, treat that root in most cases, and then judge severity: in a mild case root and branch may be managed together, in a severe case the physician concentrates on one alone. So the abstract pairing becomes a practical guide to ordering a course of treatment, asking always what came first and how grave it is before deciding where to begin. It is the difference between a cure that holds and one that unravels as soon as the surface clears.

SU WEN 78

精神不專，志意不理，外內相失，故時疑殆。診不知陰陽逆從之理，此治之一失矣。受師不卒，妄作雜術，謬言為道，更名自功，此治之四失也。

jīng shén bù zhuān, zhì yì bù lǐ, wài nèi xiāng shī, gù shí yí dài. zhěn bù zhī yīn yáng nì cóng zhī lǐ, cǐ zhì zhī yī shī yǐ. shòu shī bù zú, wàng zuò zá shù, miù yán wèi dào, gēng míng zì gōng, cǐ zhì zhī sì shī yě.

When the spirit is not concentrated, the will not ordered, the outer and inner lost to each other, then one is forever in doubt and danger. To diagnose without knowing the principle of yin and yang, of going-against and going-along, is the first failing of treatment. To receive instruction but not complete it, to dabble in mixed techniques, to call error the Way and rename it as one's own achievement, is the fourth failing of treatment.

The four failings the chapter names are not misfortunes but faults of discipline and character, lapses on the physician's own side. An unconcentrated mind, ignorance of the fundamentals, training left half-finished, and the vanity that dresses guesswork as doctrine each wreck a treatment from within. The chapter means the list to be held up as a mirror: keep the spirit concentrated and the will ordered, master yin and yang and the rules of for-and-against before practising, finish one's training, and refuse to call error the Way or rename it as one's own achievement. It places the physician's own rigour and honesty among the conditions of a cure, alongside any technique.

LING SHU 29

順者，非獨陰陽脈論氣之逆順也，百姓人民皆欲順其志也。入國問俗，入家問諱，上堂問禮，臨病人問所便。

shùn zhě, fēi dú yīn yáng mài lùn qì zhī nì shùn yě, bǎi xìng rén mín jiē yù shùn qí zhì yě. rù guó wèn sú, rù jiā wèn huì, shàng táng wèn lǐ, lín bìng rén wèn suǒ biàn.

Going along does not mean only the counterflow and compliance of qi in the discourse of yin, yang, and pulse; the common people, every one, wish their own intent to be

> gone along with. Entering a country, ask its customs; entering a home, ask its taboos; ascending the hall, ask its courtesies; coming before a patient, ask what suits them.

Going-along, the chapter says, is not only a matter of the direction of the qi; the patient's own wishes and circumstances are to be respected too. Treatment imposed against a person's grain and situation meets resistance, while care fitted to them is accepted and works, which is why the chapter tells the physician to inquire first, into custom, into the household, into what the patient finds comfortable. The regimen is then shaped to suit the person and their life rather than a textbook ideal. Attentiveness to the patient's wishes is made part of the method itself, not a bedside courtesy added on top of it, because a treatment a patient will not follow is no treatment at all.

> LING SHU 63
>
> 五味入於口也，各有所走，各有所病。酸走筋，多食之令人癃；鹹走血，多食之令人渴；辛走氣，多食之令人洞心；苦走骨，多食之令人變嘔；甘走肉，多食之令人悗心。
>
> *wǔ wèi rù yú kǒu yě, gè yǒu suǒ zǒu, gè yǒu suǒ bìng. suān zǒu jīn, duō shí zhī lìng rén lóng; xián zǒu xuè, duō shí zhī lìng rén kě; xīn zǒu qì, duō shí zhī lìng rén dòng xīn; kǔ zǒu gǔ, duō shí zhī lìng rén biàn ǒu; gān zǒu ròu, duō shí zhī lìng rén mán xīn.*
>
> When the five flavours enter the mouth, each runs to its own place and each can cause its own disorder. Sour runs to the sinews; eaten in excess it makes a person dribble urine. Salty runs to the blood; eaten in excess it makes one thirst. Acrid runs to the qi; eaten in excess it makes the heart feel hollow. Bitter runs to the bone; eaten in excess it makes one retch and change. Sweet runs to the flesh; eaten in excess it vexes the heart.

The same five tastes that nourish and treat turn injurious when overused, and this chapter is the cautionary other half of treating by flavour. Each taste runs to its own place and, taken in excess, causes its own disorder: too much sour brings dribbling, too much salty thirst, too much bitter retching, and so through the five. Since flavour is a remedy in measure and a poison in excess, the physician who prescribes by taste must also know each taste's overdose;

the practical use is to track which flavour a patient overconsumes, read the complaint against the taste that breeds it, and keep prescription and counsel within the bounds where a taste heals rather than harms. It completes the doctrine of the five tastes by marking its limits.

FROM THE AUTHOR

If the needle gate asks for patience, this one asks for humility. The classic will not let the physician forget that the patient is the root and the healer only the branch, that the best remedy fails where the spirit has gone, and that a great many faults are simply failures to ask and to listen. Arranging these chapters, I was struck by how modern that sounds, and how easily it is forgotten: that treatment is a meeting between two people, and that the most important things a physician brings are often not in the pharmacopoeia at all, but in the quality of attention paid to the person in front of them.

病為本，工為標。

The patient is the root, the physician the branch.

WHERE THIS GATE LEADS

Treatment is fitted not only to the person but to the time, and the great cycles that set the year's diseases and govern when to drain and when to supplement are the work of *Gate Nine, The Weather of the Years*. Behind every cure stand the cultivation of *Gate Ten, The Work of Return* and the nurturing of *Gate One, The Hundred Years*, for the treatments here are what remains when prevention has failed, and the surest medicine is still the life that needs none.

PART NINE

The Weather of the Years

The Movements and Qi

運氣

On the movements and qi. The classic's cosmology of time: five movements and six qi turning through the year and the great cycles, setting the climate each season brings, the diseases that follow it, and the timing that treatment must heed.

GATE NINE · THE MOVEMENTS AND QI

The Weather of the Years

運氣

> *First determine the qi of the year, and do not assault the harmony of heaven.*
>
> Su Wen 74

This gate enters the most demanding country in the Inner Classic, the doctrine of the five movements and the six qi. Where the earlier gates treat the body, these chapters treat time itself: the great rhythms by which heaven turns, the climate each season and each year brings, and the diseases that follow from them. The system is intricate, built on the stems and branches of the old calendar, and a full account of it fills the longest treatises in the book.

Its governing idea is simple even where its machinery is not. The same forces that move the seasons, cold and heat, dryness and damp, wind and fire, move the body too; and a year has a character as a season does, dominated by one qi and coloured by another, that disposes the people living through it to particular illnesses. To practise well is to know the qi of the year as one knows the weather of the day, and to treat with it rather than against it.

The chapters gathered here set out that framework, the five movements that govern the years and the six qi that rule the seasons; the variations when a movement runs to excess or falls short; the winds that blow from the eight directions and the years they leave sick or well; and, at the summit, the great treatise on the highest truths, which turns the whole cosmology back into practical rules for reading a disease and choosing a remedy. It is the classic at its most ambitious, reaching to bind medicine, calendar, and cosmos into a single science.

The Five Movements and the Six Qi

The system rests on two interlocking cycles, and the classic introduces them together: five movements that govern the years, and six qi that rule the turns of climate.

> SU WEN 66
>
> 黃帝問曰：天有五行御五位，以生寒暑燥濕風。人有五藏化五氣，以生喜怒思憂恐。論言五運相襲，而皆治之，終期之日，周而復始，余已知之矣，願聞其與三陰三陽之候奈何？
>
> *huáng dì wèn yuē: tiān yǒu wǔ xíng yù wǔ wèi, yǐ shēng hán shǔ zào shī fēng. rén yǒu wǔ zàng huà wǔ qì, yǐ shēng xǐ nù sī yōu kǒng. lùn yán wǔ yùn xiāng xí, ér jiē zhì zhī, zhōng qī zhī rì, zhōu ér fù shǐ, yú yǐ zhī zhī yǐ, yuàn wén qí yǔ sān yīn sān yáng zhī hòu nài hé?*
>
> The Yellow Emperor asked: Heaven has the five phases governing the five positions, and by them gives rise to cold, heat, dryness, damp, and wind; the human being has the five organs transforming the five qi, and by them gives rise to joy, anger, pondering, grief, and fear. The discourse says that the five movements follow one upon another, that each governs in turn, and that when the term of days is ended they circle and begin again; this much I know, but I wish to hear how they answer to the three yin and the three yang.

Heaven, the classic begins, has five phases that govern five positions and so give rise to the five climates, cold and heat, dryness and damp, and wind; and the human being has five organs that transform five qi and so give rise to the five feelings. The same five-fold order runs through the sky, the seasons, and the body alike. Because one pattern governs all three, the state of the heavens in a given year can be read forward into the climate it will bring and the disorders that climate will breed.

SU WEN 67

黃帝坐明堂，始正天綱，臨觀八極，考建五常，請天師而問之曰：論言天地之動靜，神明為之紀，陰陽之升降，寒暑彰其兆。余聞五運之數於夫子，夫子之所言，正五氣之各主歲爾，首甲定運，余因論之。鬼臾區曰：土主甲己，金主乙庚，水主丙辛，木主丁壬，火主戊癸。子午之上，少陰主之；丑未之上，太陰主之；寅申之上，少陽主之；卯酉之上，陽明主之；辰戌之上，太陽主之；巳亥之上，厥陰主之。願聞其所始也。

huáng dì zuò míng táng, shǐ zhèng tiān gāng, lín guān bā jí, kǎo jiàn wǔ cháng, qǐng tiān shī ér wèn zhī yuē: lùn yán tiān dì zhī dòng jìng, shén míng wèi zhī jì, yīn yáng zhī shēng jiàng, hán shǔ zhāng qí zhào. yú wén wǔ yùn zhī shù yú fū zǐ, fū zǐ zhī suǒ yán, zhèng wǔ qì zhī gè zhǔ suì ěr, shǒu jiǎ dìng yùn, yú yīn lùn zhī. guǐ yú qū yuē: tǔ zhǔ jiǎ jǐ, jīn zhǔ yǐ gēng, shuǐ zhǔ bǐng xīn, mù zhǔ dīng rén, huǒ zhǔ wù guǐ. zi wǔ zhī shàng, shào yīn zhǔ zhī; chǒu wèi zhī shàng, tài yīn zhǔ zhī; yín shēn zhī shàng, shào yáng zhǔ zhī; mǎo yǒu zhī shàng, yáng míng zhǔ zhī; chén xū zhī shàng, tài yáng zhǔ zhī; sì hài zhī shàng, jué yīn zhǔ zhī. yuàn wén qí suǒ shǐ yě.

The Yellow Emperor sat in the Hall of Light, first setting straight the cord of Heaven, surveying the eight far points, and examining the five constants; he summoned the Heavenly Teacher and asked: The discourse says that the motion and rest of Heaven and Earth are recorded by the bright spirit, and that the rise and fall of yin and yang are foretold by cold and heat. I have heard from you the numbers of the five movements, and what you said was only that the five qi each govern a year, with jia at the head to fix the movement; on this I have reflected. Guiyuqu said: Earth governs jia and ji, metal yi and geng, water bing and xin, wood ding and ren, fire wu and gui; over zi and wu the lesser yin governs, over chou and wei the greater yin, over yin and shen the lesser yang, over mao and you the bright yang, over chen and xu the great yang, over si and hai the reverting yin. I wish to hear where it all begins.

Upon this the classic builds its calendar of movements. Seated in the Hall of Light and surveying the heavens, the Yellow Emperor is taught how the five movements each take their turn governing a year, wood, fire, earth, metal, and water succeeding one another in order, so that each year stands under one of the five and carries its character. Knowing which movement governs a year tells the physician the climate to expect and the organ most exposed, the groundwork on which all the finer reckoning is laid.

The machinery beneath the calendar is a pairing: the ten heavenly stems with the five movements, and the twelve earthly branches with the six qi, so that the stem of a year fixes its ruling phase and the branch its ruling climate, and from the meeting of the two the character of the season is forecast. It is the oldest attempt in the tradition to read the weather of a whole year in advance, and to treat with it rather than against it. Even a reader who never works the calculations can take the plain lesson: the body is never treated in a vacuum, but always inside a particular year and a particular season.

Layered over the yearly movements run the six qi, which rule the seasons in their turn and divide further into the qi that governs the heavens above and the qi that lies in the spring below, each year carrying both. The interlocking of the five movements with the six qi, year by year and season by season, is the whole engine of the system, and the long treatises that follow are in effect its tables, working out for every combination the climate it brings and the diseases to be ready for. The physician uses these not as prophecy but as forecast, a way of anticipating a season's characteristic disorders and adjusting prevention and treatment before they arrive. Five movements through the years, six qi through the seasons, one order linking heaven and body: with this framework set, the classic can begin to read the weather of any year.

FIGURE · MOVEMENTS AND QI

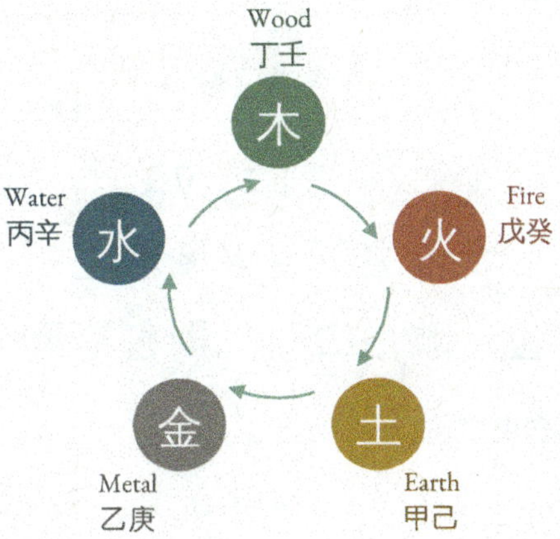

五運
The Five Movements, from the stems

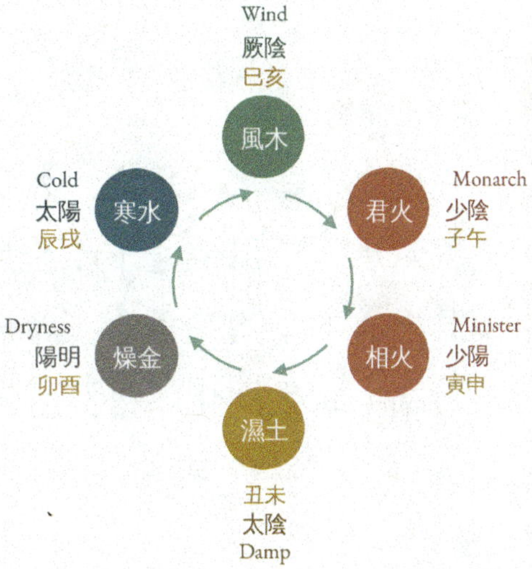

六氣
The Six Qi, from the branches

The two wheels by which a year is read. On the left, the ten heavenly stems pair into the five movements, each a phase, turning in the order one phase gives birth to the next; the pairing follows the rule of stem combination, by which the stems of a year yield a movement different from the phase of either stem alone. On the right, the twelve earthly branches pair into the six qi, the climatic powers of wind, monarch and minister fire, damp, dryness, and cold, set in the seasonal round of the host. The stem of a year fixes its movement, the branch its governing qi above, and from the meeting of the two the character of the season was forecast.

The Six Qi and the Year

With the framework set, the classic turns to the six qi themselves, and to two principles that keep the whole system in balance.

SU WEN 68

相火之下，水氣承之；水位之下，土氣承之；土位之下，風氣承之；風位之下，金氣承之；金位之下，火氣承之；君火之下，陰精承之。帝曰：何也？岐伯曰：亢則害，承乃制，制生則化，外列盛衰，害則敗亂，生化大病。

xiāng huǒ zhī xià, shuǐ qì chéng zhī; shuǐ wèi zhī xià, tǔ qì chéng zhī; tǔ wèi zhī xià, fēng qì chéng zhī; fēng wèi zhī xià, jīn qì chéng zhī; jīn wèi zhī xià, huǒ qì chéng zhī; jūn huǒ zhī xià, yīn jīng chéng zhī. dì yuē: hé yě? qí bó yuē: kàng zé hài, chéng nǎi zhì, zhì shēng zé huà, wài liè shèng shuāi, hài zé bài luàn, shēng huà dà bìng.

Below the minister fire, the water-qi succeeds it; below the position of water, the earth-qi succeeds; below earth, the wind-qi; below wind, the metal-qi; below metal, the fire-qi; below the sovereign fire, the yin-essence succeeds it. The Emperor asked: Why is this? Qibo said: When a qi runs to excess it harms, and the qi that succeeds it checks it; checked, then growth goes on, and flourishing and waning are arrayed without. But where it harms unchecked, there is ruin and disorder, and growth itself falls into great disease.

The first is the law of excess and restraint. Each qi, the classic says, is held in check by another that succeeds it: below fire stands water, below water earth, below earth wind, and so round the ring, so that none can run unchecked. When a thing grows excessive it harms, but what bears upon it then restrains it, and from that restraint generation and transformation arise. Health, in the heavens as in the body, is not the triumph of one force but the mutual checking of all, and disease comes precisely where the restraint fails and a qi runs to excess.

SU WEN 68

帝曰：何謂氣交？岐伯曰：上下之位，氣交之中，人之居也。故曰：天樞之上，天氣主之；天樞之下，地氣主之；氣交之分，人氣從之，萬物由之，此之謂也。故出入廢則神機化滅，升降息則氣立孤危。故非出入，則無以生長壯老已；非升降，則無以生長化收藏。是以升降出入，無器不有。故器者，生化之宇，器散則分之，生化息矣。故無不出入，無不升降，化有小大，期有近遠，四者之有而貴常守，反常則災害至矣。

dì yuē: hé wèi qì jiāo? qí bó yuē: shàng xià zhī wèi, qì jiāo zhī zhōng, rén zhī jū yě. gù yuē: tiān shū zhī shàng, tiān qì zhǔ zhī; tiān shū zhī xià, dì qì zhǔ zhī; qì jiāo zhī fēn, rén qì cóng zhī, wàn wù yóu zhī, cǐ zhī wèi yě. gù chū rù fèi zé shén jī huà miè, shēng jiàng xī zé qì lì gū wēi. gù fēi chū rù, zé wú yǐ shēng zhǎng zhuàng lǎo yǐ; fēi shēng jiàng, zé wú yǐ shēng zhǎng huà shōu cáng. shì yǐ shēng jiàng chū rù, wú qì bù yǒu. gù qì zhě, shēng huà zhī yǔ, qì sàn zé fēn zhī, shēng huà xī yǐ. gù wú bù chū rù, wú bù shēng jiàng, huà yǒu xiǎo dà, qī yǒu jìn yuǎn, sì zhě zhī yǒu ér guì cháng shǒu, fǎn cháng zé zāi hài zhì yǐ.

The Emperor asked: What is the meeting of the qi? Qibo said: Between the positions of above and below, in the midst where the qi meet, is where the human dwells. So it is said: above the celestial pivot, the qi of Heaven governs; below it, the qi of Earth governs; and at the dividing of their meeting, the human qi follows and the ten thousand things proceed. So when exit and entry cease, the spirit-mechanism perishes and transformation dies; when ascent and descent rest, the standing qi is left alone and in peril. For without exit and entry there is no being born, growing, maturing, aging, or ending; without ascent and descent there is no birth, growth, transformation, harvest, or storage. Thus ascent and descent, exit and entry, are found in no vessel that lacks them. A vessel is the house of growth and transformation; when the vessel scatters and parts, growth and transformation rest. So there is nothing without exit and entry, nothing without ascent and descent; transformation has its great and small, its term near and far, and these four being present, it is precious to keep them constant, for to go against the constant is for calamity to come.

The second is the law of movement. Between heaven above and earth below lies the meeting of the qi, and there, the classic says, is where the human dwells; and movement in four directions, rising and falling, going out and coming in, belongs to everything that lives. Let the going out and coming in cease, and the spirit's transformations are snuffed; let the rising and falling stop, and the standing of the qi is left in solitary peril. Life is the movement of qi, and the physician's task in every disorder is to keep that fourfold movement going, for its stoppage is death itself.

> SU WEN 71
>
> 故曰：用寒遠寒，用涼遠涼，用溫遠溫，用熱遠熱，食宜同法。此其道也。
>
> *gù yuē: yòng hán yuǎn hán, yòng liáng yuǎn liáng, yòng wēn yuǎn wēn, yòng rè yuǎn rè, shí yí tóng fǎ. cǐ qí dào yě.*
>
> So it is said: in using cold medicines, keep clear of the cold season; in using cool, of the cool; in using warm, of the warm; in using hot, of the hot; and let the diet follow the same rule. This is the Way of it.

From these laws the classic draws a plain rule of timing. In using cold medicines, it says, keep clear of the cold season; in using hot, keep clear of the hot; and let the diet follow the same rule. Because the year already leans one way, a remedy that pushes further in the same direction overshoots, so the physician times cooling and warming against the season's own qi rather than piling like upon like.

Change and Variation

A year is not always balanced. The classic devotes whole treatises to what happens when a movement runs to excess or falls short, and to naming the years by their temper.

SU WEN 69

歲木太過，風氣流行，脾土受邪。民病飧泄食減，體重煩冤，腸鳴腹支滿，甚則忽忽善怒，眩冒巔疾，上應歲星。歲火太過，炎暑流行，肺金受邪。民病瘧，少氣咳喘，血溢血泄，身熱骨痛而為浸淫，甚則胸中痛，脅支滿，上應熒惑星。

suì mù tài guò, fēng qì liú xíng, pí tǔ shòu xié. mín bìng sūn xiè shí jiǎn, tǐ zhòng fán yuān, cháng míng fù zhī mǎn, shèn zé hū hū shàn nù, xuàn mào diān jí, shàng yìng suì xīng. suì huǒ tài guò, yán shǔ liú xíng, fèi jīn shòu xié. mín bìng nüè, shǎo qì ké chuǎn, xuè yì xuè xiè, shēn rè gǔ tòng ér wèi jìn yín, shèn zé xiōng zhōng tòng, xié zhī mǎn, shàng yìng yíng huò xīng.

When the wood of the year is in excess, the wind-qi flows abroad and the spleen-earth receives the evil; the people suffer undigested diarrhoea and reduced eating, a heavy body and vexed oppression, rumbling bowels and a propped fullness of the belly, and at its worst a distracted readiness to anger, dizziness, and disorders of the crown; this answers above to the Year Star. When the fire of the year is in excess, the blazing heat flows abroad and the lung-metal receives the evil; the people suffer malaria, scant qi, cough and panting, blood overflowing and blood in the stool, a hot body with aching bones spreading into sores, and at its worst pain in the chest and a propped fullness of the flanks; this answers above to the Sparkling Deluder.

When a movement is in excess, its climate floods the world and strikes the organ it conquers. In a year of excess wood, the wind prevails and the spleen suffers, and the people fall to undigested diarrhoea, a heavy body, and rumbling fullness; in a year of excess fire, heat prevails and the lung suffers, with fevers, coughing, and bleeding. Knowing the year's excess tells the physician in advance which climate will dominate and which organ to guard, so that prevention is aimed before the season's disease arrives.

SU WEN 70

黃帝問曰：太虛寥廓，五運迴薄，盛衰不同，損益相從，願聞平氣何如而名，何如而紀也？岐伯對曰：昭乎哉問也。木曰敷和，火曰升明，土曰備化，金曰審平，水曰靜順。

huáng dì wèn yuē: tài xū liáo kuò, wǔ yùn huí báo, shèng shuāi bù tóng, sǔn yì xiāng cóng, yuàn wén píng qì hé rú ér míng, hé rú ér jì yě? qí bó duì yuē: zhāo hū zāi wèn yě. mù yuē fū hé, huǒ yuē shēng míng, tǔ yuē bèi huà, jīn yuē shěn píng, shuǐ yuē jìng shùn.

The Yellow Emperor asked: The great void is vast and boundless, the five movements turning and pressing upon one another, their flourishing and waning unalike, loss and gain following each other. I wish to hear how a balanced qi is named, and how it is reckoned. Qibo answered: An illuminating question. The balanced wood is called Spreading Harmony; the balanced fire, Ascending Brightness; the balanced earth, Complete Transformation; the balanced metal, Judging Evenness; the balanced water, Still Compliance.

And the classic names the balanced years like characters in a drama: wood's good year it calls the Spreading of Harmony, fire's the Ascending of Brightness, earth's the Complete Transformation, metal's the Examined Balance, and water's the Quiet Compliance. Each name is a forecast in a word, fixing the temper of a balanced year so that its proper climate, and any departure from it, can be recognised and met. In excess, in deficiency, or in balance, every year has a name and a tendency, and to know them is to know, before the season turns, what the body will be asked to weather.

The Highest Truths

At the summit of these treatises stands the longest of them all, the Great Treatise on the Highest Truths, where the whole cosmology is turned back into rules a physician can use at the bedside.

> SU WEN 74
>
> 帝曰：其久病者，有氣從而不康，治之奈何？岐伯曰：必先歲氣，無伐天和，無盛盛，無虛虛，而遺人夭殃。
>
> *dì yuē: qí jiǔ bìng zhě, yǒu qì cóng ér bù kāng, zhì zhī nài hé? qí bó yuē: bì xiān suì qì, wú fá tiān hé, wú shèng shèng, wú xū xū, ér yí rén yāo yāng.*
>
> The Emperor said: In a long illness, where the qi goes with the grain and yet the patient does not recover, how is it treated? Qibo said: First determine the qi of the year, and do not assault the harmony of heaven; do not make the full fuller nor the empty emptier, and so leave a person an early death.

Its first counsel is the gate's own motto: first determine the qi of the year, and do not assault the harmony of heaven; do not make the full fuller nor the empty emptier, and so hand a patient an early death. Before any remedy, the physician reckons the year's dominant qi and treats within it, neither fighting the season's grain nor worsening the patient's own excess or vacuity.

> SU WEN 74
>
> 諸風掉眩，皆屬於肝；諸寒收引，皆屬於腎；諸氣膹鬱，皆屬於肺；諸濕腫滿，皆屬於脾；諸熱瞀瘛，皆屬於火；諸痛癢瘡，皆屬於心。
>
> *zhū fēng diào xuàn, jiē shǔ yú gān; zhū hán shōu yǐn, jiē shǔ yú shèn; zhū qì fèn yù, jiē shǔ yú fèi; zhū shī zhǒng mǎn, jiē shǔ yú pí; zhū rè mào chì, jiē shǔ yú huǒ; zhū tòng yǎng chuāng, jiē shǔ yú xīn.*
>
> All wind, with its shaking and its dizziness, belongs to the liver; all cold, with its contraction and drawing-in, to the kidney; all qi, pent and stifled, to the lung; all damp,

> with its swelling and fullness, to the spleen; all heat, with its blurring and spasm, to fire; and all pain, itch, and sore, to the heart.

Then comes the most quoted passage in all of the medicine, the catalogue of disease-mechanisms, of which the classic gives a famous series: all wind, with its shaking and dizziness, belongs to the liver; all cold, with its contraction, to the kidney; all pent and stifled qi to the lung; all damp swelling to the spleen; all heat, with its blurring and spasm, to fire; and all pain, itch, and sore to the heart. Each line gathers a whole class of symptoms under one organ or element, giving the physician a first, fast sorting of any complaint, a way to find the seat of a disorder from the kind of disturbance it shows.

> SU WEN 74
>
> 謹守病機，各司其屬，有者求之，無者求之，盛者責之，虛者責之。寒者熱之，熱者寒之，微者逆之，甚者從之。
>
> *jǐn shǒu bìng jī, gè sī qí shǔ, yǒu zhě qiú zhī, wú zhě qiú zhī, shèng zhě zé zhī, xū zhě zé zhī. hán zhě rè zhī, rè zhě hán zhī, wēi zhě nì zhī, shèn zhě cóng zhī.*
>
> Hold carefully to the disease-mechanism, attending to what each sign belongs to: what is present, seek out its cause, and what is absent, seek why it is absent; what is excessive, hold to account, and what is depleted, the same. Cold, then heat it; heat, then cool it; the mild, treat against its current; the severe, treat along with it.

And from the mechanisms the classic draws its rules of treatment. Hold to the mechanism, it says, and attend to what each sign belongs to: where something is present, seek its cause; where absent, seek why; where excessive, call it to account; where depleted, the same. Then the plain reversals: cold, heat it; heat, cool it; the mild, treat against its current; the severe, treat along with it. Diagnosis and therapy are bound into one motion, the mechanism naming the seat and the principle naming the answer, opposing a mild disorder outright but, in a severe one, going along with its direction so as not to provoke it. Read the year, find the mechanism, apply the principle: the great treatise compresses the whole cosmology into a method, and it is no accident that its lines on the mechanisms have been memorised by physicians ever since.

The Winds of the Year

Two of the Numinous Pivot's chapters, with one supplement, bring the cosmology down to the wind on a given day and the health of whole populations.

LING SHU 77

風從其所居之鄉來為實風，主生長，養萬物；從其衝後來為虛風，傷人者也，主殺主害。謹候虛風而避之。

fēng cóng qí suǒ jū zhī xiāng lái wèi shí fēng, zhǔ shēng zhǎng, yǎng wàn wù; cóng qí chōng hòu lái wèi xū fēng, shāng rén zhě yě, zhǔ shā zhǔ hài. jǐn hòu xū fēng ér bì zhī.

A wind that comes from the quarter where the Grand One then dwells is a solid wind, which fosters growth and nourishes the ten thousand things; a wind that comes from the quarter opposite behind it is a vacuity wind, which harms people, ruling death and injury. Watch carefully for the vacuity wind, and keep out of it.

The wind itself, the classic says, is read by its direction. As the celestial pole-spirit moves through the eight quarters with the seasons, a wind from the quarter it occupies is a solid wind that nurtures all things, while a wind from the opposite quarter is a vacuity wind that harms, ruling death and injury; watch for the vacuity wind, it warns, and keep out of it. The same breeze is benign or dangerous by where it comes from relative to the season, so that avoidance, the oldest prevention, is made precise by direction and time.

LING SHU 79

因歲之和，而少賊風者，民少病而少死；歲多賊風邪氣，寒溫不和，則民多病而死矣。

yīn suì zhī hé, ér shǎo zéi fēng zhě, mín shǎo bìng ér shǎo sǐ; suì duō zéi fēng xié qì, hán wēn bù hé, zé mín duō bìng ér sǐ yǐ.

When the year is harmonious and its harmful winds are few, the people fall little ill and few of them die; but when a year has many harmful winds and evil qi, its cold and its warmth out of accord, then the people fall ill in great numbers and die.

And the character of a whole year can be read the same way. When the year is harmonious and its harmful winds few, the classic says, the people fall little ill and few die; but when a year has many harmful winds and evil qi, its cold and warmth out of accord, then they sicken and die in great numbers. Epidemics are understood as the meeting of a disordered year with the bodies living through it, which is why the physician watches the year's winds as a public matter and not only a private one.

> SU WEN 73
>
> 升降不前，氣交有變，即成暴鬱。至而不至，未至而至，皆為失守，而民病作矣。
>
> *shēng jiàng bù qián, qì jiāo yǒu biàn, jí chéng bào yù. zhì ér bù zhì, wèi zhì ér zhì, jiē wèi shī shǒu, ér mín bìng zuò yǐ.*
>
> When the rising and the falling of the qi do not go forward and the meeting of the qi is thrown off course, a sudden pent disorder is formed. The qi arriving when it should not, or failing to arrive when it should, is in either case a desertion of its post, and from it the diseases of the people break out.

The supplement names the mechanism behind such years. When the rising and falling of the qi do not go forward and the meeting of the qi is thrown off course, a sudden pent disorder forms; the qi arriving when it should not, or failing when it should, is a desertion of its post, and from it the diseases of the people break out. A year turns sickly when its qi-transitions miss their time, and reading those failures lets the physician anticipate a bad season and prepare against it. From the wind at the door to the temper of the year, the classic reads collective health in the heavens, and turns even epidemics into something that can be watched for and, so far as avoidance allows, met.

One Calendar, Many Arts

The reader who knows the wider tradition will already have recognised, in all this reckoning of the years, the same machinery that underlies the arts of destiny. The five movements and six qi are computed from the heavenly stems and earthly branches, the very stems and branches from which a life is read in the art of the Eight Characters (八字). The stem of a year fixes its governing movement; its branch fixes the qi that governs the heavens and the qi that lies in the spring below. This is less a resemblance than an identity: the movements and qi are the calendar of fate turned upon the season and the body rather than upon the life.

From that one root several arts branch. In reading a chart of the Eight Characters one reads not only a person's fortune but their constitution, the balance of the five phases they were born with, and from it their bodily strengths and the organs most apt to be overwhelmed, the same constitutional reading the earlier gates approached through the pulse and the complexion. The year pillars a physician consults for the season's dominant qi, a diviner consults for the temper of the year at large; and where the classic gives the broad rule, the almanacs give the particulars. The old Earth Mother Canon (地母經) sets down in verse the character of each year of the sixty-year cycle, its harvests, its floods and droughts, and the sicknesses it tends to bring; and the calculative arts, Taiyi Shenshu (太乙神數) and Qimen Dunjia (奇門遁甲), work out the qi and the disposition of a given year, or a given moment, in finer and finer detail.

The point, for a physician, is not to practise all of these but to see that they are one family. To read the qi of a year for the diseases it will bring, to read the qi of a birth for the constitution it confers, and to read the qi of a moment for the action it favours are three uses of a single literacy. This gate is where the medicine touches that wider literacy most plainly, and where the student of the Five Arts will feel most at home. Each of these arts, the reading of a life, the casting of the Yijing, the siting of a dwelling, is opened in a chapter of its own in the gate that closes the book.

READING THE YEAR

For all its complexity, the doctrine reduces at the bedside to a short routine. First, determine the year: which movement governs it, which qi governs the heavens and which lies below, and whether the movement is balanced, excessive, or deficient. From that, expect the year's dominant climate and the organ it most exposes, and watch for the season's characteristic disorders before they arrive. In treating, time the remedy against the season's own qi, keeping cold medicines from the cold season and hot from the hot, and neither feed an excess nor starve a vacuity the year has already produced. And keep an eye on the winds, the day's and the year's, for the direction and the timeliness of a wind foretell both the single illness and the epidemic. Used this way, as forecast rather than fortune, the system is a discipline of anticipation: it asks the physician to treat not only the patient and the disease but the weather of the time they share.

THE WEATHER OF THE YEARS · IN PRACTICE

Reading the Year by Hand

運氣 · 九宮八風

The classic leaves us two complete ways to read the qi of a coming year and the illnesses it favours. The first, the **Five Movements and Six Qi** (五運六氣), is the system of the Su Wen set out in this gate: it reads the year from its two calendar markers and divides it into six climatic steps. The second, the **Nine Palaces and Eight Winds** (九宮八風), comes from the Ling Shu: it reads the wind by direction and names the organ each wind harms. What follows is how to work each one by hand, with a single year, 2026, carried through as the example. Every rule here comes from the classic itself; all that has been added is a clear order of steps to follow.

GUIDE ONE

The Five Movements and Six Qi

五 運 六 氣

Two layers turn through every year. The **five movements** (五運) are the year's ground qi: an element that runs through all twelve months either too strongly or too weakly. The **six qi** (六氣) are the sky qi: the climate that rules the heavens for the first and second halves of the year and shifts through six seasonal steps. Each layer carries a fixed **host** (the season's normal weather) and a yearly **guest** (the visitor that bends it). Four steps read the whole picture.

The two markers of the year 干支

1 Name the year's stem and branch

Every year carries one **heavenly stem** (one of ten) and one **earthly branch** (one of twelve). Together they name the year, the way 2026 is the year 丙午, Bǐng-Wǔ. You need both before anything else. **The stem comes from the last digit of the year**. Read the final figure and look it up below.

THE TEN HEAVENLY STEMS, BY THE YEAR'S LAST DIGIT

Year ends in	Stem	Polarity
4	甲 Jiǎ	Yang (+)
5	乙 Yǐ	Yin (−)
6	丙 Bǐng	Yang (+)
7	丁 Dīng	Yin (−)
8	戊 Wù	Yang (+)
9	己 Jǐ	Yin (−)
0	庚 Gēng	Yang (+)
1	辛 Xīn	Yin (−)
2	壬 Rén	Yang (+)
3	癸 Guǐ	Yin (−)

EXAMPLE. 2026 ends in **6**, so the stem is 丙 Bǐng, a yang stem.

2 Find the branch from the twelve-year cycle

The branch turns in a twelve-year wheel, the same wheel as the twelve animals. Find the year below, or count forward in twelves from any year shown.

THE TWELVE EARTHLY BRANCHES, WITH TWO EXAMPLE YEARS EACH

Branch	Example year	Twelve years on
子 Zǐ	2020	2032
丑 Chǒu	2021	2033
寅 Yín	2022	2034
卯 Mǎo	2023	2035
辰 Chén	2024	2036
巳 Sì	2025	2037
午 Wǔ	2026	2038
未 Wèi	2027	2039
申 Shēn	2028	2040
酉 Yǒu	2029	2041
戌 Xū	2030	2042
亥 Hài	2031	2043

EXAMPLE. 2026 sits at 午 Wǔ. So 2026 is 丙午, Bǐng-Wǔ.

If you would rather skip the lookups, the ready-reference table at the end of this guide gives the full reading for every year from 2020 to 2043.

The five movements: the year's ground qi 五運

The **stem** fixes the element that governs the whole year and whether it runs in **excess** or **deficiency**. The two stems in each row below share one element.

3 Turn the stem into an element

Match your stem to its pair for the governing element, then read its strength: a **yang** stem makes the element **excessive** (too strong that year); a **yin** stem makes it **deficient** (too weak).

HEAVENLY STEMS TO GOVERNING ELEMENT

Stem pair	Governing element
甲 · 己 Jiǎ · Jǐ	Earth 土
乙 · 庚 Yǐ · Gēng	Metal 金
丙 · 辛 Bǐng · Xīn	Water 水
丁 · 壬 Dīng · Rén	Wood 木
戊 · 癸 Wù · Guǐ	Fire 火

The yang stems are 甲 丙 戊 庚 壬 (excess) ; the yin stems are 乙 丁 己 辛 癸 (deficiency) .

WORKED FOR 2026

The stem 丙 pairs with 辛, so the governing element is **Water**. 丙 is yang, so the **governing movement** is **Water in excess** (水運太過): the whole year carries an undertow of cold and damp.

The five seasons: host and guest movements 主運 · 客運

Beneath the single governing movement, each of the year's five seasons carries a movement of its own, just as each of the six steps below carries its own qi. These finer movements come in two kinds. The **host movements** 主運 run in the fixed generating order, the same in every year: **Wood, Fire, Earth, Metal, Water** 木 · 火 · 土 · 金 · 水, one to each season from the Major Cold onward, about seventy-three days apiece. The **guest movements** 客運 follow that same generating order, but **begin from the year's governing movement** and run round from there, so the first of them is always the governing movement itself.

WORKED FOR 2026

The governing movement is Water, so the guest movements run Water, then Wood, Fire, Earth, Metal. Set against the unchanging host movements, the five seasons read:

THE FIVE MOVEMENTS OF 2026 (丙午), HOST AND GUEST

Season	Host movement	Guest movement
Spring 20 Jan–1 Apr	Wood 木	Water 水
Summer 2 Apr–14 Jun	Fire 火	Wood 木
Late summer 15 Jun–26 Aug	Earth 土	Fire 火
Autumn 27 Aug–7 Nov	Metal 金	Earth 土
Winter 8 Nov–19 Jan	Water 水	Metal 金

The governing movement runs in excess or deficiency (Water in excess, this year), and that strength sets the year's overall tendency; the host and guest movements show which phase leads each season beneath it. For most readings the single governing movement is enough; these five are the finer grain.

The six qi: the rulers of the sky 司天 · 在泉

First, the six qi themselves, the six faces the year's weather can take, for the whole method turns on telling them apart. **Wind** (風木) stirs and scatters, restless and quick, the qi of early spring. **Monarch Fire** (君火) is mild warmth and light, the gentle ruling fire of late spring. **Ministerial Fire** (相火) is its fiercer twin, the burning, drying heat of high summer that scorches and parches. **Dampness** (濕土) is wet and heavy, slow and clinging, the close air of late summer. **Dryness** (燥金) is cool, crisp, and contracting, the qi of autumn. **Cold** (寒水) is freezing and still, the qi of deep winter. The two fires matter most: the mild Monarch Fire only warms, while the fierce Ministerial Fire dries, and that one difference can decide a year.

Each qi can be known more exactly by the way it moves. The old texts give every one a small cluster of verbs, its native gestures; and because a qi in excess only does more of what it already does, these clusters are worth holding in the mind before reading any year.

THE SIX QI AND THEIR NATIVE MOVEMENTS

Qi	Native movements	What it does
Wind 厥陰風木	升 ascending · 動 moving 散 dispersing · 搖 shaking	Initiates movement, promotes expansion and change, and sets things into motion.
Monarch Fire 少陰君火	溫 warming · 養 nourishing 明 illuminating · 主 governing	Maintains orderly warmth, supports life, illuminates the spirit, and gives stable governance.
Ministerial Fire 少陽相火	升 ascending · 散 dispersing 動 moving · 化 transforming	Drives transformation, metabolism, circulation, and dynamic physiological change.
Dampness 太陰濕土	濡 moistening · 緩 slowing 化 transforming · 載 bearing	Nourishes, receives, supports growth, and provides the medium for transformation.
Dryness 陽明燥金	收 contracting · 肅 descending 燥 drying · 斂 consolidating	Refines, contracts, dries, and gathers qi inward.
Cold 太陽寒水	寒 cooling · 凝 congealing 藏 storing · 降 descending	Preserves, conserves, quiets, stores, and directs qi inward and downward.

A PATTERN WORTH NOTING

Wind and Ministerial Fire share three of their four movements: 升 ascending, 動 moving, and 散 dispersing. They part only on the fourth. Wind ends in 搖, shaking, its gift for stirring up motion, instability, and sudden change; Ministerial Fire ends in 化, transformation, its work of driving the body's and the year's changes through warmth and activity. The same restless energy, turned to two different ends.

The **branch** fixes the climate that rules the heavens. One qi **governs heaven** (司天, Sī Tiān) and sets the weather of the **first half** of the year; its partner sits **at the spring** (在泉, Zài Quán) and sets the **second half**.

4 Turn the branch into the year's two rulers

Match your branch to its pair below to read which qi rules the first half of the year and which the second.

EARTHLY BRANCHES TO THE TWO RULING QI

Branch pair	Governs heaven (1st half)	At the spring (2nd half)
子 · 午	Monarch Fire 少陰君火	Dryness 陽明燥金
丑 · 未	Dampness 太陰濕土	Cold 太陽寒水
寅 · 申	Min. Fire 少陽相火	Wind 厥陰風木
卯 · 酉	Dryness 陽明燥金	Monarch Fire 少陰君火
辰 · 戌	Cold 太陽寒水	Dampness 太陰濕土
巳 · 亥	Wind 厥陰風木	Min. Fire 少陽相火

WORKED FOR 2026

The branch 午 gives **Monarch Fire governing heaven** (heat over the first half) and **Dryness at the spring** (dry over the second half).

The six steps: host and guest qi 主氣 · 客氣

The year divides into **six steps** of about sixty days. Each step has a **host** qi, the season's normal weather, unchanging from year to year; and a **guest** qi, the visitor for that particular year. Where host and guest agree, the season is plain; where they clash, the weather turns extreme.

The **host qi** always run in one fixed order through the six steps, the natural order of the seasons: **Wind, Monarch Fire, Ministerial Fire, Dampness, Dryness, Cold** 厥陰 · 少陰 · 少陽 · 太陰 · 陽明 · 太陽. It never changes from year to year.
The **guest qi** keep a fixed order of their own, ranked instead by the three yin and three yang: **Wind, Monarch Fire, Dampness, Ministerial Fire, Dryness, Cold** 厥陰 · 少陰 · 太陰 · 少陽 · 陽明 · 太陽. The two are nearly the same; only the middle pair differs: in the host order Ministerial Fire comes first, then Dampness; in the guest order Dampness comes first, then Ministerial Fire. Each year the guest qi are turned so that the qi that **governs heaven** and the **first half** of the year (the 司天, read from the branch in the list on the previous page) falls on the **third step** , and the qi **at the spring** that rules the **second half** (the 在泉) falls on the **sixth step** ; the other four fall in around them. For 2026 the six steps read as follows.

THE SIX STEPS OF 2026 (丙午), WITH HOST AND GUEST

Step	Solar term	Host qi	Guest qi	What it brings
1 初之氣	大寒 20 Jan–20 Mar	Wind 風木	Cold 寒水	Cold over wind: a sharp late-winter chill, spring cold-snaps.
2 二之氣	春分 20 Mar–21 May	Monarch Fire 君火	Wind 風木	Wind fans warmth: fast, windy warming.
3 三之氣	小滿 21 May–23 Jul	Min. Fire 相火	Monarch Fire (governs heaven) 君火	Two fires meet: the year's fiercest heat. The most dangerous step.
4 四之氣	大暑 23 Jul–23 Sep	Dampness 濕土	Dampness 濕土	Double damp: a long, close, humid heat.
5 五之氣	秋分 23 Sep–22 Nov	Dryness 燥金	Min. Fire 相火	Warmth lingers into a dry autumn.
6 終之氣	小雪 22 Nov–20 Jan	Cold 寒水	Dryness (at the spring) 燥金	A cold, dry winter.

THE WHOLE OF 2026 IN ONE BREATH

These are three layers of one year, not three different years. Underneath, all year long, runs a cold and wet movement (**Water in excess**). Over it, heat rules the first half (**Monarch Fire**) and dry, cool air rules the second (**Dryness**). The trouble is that the cold underneath and the heat above fight each other, water against fire. The old texts call such a year 不和, out of step with itself, its cold and heat clashing where the two meet (寒熱持於氣交而為病). So the year is not simply cold, or hot, or dry. It is **unstable**: the weather swings sharply between hot and cold, hottest in midsummer when the two fires meet, then turns damp, and ends dry and bitterly cold. For the body, protect the **Kidney** and **Heart** through the clashing first half, and the **Lung** against the dryness in the second.

A second year, worked through 癸未

Now a year on a different axis. 2003 (癸未), the year of SARS, sits on the 丑未 line: where 2026 is ruled by fire and dryness, 2003 was ruled by **Dampness governing heaven** and **Cold at the spring** (太陰濕土司天 · 太陽寒水在泉), over a movement of **weak fire** (火運不及). A different branch gives a wholly different six qi: a damp, cold-closing year with the body's own fire running low.

THE SIX STEPS OF 2003 (癸未), READ FOR A YEAR OF WEAK FIRE

Step	Solar term	Host qi	Guest qi	What it brought
1 初之氣	大寒 20 Jan–20 Mar	Wind 風木	Wind 風木	Double wind: a windy, unsettled early spring.
2 二之氣	春分 20 Mar–21 May	Monarch Fire 君火	Monarch Fire 君火	Two Monarch Fires over the damp year: warmth and wet together, the breeding ground, and SARS spread fastest here.
3 三之氣	小满 21 May–23 Jul	Min. Fire 相火	Dampness (governs heaven) 濕土	The fierce, drying Ministerial Fire arrives and burns the damp off: the turn, and SARS fell away.
4 四之氣	大暑 23 Jul–23 Sep	Dampness 濕土	Min. Fire 相火	Damp heat of deep summer.
5 五之氣	秋分 23 Sep–22 Nov	Dryness 燥金	Dryness 燥金	Double dryness: a dry autumn.
6 終之氣	小雪 22 Nov–20 Jan	Cold 寒水	Cold (at the spring) 寒水	Cold over cold: a hard, cold close.

THE WHOLE OF 2003 IN ONE BREATH

Weak fire under a damp first half, with cold to close. The danger gathered in the **second step** (春分 to 小滿), when the season's two Monarch Fires lay over the year's damp, heat and wet together over a cold undertone, the mixture in which the classics say a pestilence (瘟厲) spreads, and SARS spread fastest then. The method placed the turn at the **third step**, when 小滿 (about 21 May) brings 少陽相火, the fierce Ministerial Fire, to dry the damp off, doing what the mild Monarch Fire of spring could not, even as the damp still sat as that step's guest qi: the season's own burning heat overpowers the visitor. Practitioners of the method said so in public that April. And so it went: China's cases peaked in late April and fell away through May, all but gone by the month's end. The same 丑未 damp returned six years on in 2009 (己丑, a 太乙天符 year, where movement, sky, and branch all fall on Damp), and a second epidemic, swine flu, came on cue.

Ready reference: 2020 to 2043 速查

The method never changes from the years worked above: in every year the host qi keep the **same fixed order** and the guest qi sit by the same two rulers, and **only the year's own readings differ**. So for any year in this span, read straight across its stem-and-branch, its governing movement and whether that movement runs to excess or deficiency, and the two qi that rule its halves, then set those few readings into the same six steps.

THE MOVEMENT AND QI OF EACH YEAR, 2020–2043

Year	Stem-branch	Governing movement	Governs heaven	At the spring
2020	庚子	Metal 金, Excess	Monarch Fire	Dryness
2021	辛丑	Water 水, Deficiency	Dampness	Cold
2022	壬寅	Wood 木, Excess	Ministerial Fire	Wind
2023	癸卯	Fire 火, Deficiency	Dryness	Monarch Fire
2024	甲辰	Earth 土, Excess	Cold	Dampness
2025	乙巳	Metal 金, Deficiency	Wind	Ministerial Fire
2026	丙午	Water 水, Excess	Monarch Fire	Dryness
2027	丁未	Wood 木, Deficiency	Dampness	Cold
2028	戊申	Fire 火, Excess	Ministerial Fire	Wind
2029	己酉	Earth 土, Deficiency	Dryness	Monarch Fire
2030	庚戌	Metal 金, Excess	Cold	Dampness
2031	辛亥	Water 水, Deficiency	Wind	Ministerial Fire
2032	壬子	Wood 木, Excess	Monarch Fire	Dryness
2033	癸丑	Fire 火, Deficiency	Dampness	Cold

Year	Stem-branch	Governing movement	Governs heaven	At the spring
2034	甲寅	Earth 土, Excess	Ministerial Fire	Wind
2035	乙卯	Metal 金, Deficiency	Dryness	Monarch Fire
2036	丙辰	Water 水, Excess	Cold	Dampness
2037	丁巳	Wood 木, Deficiency	Wind	Ministerial Fire
2038	戊午	Fire 火, Excess	Monarch Fire	Dryness
2039	己未	Earth 土, Deficiency	Dampness	Cold
2040	庚申	Metal 金, Excess	Ministerial Fire	Wind
2041	辛酉	Water 水, Deficiency	Dryness	Monarch Fire
2042	壬戌	Wood 木, Excess	Cold	Dampness
2043	癸亥	Fire 火, Deficiency	Wind	Ministerial Fire

Method and figures follow the Su Wen's seven great treatises on the movements and qi (the 七篇大論).

GUIDE TWO

The Nine Palaces and Eight Winds

九 宮 八 風

This method, from the Ling Shu, reads the year by **wind**. The qi of the heavens, here called **Taiyi** (太一, the spirit of the pole star), moves through the eight directions of the **Luoshu** square across the year. A wind blowing **from the direction where the qi sits** is a **true wind** (實風) and nourishes; a wind from **the opposite direction** is a **thief wind** (虛風 · 賊風) and brings disease. The square reads two things at once, the **season's** epidemic wind and a finer **daily** wind, and it names the organ each wind strikes.

SOUTHEAST 4 陰洛 *Yīn Luò* Start of Summer	SOUTH 9 上天 *Shàng Tiān* Summer Solstice	SOUTHWEST 2 玄委 *Xuán Wěi* Start of Autumn
EAST 3 倉門 *Cāng Mén* Spring Equinox	CENTER 5 招搖 *Zhāo Yáo* Pivot · no season	WEST 7 倉果 *Cāng Guǒ* Autumn Equinox
NORTHEAST 8 天留 *Tiān Liú* Start of Spring	NORTH 1 葉蟄 *Yè Zhé* Winter Solstice	NORTHWEST 6 新洛 *Xīn Luò* Start of Winter

The nine palaces of the Luoshu, drawn in the old way with south above. Each holds a number, a direction, its palace-name, and the season it opens. The faint cross marks the rule of opposites 沖*: opposite palaces add to ten, so 1 faces 9, 2 faces 8, 3 faces 7, and 4 faces 6, while the centre 5 has none. A palace's thief wind blows from the one that completes ten with it.*

Layer one: the wind of the season 歲風 *(Seasonal / Epidemic Baseline)*

Across the year the qi keeps to each palace for a set run of days, beginning at the **Winter Solstice** and moving in the order of the seasons: North 46 days, then Northeast 46, East 46, Southeast 45, South 46, Southwest 46, West 46, Northwest 45, which is 366 days in all, returning to North. Each run covers about three solar terms, so in practice you need only know the season.

Find the palace for the season, and read its thief wind as the opposite. A wind from the palace's own direction nourishes; a wind from the opposite direction is the season's plague wind, to be sheltered from.

THE SEASON'S PALACE, AND WHERE ITS THIEF WIND BLOWS FROM

Season opens at	Its solar terms	Palace · qi sits in	Thief wind from
Winter Solstice	冬至 · 小寒 · 大寒 22 Dec–3 Feb	**1** North	South
Start of Spring	立春 · 雨水 · 驚蟄 4 Feb–19 Mar	**8** Northeast	Southwest
Spring Equinox	春分 · 清明 · 穀雨 20 Mar–4 May	**3** East	West
Start of Summer	立夏 · 小滿 · 芒種 5 May–20 Jun	**4** Southeast	Northwest
Summer Solstice	夏至 · 小暑 · 大暑 21 Jun–6 Aug	**9** South	North
Start of Autumn	立秋 · 處暑 · 白露 7 Aug–22 Sep	**2** Southwest	Northeast
Autumn Equinox	秋分 · 寒露 · 霜降 23 Sep–6 Nov	**7** West	East
Start of Winter	立冬 · 小雪 · 大雪 7 Nov–21 Dec	**6** Northwest	Southeast

WORKED EXAMPLE. Say the day falls in early April. The season comes first: early April sits just after the Spring Equinox (20 March), in the run 春分 · 清明 · 穀雨, which holds the qi in palace 3, the East. The thief wind comes next: its opposite, the palace that completes ten, is palace 7 in the West. So through that stretch a wind from the **East** nourishes, while a steady **West** wind is the season's plague wind; carried through to the eight-wind table below, that west wind strikes the **Lung** within and the **skin** without.

Layer two: the wind of the day 日游 *(Acute / Individual Threat)*

For a closer reading the qi also steps through the nine palaces **one a day**, in plain number order: palace 1 on the first day, 2 on the second, on to 9, then back to 1. The cycle is nine days long and repeats all year.

◆ Counting the day's palace, without arithmetic

Count the days from the Winter Solstice, with the solstice itself as day one. Then **count them off in nines**: the first nine days are one round (palaces 1 through 9), the next nine another round, and so on. Wherever a day falls **within its round of nine** (first place to ninth) is its palace.

EXAMPLE. Take the twentieth day after the solstice. The first nine days are round one; days ten to eighteen are round two; day nineteen opens round three at palace 1, so day twenty is palace 2 (Southwest). The day's thief wind blows from the opposite, palace 8 (Northeast).

EXAMPLE. Take the two hundred and fiftieth day after the solstice. Twenty-seven full rounds of nine reach day 243; day 244 opens round twenty-eight at palace 1, so day 250 lands on palace 7 (West). The day's thief wind blows from the opposite, palace 3 (East).

What each wind harms 八風所傷

When a thief wind strikes, the classic names exactly where it lodges, an inner organ and an outer tissue, word for word in the Ling Shu.

THE EIGHT WINDS, THE ORGAN EACH ENTERS, AND THE TISSUE IT SETTLES IN

Thief wind from	Palace	Organ harmed (inner)	Tissue harmed (outer)
South	**9**	Heart	Vessels
Southwest	**2**	Spleen	Flesh and muscle
West	**7**	Lung	Skin
Northwest	**6**	Small Intestine	Hand-taiyang channel (neck, shoulders)
North	**1**	Kidney	Bones
Northeast	**8**	Large Intestine	Ribs and the limbs
East	**3**	Liver	Tendons
Southeast	**4**	Stomach	Flesh

Reading the two layers together 虛實

Hold the season's palace and the day's palace in mind, then watch where the wind actually blows. Its meaning depends on which direction it answers to.

WHAT THE WIND MEANS, ONCE YOU KNOW THE PALACES

If the wind blows from...	It means
The season's own direction	**Safe, nourishing.** A true wind that quickens growth.
The day's opposite direction	**Caution for the day.** Shelter, and guard the organ that direction harms.
The season's opposite direction	**A seasonal plague wind.** The epidemic wind of the season; best not to go out in it.
Both opposites at once, or a sudden violent shift	**Gravely dangerous.** A doubled void; the classic warns most sharply here.

The gravest harm comes when several voids meet. The classic counts **three**: a void **year** (its qi already weak), a void **month**, and a void **day** or hour. When all three fall together and a thief wind strikes, it may bring sudden, severe collapse; where only one or two voids meet, the harm is milder. This is the old counsel to know the day, watch the hour, and shelter from the empty wind as one would shelter from flying stones.

Method, day-counts, the order of the palaces, and the eight wind-and-organ readings all follow the Ling Shu, 九宮八風 *(Treatise 77), checked against the classical commentaries (the* 類經*,* 太素*, and* 靈樞識*) and against modern scholarship.*

THE MOVEMENTS AND QI

Essential Verses

These are among the gate's most quoted lines in the classic, gathered here for study.

SU WEN 66

太虛寥廓，肇基化元，萬物資始，五運終天，布氣真靈，總統坤元。天以六為節，地以五為制。周天氣者，六期為一備；終地紀者，五歲為一周。

tài xū liáo kuò, zhào jī huà yuán, wàn wù zī shǐ, wǔ yùn zhōng tiān, bù qì zhēn líng, zǒng tǒng kūn yuán. tiān yǐ liù wèi jié, dì yǐ wǔ wèi zhì. zhōu tiān qì zhě, liù qī wèi yī bèi; zhōng dì jì zhě, wǔ suì wèi yī zhōu.

The great void stretches vast; it founds the origin of transformation, from which the ten thousand things take their start, and the five movements run their course through heaven, spreading the true and numinous qi and governing the power of earth. Heaven takes six as its measure, earth takes five as its rule. To complete heaven's qi, six periods make one round; to complete earth's reckoning, five years make one cycle.

The whole science of the movements and qi rests on two numbers, and the chapter lays them down at the start: heaven counts by six, earth by five. From six heavenly and five earthly divisions the great cycles of years are built, and within them the recurring patterns of climate and disease, so the two numbers are not numerology but the framework for reckoning the qi of any year. The work is to take the six and the five as that framework, find where a given year falls within the heavenly sixes and earthly fives, and from its place anticipate its dominant influences. It is the cosmological foundation on which the whole gate's year-by-year forecasting is raised, the grid laid down before any particular year can be read.

SU WEN 67

夫候之所始，道之所生，不可不通也。土主甲己，金主乙庚，水主丙辛，木主丁壬，火主戊癸。子午之上，少陰主之；丑未之上，太陰主之。

fū hòu zhī suǒ shǐ, dào zhī suǒ shēng, bù kě bù tōng yě. tǔ zhǔ jiǎ jǐ, jīn zhǔ yǐ gēng, shuǐ zhǔ bǐng xīn, mù zhǔ dīng rén, huǒ zhǔ wù guǐ. zi wǔ zhī shàng, shào yīn zhǔ zhī; chǒu wèi zhī shàng, tài yīn zhǔ zhī.

Where observation begins and the Way is born, one must not fail to understand. Earth governs the years jia and ji, metal governs yi and geng, water governs bing and xin, wood governs ding and ren, fire governs wu and gui. Over the zi and wu years, the lesser-yin presides; over the chou and wei years, the greater-yin presides.

This chapter supplies the key that links the calendar to the cosmos, fixing which heavenly stem governs which movement and which earthly branch carries which presiding qi. The bookkeeping is the heart of the method, because a year's movement and presiding qi follow mechanically from its stem and branch, and from them its climate and prevalent disorders are read. The physician takes the year's stem to find its governing movement and its branch to find the presiding qi, then combines the two to characterise the year and forecast its bearing on health. It is the working table by which the abstract sixes and fives are brought down to actual years, the step that turns a cosmology into a forecast.

SU WEN 69

善言天者，必應於人；善言古者，必驗於今；善言氣者，必彰於物；善言應者，同天地之化；善言化言變者，通神明之理。夫道者，上知天文，下知地理，中知人事，可以長久。

shàn yán tiān zhě, bì yīng yú rén; shàn yán gǔ zhě, bì yàn yú jīn; shàn yán qì zhě, bì zhāng yú wù; shàn yán yīng zhě, tóng tiān dì zhī huà; shàn yán huà yán biàn zhě, tōng shén míng zhī lǐ. fū dào zhě, shàng zhī tiān wén, xià zhī dì lǐ, zhōng zhī rén shì, kě yǐ cháng jiǔ.

One who speaks well of heaven must find its answer in the human; one who speaks well of antiquity must prove it in the present; one who speaks well of qi must show it in things; one who speaks well of correspondence shares in the transformations of heaven and earth; one who speaks well of transformation and change penetrates the principle of the spirit-bright. The Way is this: to know the heavens above, the earth below, and human affairs between; with this, one may endure long.

Behind all the cycles the chapter sets a test for any claim about them: whatever is said of heaven, of qi, or of the years must answer in the human body and in observable things, or it is empty. Cosmic doctrine untethered to what shows in patients and the world proves nothing, so correspondence has to be demonstrable. The discipline this imposes is to hold every principle of the movements and qi to the proof of present cases and visible signs, to unite knowledge of heaven, earth, and human affairs rather than treat any in isolation, and to verify correspondence rather than merely assert it. It keeps the most cosmological of the gates honest, demanding that its grand theories be borne out in fact before they are trusted.

SU WEN 70

化不可代，時不可違。夫經絡以通，血氣以從，復其不足，與眾齊同，養之和之，靜以待時，謹守其氣，無使傾移，其形乃彰，生氣以長，命曰聖王。

huà bù kě dài, shí bù kě wéi. fū jīng luò yǐ tōng, xuè qì yǐ cóng, fù qí bù zú, yǔ zhòng qí tóng, yǎng zhī hé zhī, jìng yǐ dài shí, jǐn shǒu qí qì, wú shǐ qīng yí, qí xíng nǎi zhāng, shēng qì yǐ zhǎng, mìng yuē shèng wáng.

Transformation cannot be replaced, the season cannot be defied. Let the channels run open and the blood and qi comply; restore what is deficient until it is even with the rest; nourish it, harmonise it, and wait quietly for the season; carefully guard the qi and let nothing tip it over. Then the body grows manifest, the life-qi lengthens, and this is called a sage-king's rule.

The chapter counsels restraint before the natural transformations: the physician must not try to stand in for what the seasons themselves accomplish, nor hurry them. The body mends in step with the turning year, and forcing it only tips the balance, so the method is patience with structure. Open the channels, restore deficiencies to the common level, then nourish and harmonise and wait for the season to finish the work, guarding the qi against disturbance rather than driving it. It tempers all the active technique of the canon with the wisdom of timing one's help to nature's own pace, on the understanding that some part of healing is done by the year and not by the hand.

LING SHU 77

太一常以冬至之日，居葉蟄之宮四十六日，明日居天留之宮。太一移日，天必應之以風雨。風從其所居之鄉來為實風，主生長養萬物；從其衝後來為虛風，傷人者也。

tài yī cháng yǐ dōng zhì zhī rì, jū yè zhé zhī gōng sì shí liù rì, míng rì jū tiān liú zhī gōng. tài yī yí rì, tiān bì yìng zhī yǐ fēng yǔ. fēng cóng qí suǒ jū zhī xiāng lái wèi shí fēng, zhǔ shēng zhǎng yǎng wàn wù; cóng qí chōng hòu lái wèi xū fēng, shāng rén zhě yě.

The Grand One always resides, from the day of winter solstice, in the palace of the hidden-burrowing for forty-six days, then on the next day moves to the palace of heaven's halt. When the Grand One shifts its day, heaven answers with wind and rain. A wind from the quarter where it dwells is a solid wind, which fosters and nourishes the ten thousand things; a wind from the opposite quarter is an empty wind, and it is what injures people.

A seasonal wind is wholesome or harmful depending on the quarter it blows from, and the chapter makes that the whole distinction. A wind out of the quarter the season favours is a solid wind that fosters and nourishes; a wind from the opposite quarter is an empty wind that wounds, the same breeze turning life-giving or dangerous by its bearing alone. So the physician tracks the season's governing quarter through the nine palaces, judges an incoming wind by whether it comes from that quarter or its opposite, and guards especially against the empty winds that strike from the wrong direction. It lets one read which winds of a given season are the ones to fear, and when shelter is worth taking.

LING SHU 79

乘年之衰，逢月之空，失時之和，因為賊風所傷，是謂三虛。故論不知三虛，工反為粗。避虛邪之道，如避矢石然，邪弗能害。

chéng nián zhī shuāi, féng yuè zhī kōng, shī shí zhī hé, yīn wèi zéi fēng suǒ shāng, shì wèi sān xū. gù lùn bù zhī sān xū, gōng fǎn wèi cū. bì xū xié zhī dào, rú bì shǐ shí rán, xié fú néng hài.

To ride the year's decline, to meet the month's emptiness, to lose the harmony of the season, and thereby to be injured by a robber wind, these are the three vacuities. One who reasons without knowing the three vacuities is, for all his skill, a crude practitioner. The way to avoid the depleting evils is to dodge them as one dodges arrows and slung stones, and then the evil can do no harm.

The three vacuities are three weaknesses that, coinciding with an evil wind, make for grave injury: a year in decline, an empty moon, and a season out of harmony. An evil that would glance off a person at full strength strikes deep when these three run low together, so the chapter turns prevention into a matter of timing. Reckon the year's strength, the moon's phase, and the season's harmony, recognise the dangerous windows when all three align, and avoid exposure to wind then as deliberately as one would dodge an arrow or a slung stone. It gives preventive care a precise rule, naming exactly when the body is most open to harm and therefore most in need of shelter.

FROM THE AUTHOR

This gate speaks the language I work in every day, though it turns that language to medicine where I turn it to other ends. When I read a person's BaZi, their Eight Characters, I am reading the same stems and branches the classic uses here, and from them I read not only the shape of a life but the make of a body, which phase is strong and which organ is apt to be overwhelmed. When I want to know the temper of a year, I turn to the pillars of that year, to the old almanacs, and to the calculative arts handed down for the purpose. So these chapters are no curiosity to me. The doctrine of the five movements and six qi is simply the calendar I use turned upon the body and the season, the one cosmology seen from the physician's side. A great deal of what the old masters set down here accords with what a careful reader of these arts comes to see, that health, like fortune, turns with the year. I have kept the framework whole and left the reader to weigh it. What I hold to is the spirit of the gate's first line, that we work within the harmony of heaven and do not set ourselves against it, which seems to me as sound now as when it was written. These arts are opened in full in the gate that closes the book.

亢則害，承乃制。

When a qi runs to excess it harms, and the qi that succeeds it checks it.

WHERE THIS GATE LEADS

The weather of the years is the outermost of the body's circles, and the innermost is the theme of *Gate Ten, The Work of Return*, where spirit and essence are cultivated at the still centre of all this turning. The daily, practical face of this cosmology is the seasonal nurturing of *Gate One, The Hundred Years*, and its bearing on when to needle and when to dose belongs to *Gate Eight, The Physician's Hand*. Its kinship with the calendar and the reckoning of fate opens, at last, onto *Gate Eleven, One Tradition, Five Gates*, where medicine takes its place among the Five Arts.

PART TEN

The Work of Return

Spirit, Essence, and Cultivation

修煉

On cultivation. Where medicine touches its own root: the shifting of essence and the transforming of qi, the spirit and the faculties that rise from it, and the wholeness the healer must cultivate within before restoring it in others.

GATE TEN · SPIRIT, ESSENCE, AND CULTIVATION

The Work of Return

修煉

> *One who keeps the spirit thrives; one who loses it dies.*
>
> Su Wen 13

The classic keeps its subtlest chapters for the level beneath the body, where healing becomes a matter of the spirit and the essence, and where medicine shades into cultivation. The earlier gates have treated the flesh, the channels, the organs, and the climate; this one treats the still centre from which all of them are governed, and which the physician must tend in themselves before they can tend it in another.

Three chapters are gathered here. The first asks why the spirit-healing of the ancients no longer suffices, and answers that the power of the spirit over illness is real but bounded by how we live. The second anatomises the inner life itself, the essence and the spirit, the two souls, and the faculties of mind, and shows how each is injured and cared for. The third names the breadth that true mastery requires, and so turns the whole book toward the cultivation of the healer.

It is called the work of return because its direction is inward and homeward: back from the symptom to the spirit, back from technique to presence, back from the turning of the outer world to the quiet at its centre. Here, more than anywhere, the classic insists that to heal others well one must first become whole oneself.

Shifting the Essence, Transforming the Qi

The gate opens on a puzzle the Yellow Emperor puts plainly, and that sets cultivation against mere technique.

> SU WEN 13
>
> 黃帝問曰：余聞古之治病，惟其移精變氣，可祝由而已。今世治病，毒藥治其內，鍼石治其外，或愈或不愈，何也？
>
> *huáng dì wèn yuē: yú wén gǔ zhī zhì bìng, wéi qí yí jīng biàn qì, kě zhù yóu ér yǐ. jīn shì zhì bìng, dú yào zhì qí nèi, zhēn shí zhì qí wài, huò yù huò bù yù, hé yě?*
>
> The Yellow Emperor asked: I have heard that the ancients, in treating disease, had only to shift the essence and transform the qi, and could heal by invocation alone, by what is called zhuyou (祝由). In the present age, disease is treated with potent drugs within and needle and stone without, yet some are cured and some are not. Why is this?

The ancients, he observes, could treat disease merely by shifting the essence and transforming the qi, healing by invocation alone, where now we use strong medicine within and needle and stone without, and still sometimes fail. Why should the inner art that once sufficed no longer do so? The question is not idle: it asks where the power of the spirit ends and the need for instruments begins.

SU WEN 13

當今之世不然，憂患緣其內，苦形傷其外，又失四時之從，逆寒暑之宜，賊風數至，虛邪朝夕，內至五臟骨髓，外傷空竅肌膚，所以小病必甚，大病必死，故祝由不能已也。

dāng jīn zhī shì bù rán, yōu huàn yuán qí nèi, kǔ xíng shāng qí wài, yòu shī sì shí zhī cóng, nì hán shǔ zhī yí, zéi fēng shuò zhì, xū xié zhāo xī, nèi zhì wǔ zàng gǔ suǐ, wài shāng kōng qiào jī fū, suǒ yǐ xiǎo bìng bì shèn, dà bìng bì sǐ, gù zhù yóu bù néng yǐ yě.

The present age is not so. Worry and care gnaw at people within, and hard toil injures them without; they have lost the following of the four seasons and gone against the fitness of cold and heat. Robber winds come again and again, and empty evils morning and evening, reaching within to the five organs and the bones and marrow, and harming without the orifices, the flesh, and the skin. So a small illness is bound to grow grave and a great one bound to kill, and invocation alone can no longer end it.

The answer is not that the old power has died but that life has changed. In far antiquity, the classic says, people lived simply, moving to flee the cold and sheltering from the heat, with no gnawing attachments within and no grinding ambitions without, and in that calm an evil could not strike deep, so a mere shifting of the spirit could turn it. The present age is otherwise: worry gnaws within and toil wears without, the seasons are defied, and harmful winds reach to the very marrow, so that ritual alone can no longer reach a disease grown so deep. The power of the spirit over illness is real but bounded, strongest where life is simple and the disease shallow, which is why the cultivation this gate teaches is also a way of living that keeps disease shallow enough to be reached.

SU WEN 13

治之要極，無失色脈，用之不惑，治之大則。閉戶塞牖，繫之病者，數問其情，以從其意。得神者昌，失神者亡。

zhì zhī yào jí, wú shī sè mài, yòng zhī bù huò, zhì zhī dà zé. bì hù sāi yǒu, xì zhī bìng zhě, shuò wèn qí qíng, yǐ cóng qí yì. dé shén zhě chāng, shī shén zhě wáng.

The utmost essential of treatment is to lose neither the colour nor the pulse; to use them without confusion is the great rule of healing. Shut the door and close the window, bind yourself to the sick one, ask again and again after their feeling, and so follow their will. One who keeps the spirit thrives; one who loses it dies.

And yet the spirit remains the hinge of everything. The utmost of treatment, the classic says, is to lose neither the colour nor the pulse; and then, in a line that has guided physicians ever since, it tells the healer to shut the door and the window, bind themselves to the sick one, and ask again and again after their feeling, following their will, for one who keeps the spirit thrives and one who loses it dies. Healing at this level is an act of complete attention, the physician shutting out the world to be wholly present to the patient, and the patient's own spirit, kept or lost, deciding the outcome more than any remedy. Shift the essence, simplify the life, and above all guard the spirit, in the patient and in oneself: the oldest medicine and the newest meet at this point, where cultivation and cure are one.

Rooting in the Spirit

If the spirit decides so much, the classic asks what the spirit is, and gives the answer in a chapter that anatomises the inner life as carefully as the earlier gates anatomised the body.

> LING SHU 8
>
> 凡刺之法，先必本於神。故生之來謂之精，兩精相搏謂之神，隨神往來者謂之魂，並精而出入者謂之魄，所以任物者謂之心，心有所憶謂之意，意之所存謂之志。
>
> *fán cì zhī fǎ, xiān bì běn yú shén. gù shēng zhī lái wèi zhī jīng, liǎng jīng xiāng bó wèi zhī shén, suí shén wǎng lái zhě wèi zhī hún, bìng jīng ér chū rù zhě wèi zhī pò, suǒ yǐ rèn wù zhě wèi zhī xīn, xīn yǒu suǒ yì wèi zhī yì, yì zhī suǒ cún wèi zhī zhì.*
>
> In all the method of needling, one must first take root in the spirit. For that which comes with life is called the essence; where two essences grapple and join, that is called the spirit; what comes and goes in the spirit's train is the cloud-soul; what goes out and in alongside the essence is the white-soul; that which takes charge of things is the heart; what the heart recalls is called the intent; and what the intent holds fast is called the will.

Needling itself, it begins, must first be rooted in the spirit; and then it lays out the spirit's household. That which comes with life is the essence; where two essences join, the spirit is born; what travels in the spirit's train is the cloud-soul, and what moves with the essence the white-soul; the heart is what takes charge of things, the intent what the heart recalls, the will what the intent holds fast. The classic gives the practitioner a working map of the mind, distinguishing essence, spirit, the two souls, and the faculties of attention, memory, and will, so that a disorder of the inner life can be located as precisely as a disorder of an organ.

The opening line is the one the whole gate is built on: in all the method of needling, one must first take root in the spirit. Then it names the spirit's members one by one and warns the needler to read them before lifting a needle, since a treatment aimed at the body while the spirit is scattered or frightened does half the work at best. It is a striking place to put such a claim, at the head of the most technical of the arts, and it is the plainest reason the reflective gates and the clinical ones belong in one book rather than two.

LING SHU 8

怵惕思慮者則傷神，神傷則恐懼流淫而不止。悲哀動中者則傷魂，喜樂無極者則傷魄，盛怒者迷惑而不治，恐懼者神蕩憚而不收。

chù tì sī lǜ zhě zé shāng shén, shén shāng zé kǒng jù liú yín ér bù zhǐ. bēi āi dòng zhōng zhě zé shāng hún, xǐ lè wú jí zhě zé shāng pò, shèng nù zhě mí huò ér bù zhì, kǒng jù zhě shén dàng dàn ér bù shōu.

Fright and anxious brooding injure the spirit, and when the spirit is injured, dread and terror stream out and will not stop. Grief that stirs the centre injures the cloud-soul; joy and pleasure without limit injure the white-soul; a towering rage confounds and cannot govern; and terror scatters the spirit so that it cannot be gathered back.

And it shows how that inner life is harmed. Fright and anxious brooding injure the spirit, until dread streams out unchecked; grief injures the cloud-soul, unbounded joy the white-soul, a towering rage confounds all governance, and terror scatters the spirit past gathering. Each excess of feeling damages a particular faculty, so the physician treats emotional disorder not vaguely but specifically, knowing which feeling has struck which part of the spirit, and that the cultivation of steady feeling is itself a medicine. Essence, spirit, soul, and will are as real to the classic as blood and qi, and as liable to injury and to care; to root medicine in the spirit is to treat the whole person, the inner life included.

The Most Exalted Teaching

The gate ends on the height the whole tradition aims at, the most exalted teaching, and on what it asks of the one who would master it.

> SU WEN 75
>
> 黃帝坐明堂，召雷公而問之曰：子知醫之道乎？而道，上知天文，下知地理，中知人事，可以長久，以教眾庶，亦不疑殆。
>
> *huáng dì zuò míng táng, zhào léi gōng ér wèn zhī yuē: zi zhī yī zhī dào hū? ér dào, shàng zhī tiān wén, xià zhī dì lǐ, zhōng zhī rén shì, kě yǐ cháng jiǔ, yǐ jiào zhòng shù, yì bù yí dài.*
>
> The Yellow Emperor sat in the Hall of Light and summoned Lei Gong, asking: Do you know the Way of medicine? As for the Way: to know the heavens above, the earth below, and the affairs of humankind between, this can endure long, and one may teach it to the multitude without fear of error.

The Way of medicine, the Yellow Emperor tells his minister, is to know the heavens above, the earth below, and the affairs of humankind between; held so, it endures, and may be taught to all without error. True mastery is not narrow but encompassing, joining the cosmology of the years, the conditions of place, and the lives of people into one understanding, and only such breadth, the classic says, lasts and is safely passed on.

This is why the gate is called the work of return. The physician who would heal at the deepest level must cultivate in themselves the very wholeness they hope to restore in others, reaching upward to the heavens and downward to the earth and inward to the spirit, until the knowledge is not merely learned but embodied. The cultivation of the healer and the healing of the patient are finally the same work, and the classic places it last because it is the ground on which all the rest stands. To know heaven, earth, and humankind, and to guard the spirit that joins them, is the return the gate is named for, the point at which medicine becomes a way of being whole.

THE INNERMOST WORK

The cultivation this gate describes can be gathered into a few commitments, as much for the physician as for the patient. Guard the spirit: protect attention and feeling from the frights, griefs, and excesses that scatter them, for a settled spirit is the ground of health. Simplify the life: keep enough of the old calm that an evil cannot strike deep, so the body stays reachable by gentle means. Be wholly present: in treating others, shut out the world and attend to the one before you, asking after their inner state as carefully as their pulse. And widen the view: reach to know the heavens, the earth, and the human world together, so that knowledge ripens into wisdom. None of this replaces the needle or the herb, but all of it decides how far they reach, and it is, the classic insists, where healing finally lives.

SPIRIT, ESSENCE, AND CULTIVATION

Essential Verses

These are among the gate's most quoted lines in the classic, gathered here for study.

SU WEN 75

而道，上知天文，下知地理，中知人事，可以長久，以教眾庶，亦不疑殆。醫道論篇，可傳後世，可以為寶。受術通明，何能不彰。

ér dào, shàng zhī tiān wén, xià zhī dì lǐ, zhōng zhī rén shì, kě yǐ cháng jiǔ, yǐ jiào zhòng shù, yì bù yí dài. yī dào lùn piān, kě chuán hòu shì, kě yǐ wèi bǎo. shòu shù tōng míng, hé néng bù zhāng.

As for the Way: to know the heavens above, the earth below, and human affairs between, with this one may endure long, may teach the multitude, and be free of doubt and danger. The discourses on the way of medicine may be handed down to later ages and held as a treasure. When one receives the art and penetrates it to clarity, how could it not shine forth?

The chapter exalts the highest reach of medical learning, a comprehension that joins heaven, earth, and human affairs, both heals and may be handed down as a lasting treasure. Such mastery is not technique alone but a clarity won through long inner discipline, which is why the chapter speaks of receiving the art and penetrating it to brightness; it belongs to cultivation as much as to study. The way to it is to observe across the three realms until correspondence becomes second nature, to refine understanding until it is clear rather than merely informed, and to hold the resulting knowledge as something to be guarded and passed on. It frames the deepest medical insight as a fruit of cultivation, and a possession worthy of transmission to those fit to receive it.

FROM THE AUTHOR

This gate is, for me, among the most personal in the book, for I came to these texts not as a scholar but as a patient. From childhood I was unwell in ways no clinic could name, a long stagnation and depletion of the spleen and stomach and a kidney that would not grasp the qi, dismissed for years under a label that fit the tests but not the illness. What turned my health was the right medicine, once it finally reached the root of the trouble rather than its surface. Its effect was profound, and it was the beginning of my recovery. But the medicine was not the whole of it. Once it had done its work, it was cultivation and a changed mind, the very work this gate describes, that let my qi and my health keep steadying and growing: shifting the essence and transforming the qi, learning to guard the spirit, to live more simply, and to attend to my own inner state as the old physicians attended to their patients. I studied the medicine while still unwell, fine-tuning it on my own body as I learned, and I came to know of the ritual side of the tradition alongside the herbal. That cultivation is not a thing I have finished. Like all such work it is the labour of a lifetime, and I am still at it. I have placed these chapters last among the medical gates because they are where medicine becomes cultivation, and because they are, in my own life, where healing took root and held. The whole of this book is written from lived experience; this gate simply tells that part of the story most plainly.

凡刺之法，先必本於神。

In all the method of needling, one must first take root in the spirit.

WHERE THIS GATE LEADS

The cultivation of spirit and essence is where medicine touches the wider tradition, and the final gate, *Gate Eleven, One Tradition, Five Gates*, carries it further than the classic itself goes: there the healing art takes its place among the Five Arts of mountain, medicine, divination, destiny, and physiognomy, and the discipline begun in this gate is opened in full in that gate's chapters on the inner elixir and on stillness, where the later art of refining essence, breath, and spirit is set out. Its daily practice is the nurturing of *Gate One, The Hundred Years*; its bearing on the needle returns us to *Gate Six, The Point of the Needle*, which must be rooted in the very spirit described here; and its stillness is the centre around which the turning of *Gate Nine, The Weather of the Years* revolves.

PART ELEVEN

One Tradition, Five Gates

Medicine and the Five Arts

五術

The last gate turns outward. It shows where this medicine sits in the larger learning, the one root it shares with Mountain, Destiny, Divination, and Physiognomy, and then opens each of those arts in turn, so the Inner Classic stands revealed as the medical gate of a single house of knowledge.

GATE ELEVEN · MEDICINE AND THE FIVE ARTS

One Tradition, Five Gates

五術

> *A person is born of the qi of Heaven and Earth and brought to completion by the law of the four seasons.*
>
> Su Wen 25

The ten gates behind us have moved through the whole of the medicine: from nurturing life and the play of yin and yang, through the organs, the diagnosis, the channels, and the needle, to the diseases and their treatment, the weather of the years, and at last the cultivation of the spirit. This final gate steps back from the medicine itself to ask where it sits, for the Inner Classic is not an isolated text but the medical face of a single great tradition, and the physician who reads it as a practitioner of that tradition reads it most fully.

That tradition is what the old learning calls the Five Arts: Mountain, Medicine, Destiny, Divination, and Physiognomy. They are five branches, but one root. All of them rest on the same few ideas, yin and yang, the five phases, the qi, and the cycles of the calendar, that the reader has met on every page of this book, and all of them are, in the end, ways of reading and harmonising the one pattern that runs through heaven, earth, and the human being alike.

This gate sets the medicine in that company. It shows how the whole of the Inner Classic grows from a single premise about the human place in the cosmos; it lays out the Five Arts and the root they share; and it shows how the classic itself already holds the seeds of all five. To gather the book this way is the purpose of the edition, and the reason its gates were arranged as they are: not as a heap of treatises but as one tradition, entered through many doors.

The One Root

Beneath the whole of the medicine lies a single claim about what a human being is, and the classic states it at the head of one of its treatises.

> SU WEN 25
>
> 黃帝問曰：天覆地載，萬物悉備，莫貴於人，人以天地之氣生，四時之法成，君王眾庶，盡欲全形，形之疾病，莫知其情，留淫日深，著於骨髓，心私慮之。余欲鍼除其疾病，為之奈何？
>
> *huáng dì wèn yuē: tiān fù dì zài, wàn wù xī bèi, mò guì yú rén, rén yǐ tiān dì zhī qì shēng, sì shí zhī fǎ chéng, jūn wáng zhòng shù, jìn yù quán xíng, xíng zhī jí bìng, mò zhī qí qíng, liú yín rì shēn, zhù yú gǔ suǐ, xīn sī lǜ zhī. yú yù zhēn chú qí jí bìng, wèi zhī nài hé?*
>
> The Yellow Emperor asked: Heaven covers and Earth bears up, and the ten thousand things are all complete, yet none is more precious than the human being. A person is born of the qi of Heaven and Earth and brought to completion by the law of the four seasons. Sovereign and commoner alike wish to keep the body whole, yet when the body falls sick, none knows the true state of it, and the lurking trouble grows deeper by the day, settling into the bones and marrow; I grieve over it in my heart. I wish to remove these diseases with the needle. How is it to be done?

Heaven covers and earth bears up, it says, and of all the ten thousand things made complete, none is more precious than the human; for a person is born of the qi of heaven and earth and brought to completion by the law of the four seasons. Everything in the book follows from this one sentence. If the human is made of the same qi as the cosmos and shaped by the same seasons, then the body can be read by the patterns of the world, and the world's patterns can be turned to heal the body, which is precisely what the ten gates have done.

Seen from here, the ten gates are one argument. Because we are born of heaven and earth, we nurture life in step with the seasons, which is the first gate; because we are made of yin and yang and the five phases, the organs, channels, and diagnoses follow, which are the gates of the body; because the qi can be reached and moved, the needle and the treatments work, which are the gates of therapy; because we live inside the turning of the calendar, the weather of the years governs our health, which is the ninth gate; and because the spirit is the finest of the qi, its cultivation is the deepest medicine, which is the tenth. One premise, unfolded ten ways: to hold the premise is to hold the whole, and to see why no gate stands alone. The precious thing, the classic says, is the human being, precisely because the human gathers heaven and earth into one form, and a medicine built on that insight is never only a medicine.

The Five Arts

The same insight founds not one art but five, and the tradition names them together: Mountain, Medicine, Destiny, Divination, and Physiognomy, the Five Arts of the old learning.

The first is Mountain, the art of cultivation: the nurturing of life, the disciplines of breath and posture, the dietary and herbal regimens, and the inner and ritual practices by which a person refines body and spirit. It is the art this book's first and tenth gates already teach, and the one nearest to medicine, for it keeps the body well before any illness begins.

The second is Medicine itself, the healing art: the diagnosis of disease and its treatment by needle, moxa, herb, and the regulating of the whole person. It is the art of the gates between, and the subject of this entire book; of the five, it is the one that meets suffering most directly.

The third is Destiny, the reading of fate: the calculation, from the time of a birth, of the pattern of a life, by the stems and branches and the five phases set out in the charts of the Four Pillars and the stars. It shares with the medicine its very alphabet, for the calendar that fixes a destiny is the same calendar that, in the ninth gate, fixes the weather of the years.

The fourth is Divination, the reading of the moment: the casting and interpreting of a situation by the Book of Changes and the arts descended from it, to know the disposition of a time and how to move within it. It is kin to the medicine's oldest layer, the invocation and ritual of the tenth gate, for both rest on the faith that a moment can be read and harmonised.

And the fifth is Physiognomy, the reading of forms: the study of face and hand, of dwelling and land, by which the qi of a person or a place is judged from its outward shape. It is the cousin of the classic's own diagnosis by complexion, for to read a life in a face and to read a disease in a face are the same skill turned to different ends. Five arts, then, each a distinct discipline, yet each a reading of the one qi by the one set of patterns; and the practitioner of the Five Arts is one who has learned to move among them as among the rooms of a single house.

One Tradition

What binds the five is not merely a shared philosophy but a shared world of texts, and the Inner Classic sits near its centre, a medical classic that already holds the seeds of the other four.

The classic's doctrine of the movements and qi is, in all but name, the art of Destiny applied to the body: the same stems and branches, the same five-phase cycles, read for their bearing on health rather than on fortune. Its diagnosis by complexion is the art of Physiognomy turned to medicine, reading the five colours on the face as the physiognomist reads them for character and fate. Its chapters on shifting the essence and healing by invocation preserve the layer the medicine shares with Divination and with the cultivation arts of the Mountain. And its whole insistence that we are born of heaven and earth is the premise on which all five arts stand. A reader who knows the Five Arts finds in the Neijing not only how to heal but a key to the entire tradition, because the classic was written from within that tradition and never pretended to stand apart from it.

This is why the gates of this edition were drawn as they were. Arranged by subject rather than by scroll, the treatises reveal the architecture beneath them, and that architecture turns out to be the architecture of the tradition itself, the same yin and yang, five phases, qi, and calendar that organise Mountain, Destiny, Divination, and Physiognomy no less than Medicine. To read the classic thematically is already to begin reading it as a practitioner of the Five Arts, which is the way it was meant to be read. The arrangement is the argument; the order of the gates is meant to let the one tradition show through the many treatises. One root, five arts, many doors: the Inner Classic is the medical gate of a single house of knowledge, and to enter it fully is to glimpse the whole house from within.

What remains is to open that house room by room. The chapters that follow take up the wider tradition in turn, beginning with the calendar of time on which all of it, the medicine included, is built, and moving through the reading of a life, the casting of the Yijing, the siting of a dwelling, the inner elixir and the practice of stillness, and the older arts of word and rite, before drawing the whole into a single field of alignment.

THE FIVE ARTS · ONE

The Calendar of Heaven

干支

> *Heaven, by the measure of six sixes, completes a single year.*
>
> Su Wen 9

Every one of these arts counts time in the same way, and reads from time the same thing, a quality. So before any of them can be opened, the calendar they share has to be set out. That shared thing is the Chinese system of stems and branches. A diviner casting a hexagram, a master siting a house, a reader of fate weighing the hour of a birth, and a physician judging the qi of a year are all consulting one clock. This chapter lays out that clock, for it is the grammar in which the rest of these chapters are written.

The medicine's own use of the calendar, its doctrine of the five movements and six qi, was given a gate of its own, the ninth, and is not repeated here. What follows is the calendar itself: how time is counted, why each unit of it carries a quality, and how that quality comes to be read in a life, a place, and a moment.

The Two Wheels

Chinese time is not counted as a single running number but as two interlocking wheels. The ten heavenly stems and the twelve earthly branches turn together, and because ten and twelve come round again only after sixty steps, they generate the sexagenary cycle, the sixty jiazi (六十甲子), a wheel of sixty named units used to mark years, months, days, and hours alike. Each stem and each branch carries one of the five phases and one polarity, yin or yang, so that any unit of time is at once a particular blend of the phases and of yin and yang. Time, in this scheme, is not empty duration. Every moment has a make-up, a specific weather of qi.

THE TEN HEAVENLY STEMS AND TWELVE EARTHLY BRANCHES WITH

THE TEN STEMS (天干)	PHASE	THE TWELVE BRANCHES (地支)	PHASE
甲乙 jiǎ, yǐ	Wood	寅卯 yín, mǎo	Wood
丙丁 bǐng, dīng	Fire	巳午 sì, wǔ	Fire
戊己 wù, jǐ	Earth	辰戌丑未 chén, xū, chǒu, wèi	Earth
庚辛 gēng, xīn	Metal	申酉 shēn, yǒu	Metal
壬癸 rén, guǐ	Water	亥子 hài, zǐ	Water

Read the table as the alphabet of every art in these chapters. The stems give the heavenly, more active layer of a moment; the branches give the earthly, more receptive one, and carry as well the twelve animals by which they are popularly known. Pair one stem with one branch and the count begins at 甲子 (jiǎ zǐ), runs through sixty distinct pairs, and returns to 甲子 again. A full life of sixty years is one complete turn of this wheel, which is why a sixtieth birthday is held to close one cycle and open the next.

The branches hold one further depth worth marking here. Concealed within each of the twelve is a heavenly stem, its dominant or root qi (本氣), and it is this hidden stem, more than the animal, that gives a branch its inner nature in the reading of a life.

FIGURE · THE STEMS AND BRANCHES

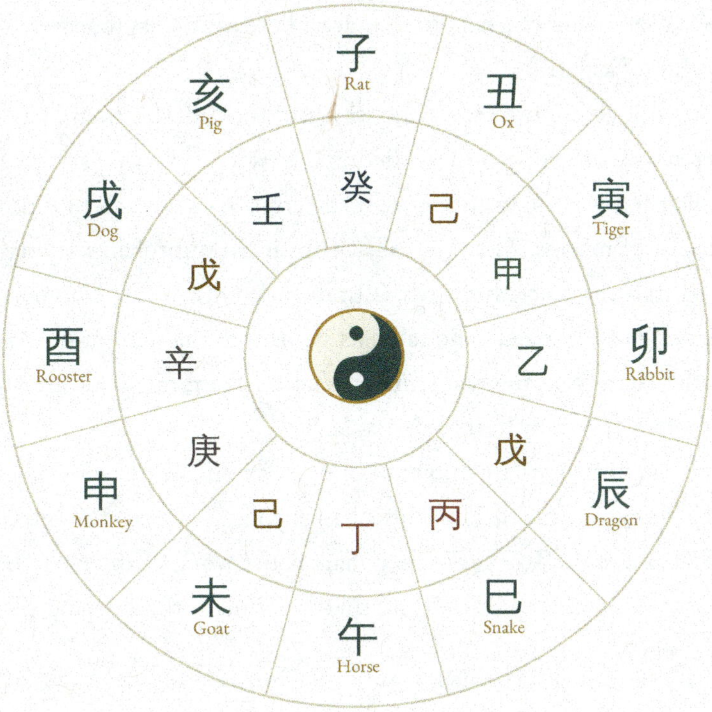

The twelve earthly branches (地支), each with its zodiac animal, form the outer ring. Hidden within every branch is a heavenly stem (天干), its dominant or root qi (本氣), set in the inner ring and coloured by the five phases. It is this concealed stem that gives a branch its inner nature, and from these hidden stems that the qi of a year and the pattern of a life are read.

The Four Pillars of a Moment

The power of the calendar, for the arts of destiny, lies in this: a single moment is stamped by the wheel not once but four times. The year, the month, the day, and the hour each receive their own stem-and-branch pair. Four pairs, two characters each, give the eight characters (八字, bāzì) from which a life is read, and the four pairs together are called the four pillars (四柱, sìzhù) of a chart.

The pillars are not all counted the same way, and the differences matter. The year's pillar turns at the beginning of spring, not at the lunar new year, for the system follows the sun. The month's pillar follows the twenty-four solar terms, so that each month is a season of qi rather than a count of moons. The day's pillar runs in an unbroken sixty-day count that has never once been interrupted across the whole of recorded history. The hour's pillar divides the day into twelve two-hour branches and takes its stem from the stem of the day. The rules that derive the month's stem from the year's, and the hour's from the day's, are old and fixed, and any practitioner carries them by heart or by table.

The result is that a birth, or any moment one cares to examine, is a small chart of the five phases: so much Wood, so much Fire, this phase strong and that one missing, this polarity crowded and that one bare. To read such a chart is the work of the next chapter. Here it is enough to see where the chart comes from, that it is simply the calendar of Heaven, read at the instant a life begins.

One Clock, Many Readings

Once it is clear that the classic itself reckons the quality of time from stems, branches, and the five phases, the other arts stop looking like foreign additions to the medicine. They are the same method turned upon different questions. The doctrine of the five movements and six qi asks what the qi of a year is and how it will fall upon the body. The art of the Eight Characters asks what the qi of the moment of a birth was and how it will shape a life. Divination asks the temper of the moment in which a question is put. The siting of dwellings asks how a place stands within the same cycles of time. The tools never change: the sexagenary stems and branches, the five phases, yin and yang.

The tradition said as much in plain words. One Ming physician held that medicine and the art of fate share a single source, because both rest on the one grammar of qi the classic lays down. Whether one reads a pulse, a year, a birth, or a hexagram, one is reading the same language in a different hand. That is the proper frame in which to receive the chapters ahead. The arts of destiny and place are not a rival system of prediction to be believed or scoffed at. They are this one cosmology, the cosmology that grounds the medicine, applied to the shape of a life, a dwelling, and a moment in time.

A NOTE ON QUALITY AND PREDICTION

The claim that survives every debate over these arts is the modest one, and it is the claim of this whole book: that time has quality, and that the quality of the time we are born into, and live through, touches the body and the life. How finely that quality can be foreseen, year by year or hour by hour, the tradition itself has long argued, and this book sets out the framework without insisting that its every forecast is exact. A chart shows where a person is naturally supported and where they must take care, much as a physician reads where a body is full and where it is empty. That is its honest use.

FROM THE AUTHOR

This is not a distant subject for me. When a client sits down, the first thing I cast is the four pillars of their birth, and from the balance of the phases in that small chart I read not only the turns of their fortune but the make of their body, which organ is well supported and which will need care across a life. The calendar in this chapter is the alphabet I work in every day. I have placed it first in these chapters because nothing that follows, the reading of a life, the siting of a house, the timing of a practice, can be understood until the way these arts count time is made plain.

THE FIVE ARTS · TWO

Reading a Life

八字 · 紫微斗數

> *At fifty, I knew the decree of Heaven.*
>
> Confucius, Analects

If the moment of a birth carries a particular weather of qi, then that weather can be read, and two great arts grew up in China to read it. The first, the art of the Eight Characters (八字, bāzì), also called the Four Pillars of Destiny, reads a life as a configuration of the five phases. The second, Purple Star Astrology (紫微斗數, zǐwēi dǒushù), reads it as a chart of stars set among the houses of a life. Both rest on the cosmology of the Inner Classic, and both are best understood not as fortune-telling in the vulgar sense but as a kind of diagnosis: a reading of where a life is strong, where it is deficient, and what it needs to come into balance.

The Eight Characters

The last chapter showed how the four pillars of a birth, the year, the month, the day, and the hour, each take a stem above a branch, and how the eight characters so formed are a portrait of the five phases at the instant a person entered the world. The art of reading them begins from that portrait. Each pillar speaks to a region of the life.

THE FOUR PILLARS OF THE EIGHT CHARACTERS

PILLAR	RECKONED FROM	READ FOR, IN TRADITION
Year 年柱	the sexagenary year of birth	ancestry and the elders; the roots and the early years
Month 月柱	the solar month, by solar term	parents and siblings; the upbringing and the family one grows in
Day 日柱	the sexagenary day; its stem is the self	the person, in the stem, and the spouse, in the branch
Hour 時柱	the two-hour branch of birth	children and juniors, the later years, the fruits of effort

At the centre of the reading stands the stem of the day, the day master (日主), which represents the person, named by one of the five phases. The whole art is then the reading of relationships: whether the day master is strong or weak amid the other characters, which phases support it and which deplete it, which it produces and which it controls. The classical vocabulary calls these relationships the ten gods, but their logic is only the generating and restraining cycles applied to a life. The phase that bears the day master is its resource and support; the phase it produces is its expression and output; the phase it controls is its wealth; the phase that controls it is its authority and its discipline. A skilled reader looks for the phase the chart most lacks or most needs to come into balance, the useful god (用神), exactly as a physician looks for the deficiency a body most needs supplied. Over this fixed birth-portrait the reader then lays the moving cycles, the great luck periods (大運) and the year-by-year flow (流年), to see when the configuration is supported and when it is strained.

What people bring to such a reading has changed little over the centuries. The old summaries gather the questioner's concerns under eight heads, and a chart is consulted to see how each one stands and when each is favoured or strained: marriage and the spouse (妻), wealth (財), children (子), rank and livelihood (祿), hardship (窮), ease and success (通), long life (壽), and an early end (夭). Between them they cover most of what a person hopes for and fears, and the art is in reading not each in isolation but how the one configuration disposes them all.

The Body in the Chart

Because each of the five phases answers to one of the five organ systems, a chart of the phases is also, read with a physician's eye, a sketch of a constitution. Wood is the liver, Fire the heart, Earth the spleen and stomach, Metal the lung, Water the kidney. The same balance of phases that a destiny reader weighs for the shape of a life, a reader trained in the medicine weighs for the make of a body. A chart that runs short of Water suggests a constitution in which the kidney and the things it governs, the bones, the will, the body's deep water and its grasp of the breath, will ask for care across a whole life. A chart in which Fire stands strong and unchecked suggests a heart and a spirit easily stirred, quick to heat and to restlessness. Wood crowded and unmoving suggests a liver apt to bind, and with it the moods and the free passage of qi.

This is the same constitution that the earlier gates read from the pulse and the complexion, approached from the other end: from the qi present at the hour of birth rather than the qi moving in the body now. It does not replace the examination, and it foretells no particular illness. What it offers is foreknowledge of terrain, a map of where a body is natively well founded and where, long before any symptom, it will reward attention and care. Read this way, the chart becomes a tool of prevention, telling the careful person which of the organ networks is theirs to guard.

The correspondence can be drawn finer than the five organs alone. The tradition assigns to each phase, and so to the stems and branches that carry it, a set of body regions as well as an organ pair, so that a chart can be read not only for which network is strong or weak but for the very parts of the body most apt to show it. The map below gathers the correspondences in common use.

THE FIVE PHASES, THEIR STEMS AND BRANCHES, AND THE BODY

PHASE	ORGANS	STEMS	BRANCHES	BODY REGIONS GOVERNED
Wood	liver, gallbladder	甲乙	寅卯	head, nape, eyes, sinews, limbs, hair
Fire	heart, small intestine	丙丁	巳午	shoulder, face, tongue, teeth, blood, throat
Earth	spleen, stomach	戊己	辰戌丑未	flank, abdomen, back, flesh, skin, mouth
Metal	lung, large intestine	庚辛	申酉	chest, nose, skin, voice, bones, navel
Water	kidney, bladder	壬癸	亥子	lower back, ears, shin, feet, essence, marrow

Read together with the chart, the map sharpens the constitutional reading. A chart heavy in one phase and bare in another points not only to an organ to support but often to the region where strain will first be felt: a thin Water may show in the lower back and the knees as readily as in the kidney itself, and an overfull Wood may bind the sinews and trouble the eyes as much as the liver. It is the same logic the medicine uses when it traces an organ's trouble outward along its channel to the surface of the body.

The correspondence can be drawn finer still, to the individual branches. The tradition gives every one of the twelve branches an organ and a region of the body it governs; a reader who knows which branches fill a chart, and where they sit, can name with some precision the organs and the very parts of the body that the chart marks for strength or for care. The table below gathers these as they are most commonly given. The ten stems carry their own such correspondences, which the verse that closes this section sets out in full.

THE TWELVE BRANCHES AND THE BODY

BRANCH	PHASE	ORGANS AND REGIONS GOVERNED
子 zǐ	Water	bladder, the urinary passages, the ears
丑 chǒu	Earth	the belly, the spleen
寅 yín	Wood	gallbladder, the hands, the channels and the hair
卯 mǎo	Wood	liver, the ten fingers
辰 chén	Earth	the skin, the shoulders, the chest
巳 sì	Fire	the face, the teeth, the throat
午 wǔ	Fire	the spirit, the eyes
未 wèi	Earth	stomach, the diaphragm, the spine
申 shēn	Metal	large intestine, lung, the channels
酉 yǒu	Metal	the essence and blood, small intestine
戌 xū	Earth	the gate of life, the legs, the feet
亥 hài	Water	the head, the kidney

NOT THE MERIDIAN CLOCK

This branch-to-organ correspondence belongs to the destiny tradition and must not be confused with the meridian clock of acupuncture, the midnight-noon ebb and flow (子午流注), which assigns the same twelve branches to the twelve two-hour periods of the day at which the qi runs fullest in each channel: 寅 the lung, 卯 the large intestine, 辰 the stomach, 巳 the spleen, 午 the heart, and so on around the clock. The two systems borrow the one set of branches for wholly different ends. The destiny reading takes the branches of a birth to weigh the make of a constitution; the meridian clock takes the branch of the present hour to time the treatment of a channel. A branch that answers to one organ here will answer to another there, and the two are not to be run together.

The whole of this was fixed long ago in a mnemonic verse, the Ziping Verse on the Origins of Illness, which physicians and destiny readers alike once committed to memory. Its couplets name, in order, the organ each stem governs and the region of the body it rules, and then the organs and regions of the twelve branches; the two tables above are simply its lines unfolded into plain speech.

THE ZIPING VERSE ON THE ORIGINS OF ILLNESS (子平病源生死訣)

甲膽乙肝丙小腸，丁心戊胃己脾鄉。庚是大腸辛屬肺，壬系膀胱癸腎藏。三焦亦向壬中寄，包絡同歸入癸方。甲頭乙項丙肩求，丁心戊肋己屬腹。庚是臍輪辛屬股，壬脛癸足一身由。子屬膀胱水道耳，丑為胞肚及脾鄉。寅膽髮脈並兩手，卯本十指內肝方。辰土為皮肩胸類，巳面齒咽下尻肛。午火精神司眼目，未土胃脘膈脊梁。申金大腸經絡肺，酉中精血小腸藏。戌土命門腿還足，亥水為頭及腎囊。午頭巳未兩肩均，左右二膊是辰申。卯酉雙肋寅戌腿，丑亥屬腳子為陰。

The Purple Star

Purple Star Astrology approaches the same moment by a different geometry. Rather than weighing the five phases, it builds a chart of twelve palaces (宮), houses that divide the domains of a life, and sets among them a company of stars, chief of which is Ziwei, the Purple Star, the imperial star the system is named after. The twelve palaces map the territories of a fate, and the positions of the major stars among them are read for the texture of each domain: where a life finds ease, where it meets obstruction, where its gifts and its trials are gathered.

The art has an imperial cast to its history as well as its name. For most of its life it was a closed system, kept within the palace and reserved for the emperor and his house, who alone were granted its readings. Only after the fall of the Qing did it pass out of private hands into the open, and it has since become one of the most widely practised arts of fate in the Chinese world.

THE TWELVE PALACES OF THE PURPLE STAR CHART

PALACE	DOMAIN	PALACE	DOMAIN
Self 命宮	character, the whole life	Travel 遷移	movement, the world outside
Siblings 兄弟	siblings, close peers	Friends 交友	associates, subordinates
Spouse 夫妻	marriage, partnership	Career 官祿	work, position, standing
Children 子女	children, creativity	Property 田宅	home, land, holdings
Wealth 財帛	money, resources	Fortune 福德	inner wellbeing, fortune
Health 疾厄	the body, its vulnerabilities	Parents 父母	parents, elders, support

The two systems differ in apparatus but agree in spirit. Both take the qi of a birth as a structured pattern; both read that pattern for tendencies rather than verdicts; both lay the moving cycles of time over a fixed chart to read the seasons of a life. And both share the cosmological grammar of the Inner Classic: yin and yang, the five phases, the stems and branches, the conviction that the influences present at a moment leave their mark on what begins in it. The Purple Star even keeps a palace for the body itself, the palace of health, where the system reads the domains in which a person is most apt to be tried.

Knowing the Decree, Not Surrendering to It

The right use of these arts turns on an old distinction the tradition guarded carefully. There is ming (命), the decree or allotment, the configuration one is born with, and there is yun (運), the moving fortune, the changing seasons that pass over it. Neither is the whole of a life. Confucius said that at fifty he knew the decree of Heaven, and the knowing was not surrender but the ground of right action; the tradition speaks of establishing one's decree (立命), taking the given configuration as the field on which character and effort do their work. A birth chart, read well, does not foretell a fixed script. It reveals the terrain: the natural strengths to be developed, the deficiencies to be guarded, the seasons of support and of trial. What one does on that terrain remains to be done.

This is precisely the stance of the physician toward the body. The constitution one is born with cannot be exchanged, but it can be known, supported where it is weak, and spared where it is vulnerable, so that a person lives well within their given nature. The diviner and the doctor offer the same gift: not the abolition of fate but a clear sight of it, and with that sight the freedom to meet it wisely. Destiny, environment, conduct, and cultivation all act upon one life; the chart names the starting configuration, and the rest of this book is concerned with what can still be done.

A NOTE ON THE RIGHT USE OF A CHART

The most useful thing a chart offers a thoughtful person is rarely a prediction. It is self-knowledge of a particular kind: a picture of one's native imbalances, the phase one runs short of, the season one is entering, the domain of life that will ask the most. Used this way, the reading is a mirror and a calendar, not an oracle. The careful practitioner resists the pull, in the client and in the self, to turn it into a script that excuses effort or breeds fear, and keeps returning it to its proper purpose: understanding, alignment, and wise timing.

FROM THE AUTHOR

This is the work I do most days. When someone comes to me, I cast their four pillars and set their Purple Star chart beside them, and read on two levels at once: the shape of the life, and the make of the body. The phase a chart runs short of tells me which organ network will ask for care long before any complaint arrives, and I have learned to trust that map. But I hold it the way I would have a client hold it. A chart is a mirror and a calendar, never a sentence. It shows where a person stands and which way the season is turning; what they build on that ground is still theirs to build. I read fate not to fix it in place, but to help a person understand their situation and navigate it with wisdom.

THE FIVE ARTS · THREE

The Book of Change

易 · 醫易同源

> *One yin and one yang: this alternation is what is called the Way.*
>
> The Great Treatise of the Yijing

Beneath the medicine, beneath the arts of fate, beneath the reading of land we will come to next, lies one book older than all of them: the Yijing (易經), the Book of Change. It is the common root, the text in which the grammar of yin and yang was first set down as a working system, and the tradition was explicit that to follow any of its branches deeply was to return, sooner or later, to the Yijing. A great physician of the Ming put the matter as a flat rule, that medicine and the Yi share one source.

One Yin and One Yang

The philosophical heart of the Yijing lies not in the hexagram texts themselves but in its appended commentary, the Great Treatise, which states the first principle in five characters that the whole tradition took as its charter.

> XICI, THE GREAT TREATISE OF THE YIJING
>
> 一陰一陽之謂道。
>
> *yī yīn yī yáng zhī wèi dào.*
>
> One yin and one yang: this alternation is what is called the Way.

The Way here is not a thing but a rhythm, the ceaseless alternation of the two phases, and the whole of the Yijing is an attempt to map that rhythm in all its configurations. The same treatise gives a cosmogony the reader will recognise at once, for it is the descent of the Daodejing told in the language of the diagram.

XICI

易有太極，是生兩儀，兩儀生四象，四象生八卦。

yì yǒu tài jí, shì shēng liǎng yí, liǎng yí shēng sì xiàng, sì xiàng shēng bā guà.

In the Yijing there is the Supreme Ultimate. This gives birth to the two forms; the two forms give birth to the four images; the four images give birth to the eight trigrams.

Here is the one breath dividing, drawn now as a branching diagram. The Supreme Ultimate (太極, tàijí) is the undivided whole, the same one that the Way gives birth to. It divides into the two forms (兩儀), yin and yang, drawn as a broken line and an unbroken one. Doubling the lines gives the four images, and trebling them the eight trigrams (八卦, bāguà), each a stack of three lines that pictures a fundamental power of nature. Pairing the trigrams in turn gives the sixty-four hexagrams, the full alphabet of situations from which the Yijing reads any moment of change. The emblem on this book's divider pages is exactly this figure: the eight trigrams ringed around the undivided whole.

FIGURE · THE ONE DIVIDING

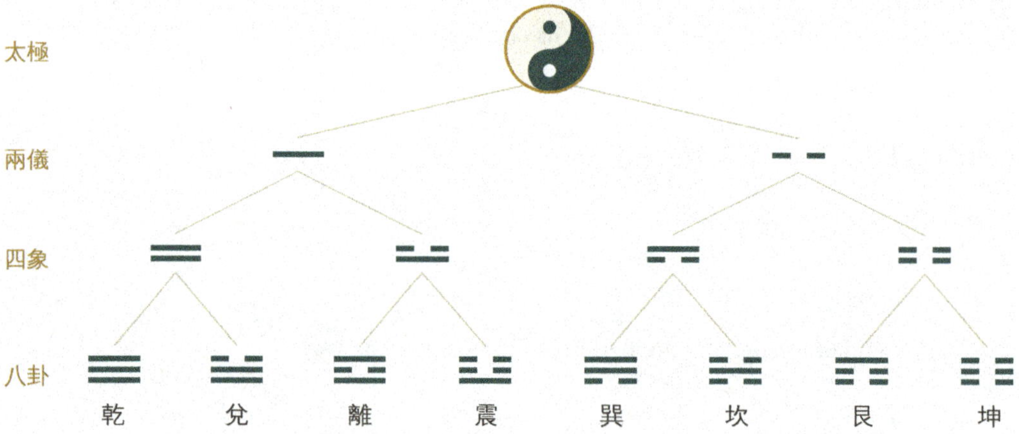

The Supreme Ultimate (太極) divides into the two forms (兩儀), the unbroken line of yang and the broken line of yin. Doubling the lines yields the four images (四象), and trebling them the eight trigrams (八卦), here in the early-heaven order. Pairing the trigrams once more gives the sixty-four hexagrams, the full alphabet of change. The whole figure unfolds from a single undivided line.

THE EIGHT TRIGRAMS, THEIR QUALITIES, AND THE BODY

TRIGRAM	NAME	IMAGE	QUALITY	BODY
☰	Qian 乾	Heaven	creative, strong	bones, heart
☷	Kun 坤	Earth	receptive, yielding	spleen, stomach
☳	Zhen 震	Thunder	arousing, movement	liver, gallbladder, voice
☴	Xun 巽	Wind	gentle, penetrating	breath, nerves, spirit
☵	Kan 坎	Water	abysmal, flowing	kidney
☲	Li 離	Fire	clinging, clarity	heart-spirit, eyes
☶	Gen 艮	Mountain	stillness, stopping	nose, back, breasts
☱	Dui 兌	Lake	joyous, open	lungs, mouth

Medicine and the Yi Share One Source

Because the Inner Classic and the Yijing rest on the same first principle, the tradition came to hold that the two were branches of a single understanding. The doctrine is gathered in the phrase yi yi tong yuan (醫易同源), that medicine and the Yi share one source. Its most famous statement comes from the Ming physician Zhang Jingyue, the same compiler whose thematic arrangement of the classic gave this edition its shape, who began as a sceptic and ended convinced.

> ZHANG JINGYUE, ON THE MEANING OF MEDICINE AND THE YI
>
> 天人一理者，一此陰陽也；醫易同源者，同此變化也。
>
> *tiān rén yī lǐ zhě, yī cǐ yīn yáng yě; yī yì tóng yuán zhě, tóng cǐ biàn huà yě.*
>
> That Heaven and the human share one principle means they share this one thing, yin and yang. That medicine and the Yi share one source means they share these same transformations.

The point is not that a physician must cast hexagrams, but that the reasoning of the medicine and the reasoning of the Yi are one reasoning. Both watch how a situation is composed of yin and yang, how it is tending, where it is full and where it is empty, and what small adjustment will turn it. To think medically is already to think in the manner of the Yi.

Reading the Moment

The Yijing is used in two ways, and the tradition kept both. As philosophy, it is the ground just described, the source of the yin and yang logic that orders medicine and every other art. As divination, it is consulted directly: by casting yarrow stalks or coins one obtains a hexagram, a figure of six lines that images the structure and the tendency of the present moment, and reads from it how the situation stands and which way it is turning. The two uses are one method at different depths. Both rest on the conviction this whole book has followed, that a moment has a structure, that the structure can be read, and that to read it rightly is to move with it rather than against it. The diviner reads the moment of a question as the physician reads the moment of a pulse, and the destiny reader the moment of a birth: three readings of the one changing pattern.

ON THE TRIGRAMS AND THE BODY

The eight trigrams are not abstractions only. The tradition assigns each one a direction, a season, a member of the family, and an organ, so that the same emblem that orders a hexagram also maps the body and the year, giving each trigram an organ, as the table earlier in this chapter set out. The reader who has come through the gates will recognise this as the same correspondence of phase, organ, season, and direction that the medicine uses throughout. The Yijing and the classic are reading one world.

FIGURE · THE EIGHT TRIGRAMS

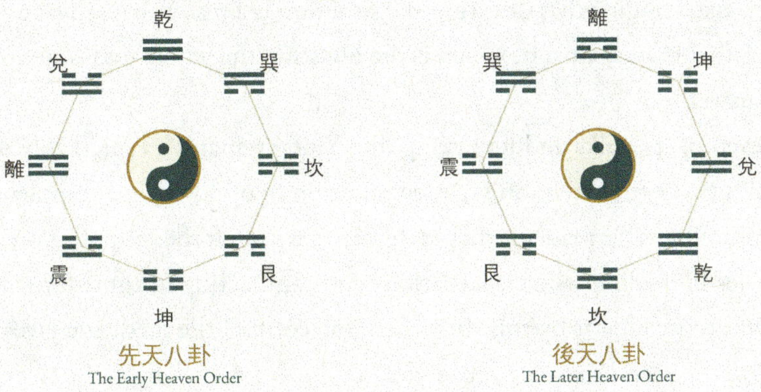

The eight trigrams in their two classical arrangements, each circling the taiji from which they unfold. In the early-heaven order, ascribed to Fuxi, the trigrams stand as pure opposites, heaven (乾) above and earth (坤) below, fire (離) and water (坎) facing across the ring. In the later-heaven order, ascribed to King Wen, they are set as forces move through the seasons and the compass, the arrangement that underlies the nine palaces and feng shui.

The Root of the Whole Tree

Seen this way, the Yijing is the root from which every art in this book grows. Its yin and yang and its five-phase logic are the medicine's own. Its eight trigrams, set to the directions and the seasons, are the compass of the one who reads a dwelling. Its stems, branches, and phases are the destiny reader's reckoning of a life. And its sixty-four hexagrams, consulted at a moment of decision, give the oldest of the arts, divination itself, the reading of the configuration of a present moment so as to act in accord with the way change is already tending. Whether the hexagrams are cast in the old manner with yarrow stalks or read through a later method, the act is the same in spirit as taking a pulse: one reads the pattern of qi as it stands now, and from the pattern infers the movement to come. To consult the Yi is to ask not what is fixed but in what direction the situation is already changing, and how one may move with it rather than against it, which is the question the whole tradition, in every branch, was built to answer.

Stripped even of its stalks and its casting, the Yijing remains a remarkably exact model of change. It holds that every situation is a configuration of opposed and complementary forces; that no configuration is permanent; that each carries within it the seed of its own turning; and that wisdom lies in reading where a situation tends and acting in time. One need not cast a single hexagram to be taught by this. It is the same counsel the medicine gives the body and the seasons give the year: know the phase you are in, and do not fight the turn already under way.

FROM THE AUTHOR

Of all the texts in this tradition, the Yijing is the one I treat as the root, and everything I do returns to it. A chart, a dwelling, the qi of a year, and above all any act of divination, are each in the end an application of the grammar it first set down. When I weigh whether a situation is full or empty, rising or falling, and what small turn will move it, I am thinking in the way the Yi taught the whole tradition to think. To study it is not to learn one more art. It is to learn the language all the arts are spoken in.

THE FIVE ARTS · FOUR

Wind and Water

風水 · 堪輿

> *The qi rides upon the wind and scatters; it meets the water and halts.*
>
> Guo Pu, the Book of Burial

We have followed the one breath through the body and through time. It remains to follow it through space, for the same qi that runs in the channels of a person and turns through the cycles of the years also moves through the land, gathering in some places and scattering in others. The art of reading and working with the qi of a place is Feng Shui (風水), literally wind and water, and its oldest source gives both the name and the principle in a single line.

The Art That Rides the Living Qi

The foundational text is the Book of Burial (葬書, Zàngshū), attributed to the Jin-dynasty scholar Guo Pu. Its argument begins from the same view of the cosmos as the medicine, and says so almost in the medicine's own words: the one qi divides into yin and yang and branches into the five phases, and this qi, running through the earth, brings forth the ten thousand things. Where it gathers and is held, a place is alive; where it races through and scatters, a place is barren.

> GUO PU, THE BOOK OF BURIAL
>
> 氣乘風則散，界水則止。古人聚之使不散，行之使有止，故謂之風水。
>
> *qì chéng fēng zé sàn, jiè shuǐ zé zhǐ. gǔ rén jù zhī shǐ bù sàn, xíng zhī shǐ yǒu zhǐ, gù wèi zhī fēng shuǐ.*
>
> The qi rides upon the wind and scatters; it meets water and halts. The ancients gathered it so that it would not disperse, and guided it so that it would come to rest, and therefore named the art wind and water.

The principle is exact and physical. Qi, like breath or warmth, is stripped away by an exposed, wind-raked site and gathered by a sheltered one; it is held and pooled where water slows and curves. A good site is one embraced by protecting land at its back and sides, so the wind cannot scour it, and met by gentle water before it, so the qi gathers and rests rather than rushing away. This is the very logic the physician applies to the body, where qi that moves freely keeps a person well but qi that scatters or stalls makes them ill. A landscape is a body, and its slopes and waters are its channels.

The Landscape as a Body

The classical art of form, xingshi (形勢), reads the land exactly as a physician reads a body. The ridgelines along which the earth's qi travels are the dragon veins (龍脈), the channels of the land, traced from far mountains down to a site as one traces a channel from its source. The ideal site sits in the embrace of four formations, named for the four celestial animals of the sky.

THE FOUR GUARDIANS OF A SITED PLACE

POSITION	CELESTIAL ANIMAL	THE GROUND IT NAMES
Left, east	Azure Dragon 青龍	rising land that shelters one flank
Right, west	White Tiger 白虎	lower protecting land on the other flank
Front, south	Vermilion Bird 朱雀	open ground and gathering water before it
Rear, north	Dark Warrior 玄武	the supporting height at its back

So sheltered, with water gathering before it, a place holds its living qi the way a sound body holds its breath. The aim is never to impose a pattern on the land but to find where the land already gathers life and to settle there, in accord with what is so of itself. It is the same restraint the first gate asked of the physician, to work within what heaven has made and not against it.

When the Qi Turns Harmful

Not all the qi of a place is benign. The same tradition that maps where the living qi gathers also maps where it turns hostile, and gives the hostile kind a name, sha (煞), the cutting or noxious qi. Sha is born of harsh, fast, and pointed forms: a straight road or corridor that rushes at a door rather than meandering toward it, so that qi strikes the dwelling instead of settling into it; the sharp corner or ridgeline of a neighbouring structure aimed like a blade at a window, what the tradition calls a poison arrow (尖角煞); the oppressive overhang of a building that looms too close and presses down on a home; and the dead, stagnant air of a sealed and lightless room, where the qi neither gathers nor moves but stalls. Where such forms bear on a dwelling, the body that lives there feels it, the tradition holds, as a low and constant pressure, an unease and a wearing that the person cannot quite name but that eases when the offending form is screened, softened, or turned aside. Much of the practical art is precisely this: not only to seat a dwelling where the qi gathers, but to guard it from the qi that cuts and the air that stagnates, so that the field a person lives in supports the body rather than pressing upon it. The same eye that reads where a body is full and where it is empty reads where a place is sheltered and where it is struck.

The Compass and the Turning Year

A second stream of the art is the school of pattern and qi, liqi (理氣). It works less with the visible form of the land than with its orientation in the cosmic grid, bringing a dwelling into line with the directions, the trigrams, and the moving influences of the time. Here the eight trigrams of the Yijing return as a compass of space, each direction carrying its phase and its character, and the geomancer's instrument, the luopan (羅盤), is in effect a portable model of the cosmos, its rings holding the stems and branches, the trigrams, and the cycles by which a place is brought into accord with the year. The two schools are not rivals but two readings of one thing: the form school asks where the qi gathers, the compass school asks how a structure should face to receive it.

FIGURE · THE NINE PALACES

S

E

SOUTHEAST 4 巽	SOUTH 9 離	SOUTHWEST 2 坤
EAST 3 震	CENTRE 5 中	WEST 7 兌
NORTHEAST 8 艮	NORTH 1 坎	NORTHWEST 6 乾

W

N

The Luoshu (洛書) arranged in the nine palaces, with the later-heaven trigrams and the five phases. Every row, column, and diagonal of the numbers totals fifteen. South is placed at the top, after the old Chinese convention, so that the chart faces the reader as a compass would: fire and the south above, water and the north below, wood to the east at the left, metal to the west at the right, and the centre held by earth.

The Luoshu is one of the two root diagrams of Chinese cosmology, the companion of the Hetu. Tradition says it rose on a turtle's shell from the Luo River and was received by Yu the Great, who read in it a square of one through nine whose every line sums to fifteen. Upon this square the later-heaven trigrams are laid, so it carries the Yijing's reading of change into number and direction; and the Neijing builds on the same grid in its Nine Palaces and Eight Winds, where the spirit Taiyi moves through the palaces with the seasons and a wind heals or harms by the quarter it blows from. The nine palaces and flying stars of feng shui, the ground of the liqi just described, come from it too.

The Dwelling as a Third Body

The deepest reason this art belongs in the book is that it completes the figure of the three powers. The body is the human realm; the offices of the organs are the small state within it; and the dwelling is the patch of Earth in which both are set. To order a dwelling is to order the immediate field of qi in which a person sleeps, eats, and works, and the tradition treats it as continuous with the ordering of the body. The placement of the bed, where a person's qi rests for a third of their life; the flow of movement through a home, as the flow of qi through channels; the gathering of light and air, and the avoidance of harsh, scattering exposures: these are read with the same eye that reads a constitution. A dwelling that gathers and holds living qi supports the body that lives in it; one that scatters or stagnates it slowly wears that body down. Place, in this view, is not a neutral container for a life but a participant in it.

The Sensible Core

Wind and water reaches the modern reader wrapped in a great deal of folklore, and an honest account must hold the refined art apart from the commercial superstition it has gathered. The enduring core is not magical. It is the recognition that a person is shaped without pause by their surroundings: that light, air, outlook, shelter, and orientation act on the body and the spirit whether or not anyone attends to them, and that a dwelling can be arranged to support the people within it or to wear them down. Much of what the classical art prescribes, a protected back and an open prospect, generous light, movement that flows rather than rushes, a bed and a hearth set in settled and commanding places, is sober observation about how people live well in a space, set down in the language of qi. Read with discernment, the art is the medicine of place: the same principle that governs the body and the year, carried to the home and the land, that life flourishes where the living breath gathers and is held.

The discipline of the practitioner is to keep the part of the art that reliably helps people clear of the part that merely trades on fear. The reliable part is close to common sense made precise: a person rests better with a solid wall behind the bed and a clear view of the door, works better in light and air, and settles in a home whose movement flows rather than snags. Where the counsel of wind and water meets what truly lets a body rest and a mind ease, it stands on firm ground. Where it leaves that to sell alarm, it has let the living qi slip from view. Stripped of the folklore, what remains is a long tradition of attention to how the shape of a place acts on the life lived in it, and that attention is worth keeping.

FROM THE AUTHOR

I have come to read a place with much of the care I bring to a chart. When I want to understand a person, I look not only at the qi they were born with but at the field they live inside: which way the home faces, where the light falls, where they sleep and where they work. The calendar tells me the qi of the year that passes over that field, and the form of the place tells me whether it gathers that qi or lets it scatter. None of this stands in for the body or the chart. It completes them. We are not sealed within our skin; we breathe the place we are set in, and to tend the place is part of tending the person.

THE FIVE ARTS · FIVE

The Inner Elixir

内丹 · 煉精化氣 · 煉氣化神

> *Follow the current, and a human being is made; reverse the current, and the elixir is made.*
>
> A maxim of the inner alchemists

The medicine of the Inner Classic guards the three treasures, essence, qi, and spirit, so that a person may live out their natural span. The Daoist art of inner alchemy takes those same three treasures and asks a bolder question: if essence can be refined into breath and breath into spirit, can a person deliberately drive that refinement, turning the ordinary descent of vitality back upon itself to distil an elixir within? This is neidan (内丹), the inner elixir, the furthest reach of the cultivation tradition, and the natural completion of this book, for it works on precisely the substances the physician conserves and the cosmology describes. Where the tenth gate gave the classic's own counsel on guarding the spirit, this chapter follows that counsel to its end.

From the Outer Elixir to the Inner

The word dan (丹), elixir, belonged first to the outer alchemists, who sought a drug of immortality in cinnabar and metals heated in a crucible. Centuries of poisonings taught a hard lesson, and the tradition turned inward: the true crucible, it concluded, is the body; the true ingredients are its own essence, breath, and spirit; and the fire is the regulated breath and gathered attention of the adept. The ancestor of the elixir writings is the Token for Joining the Three (周易參同契, Zhōuyì cāntóngqì), ascribed to Wei Boyang, which reads the work through the symbols of the Yijing; later the Chapters on Awakening to Reality (悟真篇, Wùzhēn piān) of Zhang Boduan set the inner method in verse, and the lineages of Zhongli Quan and Lü Dongbin carried it down the centuries. Through all of them runs one startling instruction, the hinge of the whole art.

> A MAXIM OF THE INNER ALCHEMISTS
>
> 順則成人，逆則成丹。
>
> *shùn zé chéng rén, nì zé chéng dān.*
>
> Follow the current, and a human being is made; reverse the current, and the elixir is made.

The current is the ordinary downward and outward flow of vitality, by which essence becomes seed and spends itself in the making of new life and the wear of daily craving. To follow it is to live as most people live, and in time to be spent. To reverse it is to turn that same flow back and upward, conserving the essence and refining it inwardly rather than expending it outwardly. The inner elixir is not a substance smuggled into the body from outside. It is the body's own treasures, gathered instead of scattered, and distilled.

The Fields of Elixir and the Refinements

The work is mapped onto the body's own landscape. Three centres called fields of elixir (丹田, dāntián) mark its stages: a lower field in the belly, below the navel, where essence is gathered; a middle field in the chest, the seat of the breath and of the heart's spirit; and an upper field in the head, between the brows, where spirit is refined. The classical sequence names a foundation and three refinements, each said to take its own season of practice, lifting the treasures of the body one degree at a time toward spirit.

THE STAGES OF THE INNER ELIXIR

STAGE	NAME	THE WORK
Foundation	築基 building the base	settle the body and the breath; gather and replenish the essence, repairing what has been spent
First	煉精化氣 refining essence into breath	conserve essence and transmute it into qi, circulating it in the lesser orbit
Second	煉氣化神 refining breath into spirit	gather the refined qi and transmute it into spirit, in the greater orbit
Third	煉神還虛 refining spirit, returning to emptiness	let the refined spirit return to the open emptiness of the Way

A final movement, refining emptiness and merging with the Way (煉虛合道), names not a further technique but the dissolving of the whole effort into its source, returning spirit itself to the formless Way from which, the Daodejing says, all things come. The ladder rises by increasing subtlety, and its last rung is to let go of the ladder. The classical teachers gave these stages a second name, calling them the three barriers or gateways through which the work must pass: the preliminary labour of building the foundation gathers and repairs the body's depleted treasures until they are whole enough to be refined; then the refining of essence into breath is the initial barrier, the refining of breath into spirit the middle barrier, and the refining of spirit toward emptiness the upper barrier. What is refined at each stage, the adepts insisted, is not the ordinary, postnatal essence, breath, and spirit that the body spends in daily living, but their prenatal sources, the Three Origins (三元): the original essence, original breath, and original spirit that were present before birth and lie buried beneath the acquired. The whole art is the recovery and refinement of these origins, which is why its language speaks so often of returning and reversing rather than of gaining.

Nature and Life, Refined Together

The mature alchemical tradition, above all the lineage of the Chapters on Awakening to Reality, framed the whole work as the joint cultivation of two things the West would keep apart. The first is nature (性, xìng), the mind, the spirit, one's inborn clear awareness. The second is life (命, mìng), the bodily endowment of essence and breath that gives vitality. To work on life alone, building energy without illumining the mind, yields vigour without wisdom; to work on nature alone, cultivating awareness while neglecting the body, yields a clear mind in a failing frame. The Daoist path insists on the dual cultivation of nature and life (性命雙修), and its teachers held that one begins with the body, with life, the doing that gathers and refines the vital forces, and lets the work of nature, the non-doing that rests in pure awareness, come to the fore as the practice ripens, so that the early stages lean toward life and the later toward nature, though neither is ever pursued quite alone. This is the alchemists' answer to a question the medicine also faced: that a human being is neither a body to be fuelled nor a mind to be freed, but a single nature-and-life to be made whole at once.

Plain Practice Beneath the Cryptic Words

It is worth saying plainly what the veiled language conceals, for the alchemical texts are written in a deliberate cipher of trigrams and furnaces, dragons and tigers, lead and mercury, the cycles of the sun and moon and the numbers of the ancient charts, so that they cannot be practised from the page alone. Beneath the cipher, the adepts themselves explained, the method is simple in outline: it takes essence, breath, and spirit as its sole materials; it gathers them in the lower field of elixir; and it refines them through quiet sitting, harmonised breathing, and the gentle direction of a focused intention (意, yì), the mind's quiet attention used as the fire that warms the work. Done rightly and patiently, the texts promise, the practice fills the organs and bones with energy, frees the flow of breath and blood, and so wards off illness and slows the body's decline. This is the point at which inner alchemy and the medicine of the Inner Classic are revealed as one study, for these are precisely the ends the physician seeks; the alchemist only carries the same conservation of the treasures past the keeping of health into the deliberate refinement of the spirit.

Why the Work Begins with the Essence

The great Ming physician Zhang Jingyue, whose Classified Classic (類經, Lèijīng) sorted the whole of the Inner Classic by subject and gave this edition its inspiration, set out plainly why the body's treasures must be kept in a particular order. The essence is the base. When the essence is kept full, he wrote, the breath grows strong; when the breath is strong, the spirit becomes whole; when the spirit is whole, the body is well; and a body that is well falls ill seldom and ages slowly. The chain runs one way only, from essence to breath to spirit, so the whole effort starts at the bottom, with not wasting the essence. This is why the texts warn so often against spending it carelessly: lose the essence and the breath has no root, and the spirit, with nothing to rest on, scatters.

The daily method that follows is not mysterious, and Zhang states it in three plain rules taken straight from the classic's opening treatise. Eat and drink with measure, which feeds the body within. Keep regular hours of waking and rest, which protects the body without. Do not wear yourself out with reckless effort, which guards the vitality you were born with. To these the classic adds the work of the mind: keep your wants few, so the heart is not pulled about; keep the heart calm and unafraid, so the breath stays settled; and let the body work without driving it to exhaustion, so that effort never turns into harm. The whole of it, in Zhang's reading, comes down to two habits, holding the fullness instead of letting it spill, and keeping the spirit at home instead of letting it run outward after every desire, for the spirit that stays within is the spirit that keeps the body whole.

How the Sitting Is Done

The systematic manuals of inner alchemy, such as Wang Mu's modern Foundations of Internal Alchemy, describe the same plain core beneath all the imagery. One takes essence, breath, and spirit as the only materials, and works on them in three simple movements: sit in stillness, harmonise the breath, and let a quiet intention be the guide. To sit in stillness is to settle the body upright and let the mind grow calm. To harmonise the breath is to let it become slow, fine, and even, drawn down toward the lower belly until it is almost unnoticed. To use the intention is to rest a light, unforced attention on the lower field of elixir, gathering the breath and the scattered spirit there. Kept up day after day, the manuals say, this fills the organs and bones with energy and frees the flow of breath and blood, which is why the same practice that refines the elixir also keeps the ordinary body well.

One principle ties the whole method together, what the texts call inverting the course (逆行, nìxíng). In ordinary life the treasures run outward and downward and are spent, the essence in desire, the breath in exertion, the spirit in the chase after things. The practice deliberately turns this current around, drawing the treasures inward and upward to be kept and refined rather than let go. This is the plain sense behind the saying that following the course makes a person while reversing it makes the elixir. Every technique that follows, the circuit of the lesser orbit, the turning of the light, the gathering of the breath, is one form or another of this single reversal.

The Lesser Orbit

The most widely taught of the practices is the circulation now usually called the microcosmic orbit (小周天, the lesser heavenly circuit). Using the two great midline vessels met in the gate on the channels, the adept guides the refined qi up the Governing Vessel (督脈) along the spine and back down the Conception Vessel (任脈) along the front, joining them into a single closed loop. The body becomes a small heaven in which the qi turns as the sun and stars turn in the great heaven, which is why the circuit is named for the rotation of the sky. The practice is built from the plainest materials, posture, quiet, and the regulated breath, but its claim is large: that the same circulation a physician studies in order to keep a patient well can be taken up consciously and turned into a path of refinement.

The detailed manuals describe the upward path as passing three gates along the spine. The qi gathered in the lower field is led first to the tail gate (尾閭, wěilǘ) at the base of the spine, by the point Changqiang (長強, GV1); then up to the spinal gate (夾脊, jiājǐ), the paired points flanking the spine known as the Huatuo jiaji (華佗夾脊), level with the gate of life (命門, GV4) between the kidneys; and on to the jade pillow (玉枕, yùzhěn), which is itself the charted point Yuzhen (BL9) at the back of the head, before it reaches the upper field in the brain; from there it descends the front of the body to return to its source, closing the circuit. These three gates are felt as the places where the ascent is hardest and where patient, unforced breathing is most needed to carry the qi through.

The manuals give the work a homely image: the lower field of elixir is a stove whose gentle inner warmth is kindled by the breath, and above it sits a cauldron in which the gathered essence is cooked and refined. As the work matures, the stove stays fixed in the lower belly while the cauldron, in a manner of speaking, rises, the refining moving upward from the lower field to the middle and at last to the upper, in step with the three refinements named above. The breath is the bellows of this fire. A slow breath drawn down to the lower abdomen rouses the warmth there and presses the essence to rise along the channel of the spine; the out-breath relaxes the belly and lets the qi sink down the channel in front, so that each full round cleanses and concentrates the essence a little further, transmuting it by degrees from the dense reproductive form into the lighter vitality of qi. Here the tradition adds a sober warning that marks the difference between a book and a teacher. The rising warmth of this inner fire is not the same as the light of the original spirit that may appear between the brows, and a practitioner who confuses the two, or who forces the breath and the attention, can drive the qi astray and lodge it where it does harm. This is why the deeper stages are never to be attempted from a page alone, and why the whole art rests, as the next chapter insists, on stillness rather than on effort.

The Fire and Its Measure

If the breath is the bellows of this inner fire, then the art lies less in the fire than in its measure, what the tradition calls the fire phases (火候, huǒhòu), the timing and degree of warmth applied at each turn of the work. The texts are unanimous that more depends on this regulation than on any other part of the practice, and equally unanimous that it is the hardest thing to set down on paper, since it must be felt rather than counted. Two degrees of fire are distinguished. The civil fire (文火, wénhuǒ) is the gentle warmth of a soft, slow breath and a light, almost resting attention; it is used to incubate and to nourish, to keep the work warm without stirring it, as one banks embers to hold their heat. The martial fire (武火, wǔhuǒ) is the stronger warmth of a deeper, firmer breath and a more gathered attention; it is used to rouse the qi at the outset, to press it through the difficult gates of the spine, and to refine with more force where gentleness alone would not move the work. The whole skill is in knowing which to apply and when, raising the fire to gather and circulate, lowering it to settle and incubate, and above all never letting it run too hot, for an unmeasured fire scorches what it was meant to refine. This is why the manuals return so often to the image of cooking: the elixir, like any fine thing on a stove, is spoiled as surely by a fierce and careless flame as by no flame at all, and the cultivator's first competence is the patient governing of heat. Here the alchemist's caution and the physician's are again one, for the classic too taught that the qi is roused by warmth and harmed by what is forced, and that a breath rightly drawn is itself a medicine, while a breath driven hard becomes its own disorder.

The Greater Orbit

When the lesser circuit is well established and the essence has been refined into a steady and abundant qi, the tradition speaks of a wider circulation, the greater orbit (大周天, the greater heavenly circuit). Where the lesser confined itself to the two midline vessels, the Governing Vessel behind and the Conception Vessel before, the greater opens the qi into the body's whole channel-system, through the eight extraordinary vessels (奇經八脈) met in the gate on the meridians and on into the twelve regular channels of the organs, until the refined qi reaches the limbs and the extremities, the arms and hands, the legs and feet, and pervades the entire frame rather than turning about a single loop. The manuals are careful to say that this is not a path forced open by the will, in the way the lesser orbit is first learned, but a circulation that arises of itself once the work has matured, the qi grown so full that it spreads through the body as warmth spreads through water, no longer pushed by the breath but moving on its own. This is the bodily side of the second refinement, the transmuting of breath into spirit (煉氣化神), in which qi and spirit are said to draw together and hold to one another inseparably; and as the qi grows full and free, the heavy labour of circulating it falls away, while the breath itself, the texts say, grows so faint that at times it seems to stop altogether, an outer stillness that is the sign of an inner fullness.

But the name reaches further than the body alone. The circuit is called the greater, and the heavenly, because at this stage the small heaven of the body is no longer a closed loop but is opened to the great heaven around it: the adept's own qi comes into exchange and accord with the qi of heaven and earth (天地之氣), the clear influences of sun and moon and the seasons drawn inward from above and the steadiness of the earth received from below, until the body is tuned to the turning of the cosmos. This is the cultivator's living enactment of the oldest principle of the medicine itself, the unity of the human with heaven and earth (天人合一). For the Inner Classic taught from the first that a human being is born of the qi of heaven and earth and brought to completion by the law of the four seasons, that the human takes part with heaven and earth and answers to the sun and moon, so that the body is a small cosmos corresponding to the great one. The greater orbit takes that correspondence, which the physician reads only in order to keep a patient in step with the seasons, and makes a path of it, deepening by deliberate work the same resonance between the human and the cosmos that the classic had observed, until the practitioner feels body and world breathing as one. This is why the tradition holds the greater orbit to be the higher and more advanced reach of the art, for it carries the circulation past the keeping of the body's own treasures into the body's conscious accord with the vast turning of heaven and earth.

FIGURE · THE TWO ORBITS

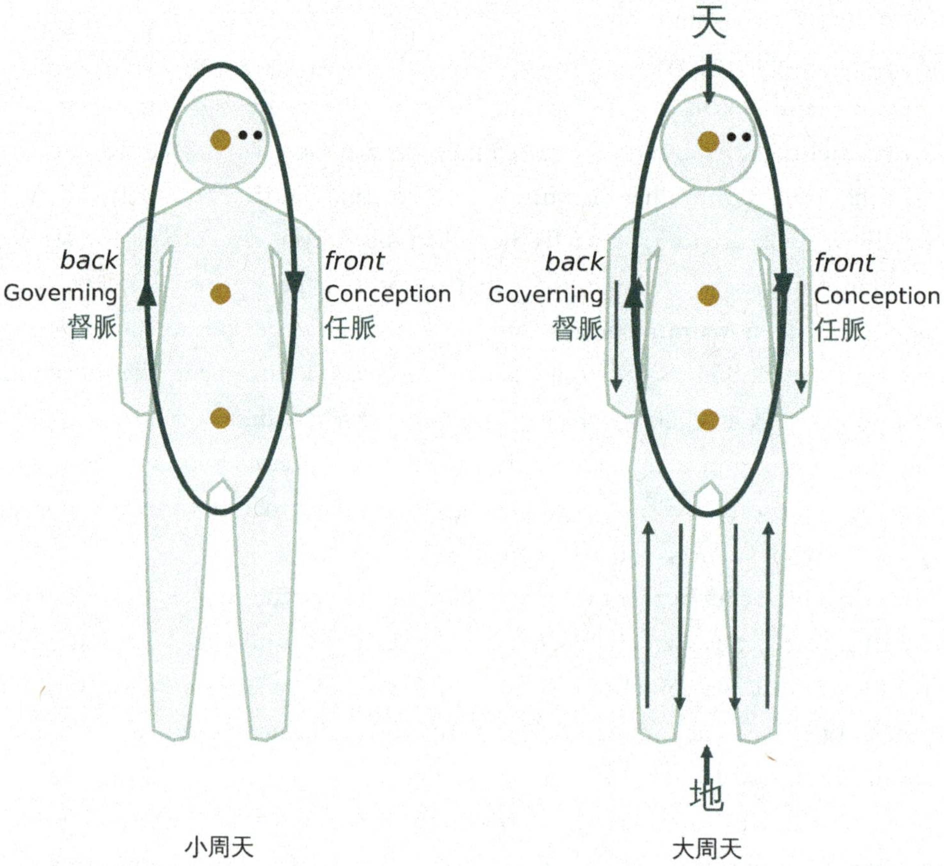

The microcosmic orbit (小周天) circulates qi up the Governing Vessel along the back and down the Conception Vessel along the front, through the three elixir fields at brow, heart, and lower abdomen. The macrocosmic orbit (大周天) widens that same circulation to the whole body: the qi ascends along the back of the trunk and limbs and descends along the front, reaching out to the hands and feet, while the body comes into resonance with the qi of Heaven (天) above and Earth (地) below.

The Crown and the Embryo

As the refinements ripen, the tradition marks their convergence with two phrases that became watchwords of the whole art. The first is the three flowers gathering at the crown (三花聚頂, sānhuā jùdǐng): essence, breath, and spirit, kept apart and spent in ordinary life, are gathered and lifted until they meet and flower together at the summit of the head, the three made one. The second is the five qi returning to the origin (五氣朝元, wǔqì cháoyuán): the qi of the five organs, each ordinarily turned toward its own season and direction as the third gate described, is drawn home and reconciled at the centre, the five made whole. The two phrases name a single event from two sides, the uniting of the body's scattered powers, the three treasures and the five organ-qi alike, into one undivided vitality, and they mark the point at which the work passes from the refining of substances toward the refining of spirit itself.

What is said to form at this convergence the texts call the holy embryo (聖胎, shèngtāi), the embryo of sagehood, an image and not a thing: the united treasures, gathered in the lower field and warmed by the gentle civil fire, are spoken of as a seed conceived within, which the adept tends as a mother tends the child in her womb, through long and quiet incubation. Refined and ripened, this embryo is said at last to issue forth as the yang spirit (陽神, yáng-shén), the pure and illumined spirit that is the fruit of the whole work, the spirit returned to its original wholeness and no longer bound to the body's spending. Here the language of alchemy reaches its furthest and most figurative pitch, and it is honest to say plainly that these are the tradition's accounts of its own highest attainment, set down in images that point past what plain words can hold. This book records them not as claims to be tested but as the far horizon toward which the whole path leans, so that the reader may see the shape of the road entire, from the keeping of a single drop of essence to the return of the spirit to its source.

Already in the Classic

It would be a mistake to think of inner alchemy as a later system imposed upon the medicine, for its seeds are in the Inner Classic itself. The True Person of the first treatise breathed the pure essence and stood alone, guarding the spirit, which is the whole of cultivation in a single line. The thirteenth treatise of the Su Wen is titled On Shifting the Essence and Transforming the Qi. The counsel to keep the essence and the spirit guarded within is at once a physician's hygiene and an adept's first instruction. The inner elixir simply takes the conservation that medicine prescribes for health and carries it to its furthest conclusion, turning the keeping of the treasures into their refinement. Medicine and alchemy are the same road walked to different distances: one to wholeness and a long life, the other to the return of the spirit to its source.

A CAUTION AND A CLARIFICATION

The inner alchemical literature is deliberately veiled, written in dense symbol so that it cannot be practised from a book alone, and the tradition is unanimous that its deeper stages require a living teacher and a sound foundation, lest forced effort disturb rather than refine. This chapter describes the art to show its place in the whole, not to instruct in it. What can be said plainly and safely is that its foundation, the settling of the body, the quieting of the breath, the gathering of a scattered attention, and the conservation of vitality, is continuous with everything the earlier gates counselled for health, and is sound ground for anyone.

FROM THE AUTHOR

Cultivation, for me, is less a practice one completes than a direction one keeps, a constant refining and steadying of the self that has no final day; in that sense it is the quiet work of a life, my own included. But I want to be exact about what this chapter is. I have set the inner elixir down for the reader's knowledge, because no honest map of this tradition could leave it out, and not as an account of my own daily discipline. The growing of my qi I have pursued largely through other systems of energy work; where the inner elixir has served me is in the processing of that qi once it is raised, and in the settling and storing of it, so that what is gathered is kept rather than spent. I write of the art, then, with respect and from its threshold, and chiefly to show the reader how the whole of this tradition, the medicine not least, leans toward this one work: the refining of what we already are.

THE FIVE ARTS · SIX

Stillness and the Return

致虛極 · 守靜篤 · 歸根

> *Reach the utmost emptiness; hold fast to deep stillness. The ten thousand things rise together, and in them I watch the return. The things in all their profusion each return again to their root. To return to the root is called stillness.*
>
> DAODEJING 16

Beneath every technique of cultivation lies one practice, and it is the simplest and the hardest: to grow still. The refinements of the inner elixir, the circulations of the breath, the regimens of nourishing life, all rest on a foundation of quiet, and without it none of them reach very far. The last chapter ended by saying that the whole art of the elixir rests not on effort but on stillness; this chapter is that stillness, the quiet ground on which the tenth gate's cultivation and the elixir's refinement alike are built. The Daodejing states the practice in two lines that the whole tradition took as its meditation manual in miniature.

Two movements are named here, and they are the whole of the contemplative path. The first is emptying, the laying down of the clutter of craving and thought until the mind is open and still. The second is the return, gui gen (歸根), the homecoming of all things to their root, which the stilled mind is at last quiet enough to witness. Cultivation, in this tradition, is not the acquisition of powers but a returning: the reversal of the outward, scattering current of an ordinary life back toward the source from which it came. This is the same reversal the alchemists meant by turning the current, now seen from within, as the felt movement of a mind coming home.

The Breath of the True Person

Zhuangzi, the second great voice of Daoism, describes the bodily sign of this stillness in an image the cultivators never forgot.

> ZHUANGZI, THE GREAT AND VENERABLE TEACHER
>
> 真人之息以踵，眾人之息以喉。
>
> *zhēn rén zhī xī yǐ zhǒng, zhòng rén zhī xī yǐ hóu.*
>
> The True Person breathes from the heels; the common run of people breathe from the throat.

The contrast is between a breath that is shallow, quick, and caught high in the throat, the breath of agitation, and a breath so deep, slow, and settled that it seems to reach the very soles of the feet, the breath of profound calm. To breathe from the heels is to be wholly at rest, the qi sunk to its root in the lower field of elixir rather than floating restless at the surface. Here the cultivator's instruction and the physician's meet again, for the Inner Classic said the same thing in its own way, that in calm detachment and open emptiness the true breath follows. A settled breath is at once the means and the sign of a settled spirit.

Fasting the Heart, Sitting in Forgetfulness

Zhuangzi gives the inner method two names that became permanent in the tradition. The first is the fasting of the heart-mind (心齋, xīnzhāi). This is not a fasting of the body but an emptying of the mind. One stops grasping at things with the senses and the intellect and listens instead with the open emptiness of qi, until the noise of the self grows quiet. The second is sitting in forgetfulness (坐忘, zuòwàng), in which one lets fall limb and body, dims hearing and sight, and merges with the great pervading Way. Both name the same emptying the Daodejing prescribed, and both produce the same fruit: a mind no longer scattered across its wants, gathered back to its root, from which it can act with the spontaneous rightness the Daoists called moving with the Way. To embrace the One, in the Daodejing's phrase, and to guard the One, in the cultivators', is to rest the whole of oneself on that single recovered stillness. First empty, then return: the path is not forward into more, but back into the source.

The Clearing of Desire

A later scripture, short enough to be learned by heart and recited as the Daodejing and the Zhuangzi were, gathered this whole teaching into a single thread and gave the tradition its plainest account of why stillness is so hard to hold and how it is won. It is the Classic of Purity and Stillness (清靜經, Qīngjìng jīng), and it opens not with a technique but with a diagnosis of the trouble.

> CLASSIC OF PURITY AND STILLNESS
>
> 夫人神好清，而心擾之；人心好靜，而欲牽之。常能遣其欲，而心自靜，澄其心，而神自清。
>
> *fú rén shén hào qīng, ér xīn rǎo zhī; rén xīn hào jìng, ér yù qiān zhī. cháng néng qiǎn qí yù, ér xīn zì jìng, chéng qí xīn, ér shén zì qīng.*
>
> The human spirit loves clarity, but the mind disturbs it; the human mind loves stillness, but desire pulls it about. If one can constantly dispel desire, the mind stills of itself; settle the mind, and the spirit clears of itself.

The diagnosis is exact and, to a physician's ear, familiar. The spirit by its own nature wants to be clear and the mind by its own nature wants to be calm; what unsettles them is not some flaw in their making but the steady tug of craving, the wanting that will not let the water's surface lie still. The cure follows from the cause. One does not force the mind quiet, which only lays a further agitation on top of the first, but loosens the grip of desire, and the stillness that was native to the mind all along returns of its own accord, as a pond clears the moment one stops stirring it. The scripture carries this clearing through by degrees, observing the mind until no mind is found, the form until no form is found, the things of the world until they too are seen to be empty, and so passing from the stilling of a particular desire to a stillness that nothing can disturb, which it calls the true and constant (真常, zhēncháng). What the medicine names a heart at rest, ruling a quiet country, the scripture names from within, as a spirit grown clear because the wanting that had muddied it has been set down.

Turning the Light Around

One late and beautiful current of the tradition, gathered in the text known as the Secret of the Golden Flower, gave this return a precise inward image: the turning of the light around (回光, huíguāng). Ordinarily the light of awareness streams outward through the senses, spent upon things desired and feared, scattering the spirit into the world until it is exhausted. The practice reverses this outward flow, turning the light back upon its source, so that attention, instead of pouring out through the eyes, is gently gathered inward and downward to rest in the body's centre. The same backward turning the alchemists called reversing the current is here felt from within, as the simple act of letting the gaze and the mind fall quiet and return home. Done steadily, the tradition teaches, this gathering of the scattered light kindles within a stable centre of awareness, the golden flower that is nothing other than the spirit no longer leaking outward but collected and bright.

Said plainly, the method has only a few parts. One sits upright and still in a quiet place and lets the breath grow slow, soft, and even until it is barely felt. The eyes are lowered and half closed, the gaze resting lightly along the line of the nose rather than fixing on anything, so that sight is drawn inward instead of out. A gentle attention is then laid at the body's centre and kept there without strain, brought back each time the mind wanders off. Breath and attention are held together, the mind riding the breath as it settles, so the two grow quiet as one. The manuals are firm that the touch must be light: one neither forces the breath nor stares hard at the centre, since effort scatters the very stillness it is meant to gather. A little of this each day, kept up patiently, does more than long sittings strained after.

Behind this practice lies a distinction the Daoists drew within the mind itself, between two kinds of spirit. There is the conscious or cognitive spirit (識神, shíshén), the busy, calculating, grasping mind that sorts and names and wants, the mind of the ordinary waking day; and beneath it the original spirit (元神, yuánshén), the still, prior awareness that was there before thought, clear and undivided, akin to the open emptiness of the Way. The cognitive spirit is not an enemy but a servant that has usurped the throne; the work of stillness is to let it grow quiet so that the original spirit, which it had drowned out with its chatter, may come forward of itself. This is why the tradition prizes silence above striving: the deeper awareness cannot be manufactured, only uncovered, and it appears only when the grasping mind consents to rest. Here the contemplative path and the medicine meet once more, for the heart that the Inner Classic calls the sovereign, when it is clear and at rest, is precisely this original spirit restored to its throne, ruling a peaceful country from a quiet centre.

The Virtue of Stillness

The reach of this stillness runs back through the entire book. It is the medicine's quiet heart, from which the seven feelings rise and pass without lodging. It is the foundation of the inner elixir, without which no refinement holds. It is the steadiness the diviner needs to read a moment clearly and the calm the physician needs to feel a pulse truly. And it is the ground of virtue itself, for a still mind is an undistorted one, able to see what is actually before it and to respond without the warping of fear and craving. The cultivation of stillness is therefore not a withdrawal from life but the condition of living it well, the inner alignment that makes the outer alignments, of body, of time, of place, of conduct, possible. It is the human being's own contribution to the harmony of the three powers: Heaven turns, Earth abides, and the human, grown still, can at last move in time with both.

IN MODERN LIFE

The practices the tradition gathered under stillness, slow breath, settled attention, the deliberate quieting of a racing mind, are now among the most studied interventions in medicine, shown to lower the body's stress response, steady the heart, and ease the very disorders the gate on the seven feelings described. The framework offered here adds only this: that such practice is not a technique bolted onto a busy life to make it bearable, but a return to the baseline from which a whole life is meant to be lived. The stillness is not the exception. It is the root, and the noise is the departure from it.

FROM THE AUTHOR

Of everything in these chapters, stillness is the one I would most want a reader to try, for it asks for nothing rare. It is the plainest practice there is, and anyone can begin it: to sit, to let the breath grow slow, to let the grasping mind settle, and simply to rest there with the breath and nothing more. In an age as crowded and noisy as ours, where information presses in without pause, the simple act of returning to that quiet may be the most useful thing in this whole book, and it is open to everyone. I come back to it each day, beneath the reading of charts and dwellings and years, and beneath the medicine itself. The tradition is right that it is at once the simplest thing and the hardest, and right that it is the root a life departs from and, now more than ever, needs to return to.

THE FIVE ARTS · SEVEN

Word and Rite

道醫 · 祝由

> *The way of medicine opens onto the way of the immortals.*
>
> A saying of the Daoist physicians

Behind the medicine set out in this book stands an older root. Long before there was a settled profession of medicine, there were people who cultivated the Dao, and for whom healing was simply one of the things that cultivation made possible. Their medicine and their practice of the Way were not two pursuits but one: a person first worked on themselves, and the power to help others followed of its own accord. From this older Daoist medicine (道醫) the later and more public art we now call Chinese medicine slowly grew, drawing off its theory and its methods while leaving much of its inner discipline behind. Mainstream Chinese medicine narrowed itself, over the centuries, to the body that can be seen and measured and to the disorders that can be named and treated by herb and needle; Daoist medicine kept a wider view, working with the sacred and with what the eye cannot see, and it is just this dimension that the popular practice has largely lost. At its heart lies one conviction: that the Dao and medicine cannot be parted. One does not set out to become a healer; one sets out to cultivate the Way, and healing follows as a natural fruit.

A Cure as a Turning Point

It was always stressed that to be cured of an illness is not a licence to return to the life that bred it. The old habits and the old turns of thought were what made a person ill in the first place, and to take them up again is to call the illness back. One is healed for a purpose: to make a new self and a new life. The cure of the body is meant to be a turning point, a chance for a clearer perception and a steadier conduct than before, so that a new person emerges along with the new health. Seen this way, healing is a kind of sacred change, and the medicine is only its occasion, one of the many roads that lead toward a deeper understanding of the Dao.

The Seen and the Unseen

Daoist medicine attends to two bodies at once. There is the body of form (有形), the flesh the physician can touch and treat, and there is the formless body (無形, the 虛體) that the flesh is built upon. The tradition even ranks the degrees of the formless: its lower reaches are counted as yin, its higher reaches as a mixture of yin and yang, and its very highest as pure yang (純陽). Because it reckons with the unseen as well as the seen, the reach of its diagnosis is far wider than that of mainstream medicine, for it reads three orders of cause at once: the causes of Heaven, of the human, and of Earth (天因, 人因, 地因).

The Causes of Heaven

The causes of Heaven are the ones a person carries into the world before they draw a breath. They take in what is given before birth (先天), the workings of cause and effect across a life and beyond it (因果), and the spiritual and psychological factors that shape a person from within. Some are born already leaning toward a particular illness, and the tradition traces this to what was inherited and to what was set before birth, a tendency handed down from parents and ancestors, or a reckoning carried over from before this life. Such an inheritance is the inheritor's own to resolve or to repay, and it is often not the physician's place to interfere with it, or only with great care, for to lift from a person what they were meant to work through is not always a kindness. To this order belong, too, the disturbances of feeling and the burdens of a life: the seven feelings and the six desires, the press of society, the strain of unhappy bonds, the weight of money and circumstance, all of which leave their mark on the formless body before they reach the flesh. So does the pattern a person is born under, read in the eight characters of the four pillars (八字四柱), which fix at the moment of birth a particular share of the five phases; and even what the tradition calls a person's reason for coming (來因), the purpose of their being here at all, is counted among the deeper causes that may shape a life of health or of illness.

The Hun and the Po

Here the two souls come into their own. The ethereal soul (魂) and the bodily soul (魄) are named in ordinary Chinese medicine but little used in its clinic; Daoist medicine makes far more of them. The po is the more yin and the hun the more yang, yet the two cannot be separated, and may be likened to the north and south poles of the earth, distinct but bound in one body. They are, in this understanding, a kind of channel between a person and the unseen, and they keep their work only where the life within and the life around are at peace. They are worn by grief and fear, and injured by deeper faults as well, by harm done to other living things, an injury that may even be carried down a line. A Daoist physician weighs all of this, for such hidden wounds are often the root of an illness that will not yield to ordinary treatment, and learns with time when such a debt (業障) may rightly be eased and when it must be left to run its course. Compassion is always required, but so is the humility to see when a force higher than oneself is at work.

When the Cause Is Unseen

At its furthest reach Daoist medicine treats afflictions that have no bodily cause at all. The tradition holds that there are formless influences, presences of a yin nature and old by the measure of human time, that fasten onto a person on the unseen level and draw on their vitality. Such an attachment is said to settle often at the gate of life and to leach the essence of the kidney, so that it shows in the body as a leaking of essence. These influences are said to work most easily at night, when the guarding and nourishing layers of qi (營衛) run low, though they may also act by day in a slower way, as a magnet left beside iron will in time draw the iron to its own charge. The healing rites of the tradition are aimed at causes such as these, and are said to put the weaker of these presences to flight. This is the precise place where the rites described below have their work, and it is why a tradition that begins in the cultivation of the self comes, at its edge, to the spoken word and the drawn sign.

The Causes of the Human, and of Earth

The causes of the human are the everyday ones, and these mainstream medicine knows well, for they are the very matter of the Inner Classic: the daily round of habit (日常生活習慣), food and drink (飲食), the spending of desire (縱慾), and the labour of the body (勞作). Here the Daoist physician adds a particular stress on prohibitions (禁), plain rules that forbid, for a time, the very things that fed the disease, their aim being not only to remove the cause but in time to shift the mind of the patient, so that a healthier way of living is taken up willingly rather than merely imposed.

The causes of Earth are those of place, and here medicine and the art of wind and water are one work. Where a house stands, and how it is arranged within, presses on a body over years until it leaves its mark: the lie of mountains and rivers, the run of roads and buildings, the quality of the light and the air, the nearness of graveyards and of the lines that carry power, all of these may bear on health for good or ill. The Daoist physician must be able to read such features of a place as causes of illness, and to set them right, exactly as the chapter on wind and water reads them.

The Physician's Own Cultivation

What most sets the Daoist physician apart is that their skill rests first on their own cultivation. Before they are a healer they are a person who has worked, through breathwork and the fostering of life, through sitting and stillness and guided movement, to build and settle a strong field of qi (氣場) about themselves. So prepared, the tradition holds, a healer can reach the root of a disorder almost regardless of the technique they use, because the qi and the steadiness they bring are themselves part of the cure. The same teaching explains a thing every careful practitioner notices, that the same formula written by two different healers does not act the same way, for something of the healer's own qi and intent attaches to the prescription. For the same reason Daoist medicine prefers fresh and local herbs, in which the whole virtue of the plant is still present, to herbs long dried and mass-produced, and it keeps words of thanks to be said over the herbs as they are gathered.

The Seven Skills, and the Methods Set Aside

Beyond herb and needle, Daoist medicine held a body of methods that mainstream medicine has largely let go. They are counted as seven: the hand-seal, the rite, the incantation, the talisman, the prohibition, the working of qi, and technique itself (訣, 法, 咒, 符, 禁, 氣, 術). These were not a folk superstition grafted on from outside; they stood near the centre of the canonical tradition. The Inner Classic itself records that the ancients could cure by the spoken rite of zhuyou (祝由) alone, shifting the essence and turning the qi; the imperial medical academy long taught zhuyou as one of its departments; and the great Sun Simiao, whose oath on the conduct of the physician closes this book, set down a book of prohibitions and incantations within his Supplement to the Essential Prescriptions Worth a Thousand Gold (千金翼方), and is remembered for the thirteen ghost points (十三鬼穴), once used in exorcism to drive out possessing spirits and now classified, in modern practice, for the treatment of mental and emotional disorders.

Every one of these skills rests on the practitioner's own training. Their root lies in the body of the one who works them, who must first have opened a line of communication with the higher reaches of Heaven and Earth, and they must be founded on compassion, love, and mercy, on a great compassion (大慈悲) that reaches beyond the human scale of thought and desire. The skills are not used singly but woven together; one cannot apply a rite without the incantation and the hand-seal that belong to it. Each is gained by a season of intense study and then kept by steady practice, so that the power built into it is not lost. A talisman, to take one example, must be trained day after day under strict conditions, with incantations passed by word of mouth, before it carries any power at all. The talismans that lie scattered through old books are cut off from their lineage and their oral tradition, and are often altered so that their force is curbed, a safeguard against the harm their misuse could do; their proper use is hedged about with conditions, to be drawn only when a patient begs for help, sets aside every preconception, and gives the healer their full trust, and only where the healer feels a true bond of destiny (緣分) with the one before them.

Many of the plainer techniques are shared with ordinary Chinese medicine: acupuncture and moxibustion, massage and cupping, steaming and fumigation, herbal medicine in its pills and decoctions and plasters, dietary regulation, healing with music, the work of qi, and the arts of wind and water and of the Yijing. Much of this was pared away in the last century. As the tradition was reorganised along clinical and material lines, the ritual methods were dropped from the schools and struck from the textbooks, and what is now taught as the whole of the tradition is in truth only a part of it, with the older and stranger half quietly removed. To return to the root of the medicine is, in some measure, to remember what was left out, and that remembering is among the reasons this book exists.

Time, the Needle, and the Yi

For all its reach into the unseen, Daoist medicine takes its theory of the needle from the same source as mainstream medicine, the Inner Classic, and in practice it leans on the reckoning of time. Methods such as the Eight Methods of the Sacred Tortoise (靈龜八法) open a given point according to the hour, read from the stems and branches, so that the body is treated as a part of the wider turning of Heaven, Earth, and time. Mainstream medicine has largely set the Yijing aside, but in Daoist medicine it has stayed central; the bond between the Yi and medicine was held to be so near that, in Sun Simiao's words, one who does not know the Yijing is not fit to be called a great physician (不知《易》，不足以言太醫). The Yi sets down the flux of change that runs through all things, the changes of health and illness among them, and so it serves in diagnosis and in the planning of treatment, exactly as the chapter on the Yijing described.

FROM THE AUTHOR

This older root of the medicine is one I hold in deep respect. The Heaven-given causes, the constitution a person is born with, I do read, from the eight characters of a birth, as the earlier chapters set out, and much of what I do for those who come to me begins there. The ritual heart of this tradition, the rites and incantations and talismans, is another matter: an art of living transmission, passed from teacher to student under conditions a book cannot supply. I have long known of the old texts of prohibition and incantation, Sun Simiao's among them, and I set the art down here for the reader's knowledge, so that the wider and stranger half of the medicine, the half so nearly lost, is at least remembered and given its place.

THE FIVE ARTS · EIGHT

One Field of Alignment

大醫精誠

> *A human life is of the heaviest weight, more precious than a thousand pieces of gold; to save it with a single prescription is to bestow a kindness beyond that.*
>
> Sun Simiao

The arts gathered in these chapters all converge on a single figure: the person fit to wield them. The book began with a question about how to live a whole life, and it ends with a portrait of the one fit to guide others toward it, the great physician, in whom the whole of this tradition is gathered into a single character. Before that portrait can be drawn, one thing must be said about where the healing art itself stands within the larger work of the Way.

Medicine as a Stage of the Way

For all its dignity, the rank of healer is, in the larger scheme of Daoist cultivation, still a modest one. It belongs to the work of refining the self and laying a foundation (煉己, 築基), the preparation for the later stages of the inner elixir. Medicine is a way of using what one has gained in order to help others, and so of gathering virtue (積累功德); practised in this spirit it becomes one of the roads toward the Dao, and the old phrase holds that the way of medicine opens onto the way of the immortals (醫道通仙道). Yet the tradition is firm that the healer who would go further must in time lay even these hard-won skills down. To cling to them is to take a wrong turning, a detour on which all further cultivation comes to a halt. Medicine is a true path, but it is a path through, not a place to stop.

The Ranks of the Healer

The tradition ranks physicians in an old order: the highest tends the realm, the middling tends people, and the lowest tends disease (上醫醫國, 中醫醫人, 下醫醫病). Above even the highest of these the Daoist scheme sets the great physician (大醫), to make room for the rare and miraculous healings of the great spiritual sages, who are said to lift the karmic burden at the root of an illness with a single word or thought. Below it, the upper physician can cure what seems incurable, drawing on the seven skills as well as the ordinary techniques, treating the illness that has not yet arisen and setting right the habits behind the one that has. The middle physician, the rank in which most able doctors fall, is named not only for the realm but for harmony itself (中和), and is one who can bring the body's yin and yang back into balance. The lower physician keeps rigidly to the protocols they were taught, treating the named complaint by rote, without flexibility or art. Lower still, and outside this honourable order altogether, stand the false physicians and the scam artists, who have neither skill nor care, and who exist only to part people from their money by fraud.

The Great Physician: Compassion First

No one drew the portrait of the great physician (大醫) more memorably than Sun Simiao, the Tang physician later honoured as the King of Medicine, whose essay On the Absolute Sincerity of the Great Physician remains the conscience of Chinese medicine. Its argument is that skill, however great, is not enough; the root of a true healer is virtue. Sun opens not with technique but with the state of the healer's heart, which must first settle the spirit and steady the will, free of craving and demand, and bring forth a heart of great compassion. Before such a physician, all who come are equal.

> SUN SIMIAO, ON THE ABSOLUTE SINCERITY OF THE GREAT PHYSICIAN
>
> 若有疾厄來求救者，不得問其貴賤貧富，長幼妍媸，怨親善友，華夷愚智，普同一等，皆如至親之想。
>
> *ruò yǒu jí è lái qiú jiù zhě, bù dé wèn qí guì jiàn pín fù, zhǎng yòu yán chī, yuàn qīn shàn yǒu, huá yí yú zhì, pǔ tóng yī děng, jiē rú zhì qīn zhī xiǎng.*
>
> If any come in sickness and distress seeking help, the physician must not weigh whether they are noble or humble, rich or poor, old or young, beautiful or plain, enemy or kin, friend or stranger, of this people or another, clever or dull. The physician must regard them all alike, holding every one as close kin.

From this root of compassion the rest follows: the tireless mastery of the art, for Sun also demands that the physician exhaustively master the sources of medicine and labour at them without rest, never claiming a knowledge they do not have; and the integrity to refuse the corruptions of greed and display. The physician who heals for compassion he names a great healer of the common people; the one who heals for gain and reputation he calls, in a phrase meant to sting, a great thief among living beings. Skill without virtue, in this teaching, is not a lesser good but a danger.

The Physician Must Know the Whole

It is Sun Simiao, too, who states most plainly the thesis this entire book has followed: that the great physician cannot be a narrow specialist, because the body cannot be understood apart from the cosmos it belongs to. In his chapter on the great physician's course of study, he sets out a curriculum that would daunt any modern professional.

> SUN SIMIAO, ON THE PRACTICE OF THE GREAT PHYSICIAN
>
> 又須妙解陰陽祿命，諸家相法，及《周易》六壬，並須精熟。如此乃得為大醫。
>
> *yòu xū miào jiě yīn yáng lù mìng, zhū jiā xiàng fǎ, jí Zhōuyì liù rén, bìng xū jīng shú. rú cǐ nǎi dé wéi dà yī.*
>
> The physician must also have a fine understanding of yin and yang and the reckoning of fate, of the various methods of reading signs, and of the Zhouyi and the liuren divination, all of which must be thoroughly mastered. Only one who is like this may be called a great physician.

He goes further still, requiring that the aspiring healer read the classics, the histories, and the philosophers, Laozi and Zhuangzi among them, and grasp the waxing and waning of the five phases and the movements of the heavenly bodies. Without the classics, he says, one will not know the virtue of compassion and acceptance; without the philosophers, one cannot act with quiet spontaneity; without the reckoning of the five phases and the stars, one will meet disaster blindly. Here, from a physician of the seventh century, is the whole programme of this book set down as a professional requirement. Medicine, the reckoning of destiny, the divination of the Yi, the movements of the heavens, the cultivation of Daoist stillness, and the virtue of the classics are not separate competencies. They are the single education of one who would understand a human being, and Sun Simiao made their union the very definition of greatness in the art.

Virtue as the Root

Why should virtue be the root, and not merely an ornament, of skill? The answer reaches back to the making of the human being in the gate on the three treasures, where the Inner Classic said that what Heaven gives to a person is its de, its power or virtue, the very thing that, streaming down to meet the breath of Earth, brings a person to life. De (德) is at once moral virtue and the active power of the Way working through a thing. To cultivate virtue, then, is not to obey an external rule but to keep oneself aligned with the source from which life and clarity flow. A physician whose heart is disordered by greed and fear sees a distorted world and acts on it crookedly, however much technique they possess; a physician whose heart is still and compassionate sees truly and acts in accord with the way things are. Virtue is the inner alignment on which all the outer alignments depend, and it is why the cultivation of the self and the practice of the art are, in the end, one work.

One Field of Alignment

Here the whole book gathers to a point. Every art it has set out is a form of alignment: the nurturing of life aligns the body with the seasons; the reading of a chart aligns a person with the qi of their birth; wind and water aligns a dwelling with the land; divination aligns a choice with the way a moment is already turning; cultivation aligns the spirit with its own still source. And beneath them all lies the one alignment that makes the rest possible, the inner accord of a settled and compassionate heart with the power of the Way, which the tradition calls virtue and which the contemplative calls stillness. This is why the great physician and the accomplished adept turn out, in the end, to be the same person seen from two sides. The outer alignments, of body, of time, of place, of conduct, are the work of the arts; the inner alignment is the work of a life, and the arts are sound only when they rest upon it. Heaven turns and Earth abides; the human being, aligned within and so able to align without, is the third power that joins them, and the field in which all these alignments meet is a single human life lived well.

FROM PRACTICE

The old teachers held that a student's character was watched as closely as their knowledge, on the conviction that a clear remedy in a clouded hand goes wrong. The great physicians are remembered less for any single cure than for a quality patients felt in their presence: an attention undivided by self-interest, a calm that steadied the room. That quality cannot be examined for or bought. It is grown, slowly, by the same cultivation this whole book describes, which is why the great physician and the accomplished adept turn out, in the end, to be the same person seen from two sides.

READING THE CLASSIC AS A WHOLE

This edition was made to be read in more than one way. Followed from the first gate to the last, it traces an arc from the nurturing of life to the cultivation of the spirit, the whole of the medicine in order. Consulted by theme, each gate stands as a complete treatment of its subject, the organs or the channels or the needle gathered in one place. And read by a student of the wider tradition, the gates open onto the Five Arts, the medicine showing its kinship with destiny, divination, physiognomy, and the disciplines of cultivation. However it is entered, the aim is the same: to let the reader meet the Inner Classic not as a thicket of ancient chapters but as one coherent body of knowledge, as alive and as ordered as the body it describes.

FROM THE AUTHOR

I made this book because the knowledge it gathers came near to being lost, and because it gave me back my life. Under the name Destiny and Alchemy I have tried to keep the old learning whole, the Five Arts together rather than scattered, and the medicine at their heart rather than cut off from its roots. The Inner Classic is the oldest and deepest of the medical texts, and arranging it by theme is my attempt to make it not only readable but usable, by physicians, by students of the Five Arts, by the ordinary reader who simply wishes to understand and improve their own health, and by anyone who suspects, as I have come to, that the body and the cosmos are written in one hand. If this edition helps even a few readers enter that tradition and carry it forward, it will have done what I hoped.

法於陰陽，和於術數。

Pattern yourself on yin and yang, and accord with the arts of number.

THE CIRCLE CLOSES

And so the book returns to where it began. The first gate opened with the ancients who patterned themselves on yin and yang and accorded with the arts of number, and lived out their hundred years; this last gate closes with the same counsel, now seen as the root not only of medicine but of the whole tradition it belongs to. Gate One, The Hundred Years and this eleventh gate are the two ends of one circle, the practical and the philosophical faces of a single teaching: that to live well and to heal well are to move in step with the pattern of heaven and earth. The reader who has passed through all eleven gates has walked that circle once; the tradition asks only that we keep walking it.

A PRACTICAL CLOSE

Living Well

養生指要

The gates have set out, at length, what the classic teaches of the body, the seasons, the feelings, and the inner work. This closing chapter gathers that teaching into a plain practice, so that the reader who wants none of the theory and only the living of it may begin today. Nothing here is new. It is the classic's own counsel on nurturing life, set down as a handful of habits a person can actually keep. None of it asks for special equipment or belief, only attention and a little steadiness. Begin with one part of it, hold to that until it is second nature, and add the next. A small practice kept for years outweighs a large one abandoned in a month.

Living with the Day

The body's qi rises with the morning, crests by midday, and sinks toward night, and a life ordered to that tide tires far less than one set against it. Rise near dawn and rest not long after dark, letting your waking and sleeping follow the light through the year. Keep your hours regular, for the body thrives on rhythm more than on any single virtuous act; rising, eating, and sleeping at steady times is itself a medicine. Take your largest meal when the sun is high, when the stomach and spleen are at their strongest, and eat lightly in the evening, never to fullness, for a heavy stomach late at night burdens the middle and breaks the sleep. Spend your effort in the active hours of morning and afternoon, and let the evening be for winding down, dim and quiet, so that the spirit settles before you lie down. Sleep before midnight where you can, for it is in the deep of the night that the liver stores the blood and the body does its mending.

Living with the Seasons

The oldest counsel in the classic is to live differently in each season, nourishing in spring and summer the rising yang, and in autumn and winter the gathering yin, so that each season builds the root for the one to come. In spring, sleep a little less and rise early; walk in the open with the body loose and the mind generous and unhurried, giving rather than holding, for spring is birth and asks to be let grow. In summer, rise early and do not resent the long days or the heat; stay active, let the qi flow outward, and do not bottle up what you feel, for summer is flowering and asks for openness. In autumn, sleep and rise early with the light; draw the mind inward and keep it calm and collected, gathering yourself as the year gathers its harvest. In winter, sleep early and rise late, after the sun; keep warm and do not sweat the qi away, and hold the will quiet and inward as though guarding something precious, for winter is storage and asks for stillness. To force the body's openness in winter or its rest in spring is to plant against the season, and the cost is paid later, when the next season finds the root unmade.

At the Table

Eat to the season and to the body's warmth: warming food in the cold, cooling food in the heat, and through the year more of what is cooked and warm than what is raw and cold, which taxes the gentle fire of the spleen on which the whole of digestion rests. Keep the five flavours in balance, none of them to excess, for the classic warns that a flavour overindulged injures the organ it belongs to, the salt that hardens the blood and the rich that clogs as surely as too little nourishes too poorly. Eat to about seven parts of fullness and stop, leaving the stomach a margin to work; rising from the table still light is worth more than any tonic. Take your food at regular times and eat it calmly, without haste, anger, or distraction, for the state of the heart at the table passes into the meal. Drink warm rather than iced, and let plain water, taken through the day, be most of what you drink.

The Feelings

The feelings are not separate from the body in this medicine; each of the seven, joy and anger, anxiety and brooding, grief, fear, and fright, moves the qi in its own direction, and any of them, held too long or felt too hard, injures the organ it answers to. Anger drives the qi up and harms the liver; unbridled joy scatters the heart; worry and brooding knot the spleen; grief wears down the lung; fear and fright drain and unsettle the kidney. The counsel is not to feel nothing, which is neither possible nor healthy, but to let no feeling rule you or take up lasting residence: let it rise, be felt, and pass, the way weather crosses a sky. Cultivate evenness and contentment as the ground state to which you return, for a settled heart keeps the qi orderly and the body well. When a strong feeling takes hold, come back to the breath and let a few slow breaths settle the qi before it does its damage; this small act, done in the moment, is among the most protective in the whole regimen.

Movement and Rest

Qi and blood are meant to flow, and where they pool, illness gathers, so the old saying holds that running water never grows stale and a turning hinge never rusts. Move every day, but gently: walking, easy stretching, and the slow forms such as the shadow-boxing and the breathing exercises suit the nurturing of life far better than violent or exhausting effort, which spends the very qi it means to build. Do not drive yourself to exhaustion, for over-exertion scatters the qi; nor sit idle and unmoving for long hours, for that too has its harm, wearing the flesh and letting the qi stagnate. Match work with rest in the day and across the week, and treat tiredness as information rather than weakness, resting before you are wrung out rather than after. A body kept supple and lightly worked, then properly rested, is the aim, not a body driven hard and then collapsed.

Breath and Stillness

A few minutes of quiet each day, kept up over years, does more for the spirit than long sessions taken up and dropped. Set aside a regular time, in the early morning or before sleep, and a quiet place. Sit upright and at ease, the spine straight without stiffness, the shoulders soft, the hands resting and the eyes lightly closed or lowered. Let the breath slow of its own accord and deepen, drawn down toward the lower belly rather than held high in the chest, the out-breath long, soft, and unhurried. Rest the attention lightly on the breath, and each time the mind wanders, as it will, bring it back without irritation or strain; the returning is the practice. Begin with five or ten minutes and let it lengthen naturally as it becomes a habit rather than a task. This simple sitting steadies the spirit, gathers the qi, and quiets the feelings; for the fuller inner work that grows from it, the gate on cultivation and the chapter on the inner elixir carry it much further.

Guarding the Root

Beneath the daily and seasonal habits lies one deeper principle: the essence stored in the kidney is the body's root and its capital, the stuff of growth, vigour, and long life, and it is to be spent sparingly and guarded well. Keep moderation in all the appetites, and do not exhaust yourself in work, in pleasure, or in endless worry, for each of these, carried to excess, draws on the same reserve. Sleep enough and sleep well, for it is rest above all that restores the essence and the spirit. The classic is plain that those who burn through their reserve early, however vigorous they seem, fade before their time, while those who husband it live out the full span their nature allowed. The long life is not won by any tonic or feat but by this patient conserving of the root, year upon year.

The Quiet Mind

The classic opens by asking why the ancients lived a hundred years with vigour while later people aged by fifty, and answers that the ancients were tranquil and content, empty of grasping, so that the true qi followed easily and the spirit was kept within. This calm of mind is not the last item on the list but the ground of all the rest, for without it no regimen holds and with it even an imperfect one goes far. Keep your desires few and your heart at peace; want little, fear less, and find contentment in what is enough rather than in always more. Let go of what you cannot change, and do not let the mind run ahead into dread or back into regret, for a restless, grasping mind wears the body faster than any labour. To be content, unhurried, and inwardly quiet is, in the end, the whole secret the classic offers; the habits of the day, the season, the table, and the breath are only the ways that quiet is made daily and kept.

恬淡虛無，真氣從之。

In stillness and contentment, empty of grasping, the true qi follows of itself.

These are not many rules but one practice in many forms: to live in step with the way things are, by the day and by the season, in the body and in the heart. Take up a little of it, hold to that, and let the rest follow in time. Done steadily, and without strain, it keeps the body whole and lets the years come full, which is all the classic ever promised and all, in the end, that it asks.

REFERENCE

Concordance of the Treatises

索引

The thematic arrangement of this edition gathers the treatises by subject rather than by their traditional order, so that any one of them may be found at some distance from its neighbours in the original scrolls. This concordance restores the bridge. It lists all one hundred and sixty-two treatises in their canonical sequence, the eighty-one of the Plain Questions and the eighty-one of the Numinous Pivot, and gives for each its title, the gate in which it is gathered here, and the page on which its passages begin. A reader who knows a treatise by its received number or name will find, in a glance down these columns, exactly where in the eleven gates it now lives.

Su Wen 素問 · The Plain Questions

33	評熱病論	A Discussion of Heat Diseases	*VII*	193, 226
34	逆調論	On Counter-Regulation	*VII*	213
35	瘧論	On Malaria	*VII*	195, 196
36	刺瘧	Needling Malaria	*VII*	197
37	氣厥論	On the Qi Reversal	*VII*	206
38	欬論	On Cough	*VII*	198
39	舉痛論	On the Various Pains	*VII*	199, 200
40	腹中論	On Disorders Within the Abdomen	*VII*	209
41	刺腰痛	Needling Lumbar Pain	*VII*	200
42	風論	On Wind	*VII*	189
43	痺論	On Impediment	*VII*	202
44	痿論	On Wilting	*VII*	203, 204
45	厥論	On Reversal	*VII*	205
46	病能論	On the Forms of Disease	*VII*	221, 227
47	奇病論	On Strange Diseases	*VII*	220, 228
48	大奇論	The Greater Discourse on Strange Pulses	*IV*	94
49	脈解	Explaining the Channel Symptoms	*VII*	223, 229
50	刺要論	Essentials of Needling	*VI*	149
51	刺齊論	On the Depths of Needling	*VI*	150
52	刺禁論	Prohibitions in Needling	*VI*	151, 170
53	刺志論	On the Intent in Needling	*VI*	150
54	鍼解	Explaining the Needles	*VI*	154
55	長刺節論	On the Extended Needling Methods	*VI*	152
56	皮部論	On the Cutaneous Regions	*V*	112, 125
57	經絡論	On the Channels and Collaterals	*V*	113, 126

Ling Shu 靈樞 · The Numinous Pivot

REFERENCE

Topical Index

通檢

This index points to where the book treats its principal subjects, gathered by theme rather than by chapter, so that a reader may enter at a concern, a symptom, an organ, or an art and find it at once. The page numbers mark the main discussions of each subject, not every passing mention. The terms themselves are defined in the Glossary that follows, and the treatises of the classic are listed by their canonical number in the Concordance above.

REFERENCE

Glossary of Key Terms

詞彙

The terms below are central to this book, arranged alphabetically by their English or romanised heading. Characters are given in traditional form, with the Mandarin sound in pinyin. Definitions are brief; the fuller sense of each is drawn out in the chapters.

Bagua 八卦 *bā guà*

The eight trigrams, each three lines imaging a power of nature; paired, they form the sixty-four hexagrams.

Bazi 八字 *bā zì*

The Eight Characters, or Four Pillars; a life read as a configuration of the five phases at the moment of birth.

Blood 血 *xuè*

The red and nourishing fluid that, moving with the qi, moistens and feeds the whole body; it is ruled by the heart, stored by the liver, and drawn from the essence of food.

Cold and heat 寒熱 *hán rè*

One of the eight guiding distinctions: whether cold or heat predominates in a pattern of illness, and so whether the body is to be warmed or cooled.

Dantian 丹田 *dān tián*

The fields of elixir; three centres, lower, middle, and upper, where the treasures are gathered and refined.

Dao 道 *dào*

The Way; the source and pattern of all things, known by its manner rather than by description.

Daoyi 道醫 *dào yī*

Daoist medicine; the older, cultivation-based healing from which Chinese medicine descends, reading the causes of Heaven, the human, and Earth.

De 德 *dé*

Virtue; also the active power of the Way working through a thing. Heaven's gift that, meeting Earth's breath, brings life.

Eight Extraordinary Vessels 奇經八脈 *qí jīng bā mài*

The eight reservoir channels, the Governing Vessel and the Conception Vessel among them, that hold and regulate the qi of the twelve regular channels and serve as the principal pathways of the inner work.

Evil 邪 *xié*

A harmful influence that disturbs the right qi of the body, whether a wind, a cold, a damp, a heat, or another excess from without; illness takes hold where an evil meets an opening within.

Exterior and interior 表裏 *biǎo lǐ*

One of the eight distinctions: the depth at which a disorder lies, at the surface of the body or within its organs, which tells how far the trouble has gone.

Feng Shui 風水 *fēng shuǐ*

"Wind and water"; the art of reading and gathering the living qi of a place.

Fire phases 火候 *huǒ hòu*

The measure of warmth and effort in cultivation, the breath now gentle as a civil fire, now urgent as a martial one, by which the work is brought to its right degree.

Five Movements, Six Qi 五運六氣 *wǔ yùn liù qì*

The classic's cosmology of time, reckoning the qi of each year from the stems and branches.

Five Phases 五行 *wǔ xíng*

Wood, Fire, Earth, Metal, Water; the five movements through which any complete process passes, bound by cycles of generation and restraint.

Fluids 津液 *jīn yè*

The thin and thick waters of the body, the light and spreading and the dense and still, which moisten the skin and orifices, the joints, the marrow, and the organs.

Gate of life 命門 *mìng mén*

The life gate; the root of the source qi and original fire of the body, tied to the kidneys, from which warmth, vitality, and the power of generation arise.

Hun and Po 魂魄 *hún pò*

The ethereal soul, which travels with the spirit, and the bodily soul, bound to the flesh.

Jing 精 *jīng*

Essence; the dense, fluid reserve of vitality, stored chiefly in the kidney, both inherited and replenished.

Jingluo 經絡 *jīng luò*

The network of channels and connecting vessels through which qi and blood travel.

Ling Shu 靈樞 *líng shū*

The "Spiritual Pivot," the second of the two books of the Inner Classic, on the channels and the needle.

Longmai 龍脈 *lóng mài*

The dragon veins; the ridgelines along which the earth's qi travels.

Macrocosmic orbit 大周天 *dà zhōu tiān*

The greater circulation that opens beyond the two midline vessels, the Governing and the Conception, into the whole channel-system and brings the body into accord with the qi of heaven and earth; the work of the second refinement.

Microcosmic orbit 小周天 *xiǎo zhōu tiān*

The circulation of refined qi up the Governing Vessel and down the Conception Vessel in a closed loop.

Ming and Yun 命運 *mìng yùn*

The decree or allotment one is born with, and the moving fortune that passes over it.

Neidan 內丹 *nèi dān*

The inner elixir; Daoist cultivation that refines essence into breath, breath into spirit, spirit into emptiness.

Qi 氣 *qì*

The vital breath; the one active substance of the world, at once matter and force, of which Heaven, Earth, and the body are all made.

Qi mechanism 氣機 *qì jī*

The dynamic of qi in four movements: rising, falling, entering, exiting. Health is their free play.

Root and branch 標本 *biāo běn*

The root of an illness and its branch, the underlying cause and the outward signs; treatment attends now to one and now to the other, the branch when it is urgent, the root when there is time.

Seven Feelings 七情 *qī qíng*

Joy, anger, anxiety, brooding, grief, fear, and fright; the emotions that, in excess, disturb the qi and injure the organs.

Shen 神 *shén*

Spirit; the conscious brightness and coherence of a person, housed in the heart.

Stems and Branches 干支 *gān zhī*

The ten heavenly stems and twelve earthly branches; the interlocking wheels that mark time and carry its quality.

Su Wen 素問 *sù wèn*

The "Basic Questions," the first of the two books of the Inner Classic, on theory.

Taiji 太極 *tài jí*

The Supreme Ultimate; the undivided whole from which yin and yang arise.

Three Powers 三才 *sān cái*

Heaven, Earth, and the human being; the frame within which all process unfolds.

Three Treasures 三寶 *sān bǎo*

Essence, breath, and spirit (jing, qi, shen), the wealth of the body and the material of cultivation.

Tiangui 天癸 *tiān guǐ*

The reproductive essence released by the kidney, governing the cycles of growth and decline.

Triple burner 三焦 *sān jiāo*

The three burning-spaces, upper, middle, and lower, that move and transform the qi, the food, and the waters; counted among the bowels, it is said to have a name but no form.

Yangsheng 養生 *yǎng shēng*

The fostering of life; the art of living in accord with the rhythms of the body and the world.

Yi yi tong yuan 醫易同源 *yī yì tóng yuán*

"Medicine and the Yi share one source"; the doctrine that both rest on yin, yang, and change.

Yidao tong xiandao 醫道通仙道 *yī dào tōng xiān dào*

"The way of medicine opens onto the way of the immortals"; medicine practised as a stage of Daoist cultivation and a gathering of virtue.

Yijing 易經 *yì jīng*

The Book of Change; the root text of yin-yang and the eight trigrams.

Yin and Yang 陰陽 *yīn yáng*

The two complementary phases of every process: receptive and active, dark and bright, quiet and moving. The first division of the one breath.

Ying and Wei 營衛 *yíng wèi*

The nutritive qi within the vessels and the defensive qi outside them.

Zang and Fu 臟腑 *zàng fǔ*

The five storing depots and six hollow palaces; the organs as makers, keepers, and movers of the vital substances.

Zhenren 真人 *zhēn rén*

The True Person; the highest of the ranks of attainment, wholly in accord with the Way.

Zhi wei bing 治未病 *zhì wèi bìng*

Treating what is not yet ill; preventing disorder before it forms.

Zhuyou 祝由 *zhù yóu*

The old art of healing by word, sign, and rite, without drug or needle; named in the Inner Classic and once a department of the imperial medical academy.

Ziran 自然 *zì rán*

"Self-so"; the spontaneous way a thing is when nothing forces it. The Way's own manner.

Ziwei Doushu 紫微斗數 *zǐ wēi dǒu shù*

Purple Star Astrology; a life read as stars distributed through twelve palaces.

REFERENCE

Sources and Further Reading

書目

All translations of classical passages in this book are the author's own, prepared for this volume from the public-domain original texts. The works below are the classical sources drawn upon and a selection of modern studies and translations consulted for interpretation and offered for the reader who wishes to go further. Mention here is acknowledgement of scholarship, not reproduction of it.

CLASSICAL SOURCES

Huangdi Neijing 黃帝內經 , in its two books, the *Su Wen* 素問 and the *Ling Shu* 靈樞 . The foundational text, quoted throughout. The received order follows the eighth-century recension of Wang Bing 王冰 .

Daodejing 道德經 , attributed to Laozi 老子 . Source of the cosmology of the Way and the one breath.

Zhuangzi 莊子 . Source of the teachings on stillness, the fasting of the heart, and the breath of the True Person.

Yijing 易經 , with its appended *Great Treatise* (Xici 繫辭). Root of yin-yang, the trigrams, and the philosophy of change.

Zhouyi cantong qi 周易參同契 , attributed to Wei Boyang 魏伯陽 . The ancestral classic of alchemy.

Wuzhen pian 悟真篇 , by Zhang Boduan 張伯端 . A central text of the inner elixir.

Taiyi jinhua zongzhi 太乙金華宗旨 , the Secret of the Golden Flower. A later classic on turning the light around and the original spirit.

Qingjing jing 清靜經 , the Classic of Purity and Stillness. A short Daoist scripture on stilling the mind and clearing desire, drawn upon in the chapters on cultivation and stillness.

Huiming jing 慧命經 , the Classic of Wisdom and Life, attributed to Liu Huayang 柳華陽 . Drawn upon for the fire phases, the circulation of the orbits, and the forming of the spiritual embryo.

Zangshu 葬書 (the Book of Burial), attributed to Guo Pu 郭璞 . The classical source of Feng Shui and of its defining line.

Beiji qianjin yaofang 備急千金要方 , by Sun Simiao 孫思邈 , including the essays "On the Absolute Sincerity of the Great Physician" and "On the Practice of the Great Physician," and the chapter on nourishing nature.

Qianjin yifang 千金翼方 , Sun Simiao's later supplement, which preserves the *Book of Prohibitions* 禁經 , the talismanic and incantatory healing of the zhuyou tradition.

Leijing 類經 and *Leijing fuyi* 類經附翼 , by Zhang Jingyue 張景岳 (Zhang Jiebin), the great Ming reorganisation of the whole *Inner Classic* by subject, with commentary. Drawn upon throughout for the classical explanation of the text and of the methods of nurturing life, as well as for the doctrine that medicine and the Yi share one source.

MODERN STUDIES AND TRANSLATIONS

Paul U. Unschuld, translations and studies of the *Huang Di Nei Jing Su Wen* and *Ling Shu* , and his broader histories of Chinese medicine, valuable for the dating and textual history of the classic.

Ilza Veith, the first English translation of the opening treatises of the *Su Wen* , of historical importance.

Standard reference works on the foundations of Chinese medicine, on the theory of the channels and organs, and on the materia medica, for the clinical framework summarised here.

Modern scholarship on Chinese cosmology, the *Yijing* , Daoist internal alchemy, and the history of the arts of fate and of Feng Shui, for the wider context of the synthesis.

For the chapters on cultivation and stillness, modern studies and translations of Daoist internal alchemy were consulted, including Wang Mu's outline of the practice of *Neidan* drawn from the *Wuzhen pian* ; Lu K'uan Yü's rendering of the Daoist alchemical and meditative texts; the Wilhelm and Jung edition of the *Secret of the Golden Flower* ; and modern manuals on cultivating stillness. Their ideas are summarised here in the author's own words.

Readers are encouraged to seek out full scholarly translations of the *Inner Classic* for study of the complete text, and to learn the practices of cultivation, where they wish to take them up, from a qualified living teacher.

ABOUT THE AUTHOR

The Road to This Book

元遇五行館 · DESTINY AND ALCHEMY

> *What began in suffering became a calling.*

I am Zachery Chionch, the founder of Destiny and Alchemy (元遇五行館), a practice in Singapore given over to the ancestral Chinese arts of healing, destiny, and cultivation. This book did not begin as a scholar's project, nor as a labour of leisure. It began as a matter of survival, in a body that for most of my life did not seem to want to keep me.

From my earliest years I was weak and often ill (體弱多病). Where friends went to school, studied and played, I watched. Sickness kept me to one side of things, and what sickness did not take from me, the years of being bullied did. For more than twenty years misfortune seemed to follow me without pause, as though some weight I could not see had been laid across my shoulders at birth. In the end I left school without finishing, and in a society that reads a person's worth from their certificates, a young man with no papers and no health finds very few doors open to him. I learned early what it is to be counted as nothing.

Then came the illness that nearly ended it. I could not breathe. Every day was a struggle for air, my chest locked tight, each breath shallow and hard-won, and the fear that came with it was worse than the breathlessness itself: the quiet terror of a body that will not do the one thing it must. The doctors of modern medicine examined me and found nothing wrong. They named it acid reflux, handed me antacids, and sent me home. The antacids did nothing, because the trouble was never about the acid of the stomach. Their instruments photographed my organs and found no issues, but none of them can photograph qi (氣), and it was in the qi that my illness lay.

I went from doctor to doctor and spent what little my family had. It was not only that the money ran low; no one seemed to know how to help me, or even to understand what was happening to my body. I went to the Accident and Emergency department (A&E) of the hospital as well, and even there the doctors could not help. I remember being taken, gravely weak, to a Chinese physician who saw patients from his home. My parents had taken leave from their work and travelled a long way to bring me there, carrying their hope as much as they carried me. He would not see me. They stood at his gate and pleaded for nothing more than a single reading of the pulse, and he turned them away. I have never forgotten it. What wounded me was not my own sickness, which I had long grown used to, but the sight of my parents lowering themselves to beg a stranger who simply did not care. Something in me broke that day, and in breaking, it hardened into a vow: that never again would I leave my life, or my family's hope, at the mercy of someone else. If no one in the world would help me, then I would learn to heal myself, and I would never turn away another soul who came to me in need. I enrolled at a college of Traditional Chinese Medicine (中醫) and gave myself wholly to the study.

Slowly, studying by day and testing the medicine on my own body, I found the root of my illness. It was a deep weakness and stagnation of the spleen and stomach qi, joined to a kidney that could no longer grasp the breath: in the language of the tradition, an insufficiency of the middle qi with qi held and stagnant (中氣不足、 氣滯), and a kidney failing to grasp the qi (腎不納氣). Simply to name the thing truly was already half the cure. For the first time, I was not helpless.

But the deeper I went, the more clearly I saw that medicine alone was not enough. Many illnesses, and many of the obstacles, the roadblocks, and the dead ends that shape a life, cannot be fully resolved by medicine or by ordinary knowledge; some of them ask for a higher order of wisdom and power before they will yield. Among these are disorders such as the strange diseases (怪病), and afflictions such as gu (蠱).

My questions led me somewhere I had not expected. One day my acupuncture teacher mentioned, almost in passing, things that were never written in our textbooks: the eight-trigram (八卦) methods of needling, and Sun Simiao's thirteen ghost points (十三鬼穴). After the class I stayed behind and asked him about gu. He smiled, as though surprised that anyone still asked, and said: have you heard of the department of zhuyou (祝由十三科)? I had not. When I searched further, I found that within Chinese medicine there is a whole syllabus and tradition of healing that does not require a single drug or needle: a healing by talisman, by incantation, and by rite. My teacher told me that even Sun Simiao's Supplement to the Essential Prescriptions Worth a Thousand Gold (千金翼方) had once held such talismans, before they were removed from what was taught. It shook me to realise that what I had been given, and what the world now calls Chinese medicine, was only a fragment of the whole. The deeper knowledge of our ancestors had been pared away in the upheavals of the last century, and the living tradition remade along narrow, clinical lines. That discovery, more than any other, is why this book exists: so that what was almost lost would not be lost completely.

Searching back through our history for what had been taken, I came upon the Five Arts (五術：山醫命卜相 , Mountain, Medicine, Destiny, Divination, and Physiognomy). Above all I wanted to understand my own fate, to know why I had been born into such frailty, and why misfortune had shadowed me for over twenty years. In the year of the water tiger (壬寅年 , 2022) I gave myself fully to the study of destiny, to the Eight Characters (八字), Purple Star astrology (紫微斗數), and the wider arts of Chinese metaphysics, and I have been deepening and refining that study every day since.

What began in suffering has become my life's work: to help others understand themselves, to resolve what conventional means cannot reach, to carry a little light to those who can see none, and, beyond all of this, to recover and preserve the original knowledge and wisdom of our ancestors, and to keep it safe for the generations still to come. It is the ground on which I built Destiny and Alchemy (元遇五行館), and it is the spirit in which I offer this, my first book, to you. Whoever you are, and whatever has brought you to these pages, I wish you Love, Light, and good health.

Destiny and Alchemy
元遇五行館

天地人合一

The Yellow Emperor's Inner Classic: A Thematic Edition, with Translation and Commentary. All one hundred and sixty-two treatises of the two books, reorganised by theme into eleven gates, each opened through its essential passages.
Curated, arranged, translated, and annotated by Zachery Chionch.
Published in Singapore by Zachery Chionch. Designed by Destiny and Alchemy (元遇五行館).
The Chinese text is the public-domain original; the English translations and all commentary are the author's own.

© 2026 Zachery Chionch

www.ingramcontent.com/pod-product-compliance
Lightning Source LLC
LaVergne TN
LVHW060439061126
851857LV00016B/1665